Ultrasound

Editor

JASON M. WAGNER

RADIOLOGIC CLINICS OF NORTH AMERICA

www.radiologic.theclinics.com

Consulting Editor
FRANK H. MILLER

May 2019 • Volume 57 • Number 3

ELSEVIER

1600 John F. Kennedy Boulevard • Suite 1800 • Philadelphia, Pennsylvania, 19103-2899

http://www.theclinics.com

RADIOLOGIC CLINICS OF NORTH AMERICA Volume 57, Number 3
May 2019 ISSN 0033-8389, ISBN 13: 978-0-323-67831-5

Editor: John Vassallo (j.vassallo@elsevier.com)
Developmental Editor: Donald Mumford

Radiologic Clinics of North America (ISSN 0033-8389) is published bimonthly by Elsevier Inc., 360 Park Avenue South, New York, NY 10010-1710. Months of issue are January, March, May, July, September, and November. Periodicals postage paid at New York, NY and additional mailing offices. Subscription prices are USD 508 per year for US individuals, USD 933 per year for US institutions, USD 100 per year for US students and residents, USD 594 per year for Canadian individuals, USD 1193 per year for Canadian institutions, USD 683 per year for international individuals, USD 1193 per year for international institutions, and USD 315 per year for Canadian and international students/residents. To receive student and resident rate, orders must be accompanied by name of affiliated institution, date of term and the signature of program/residency coordinator on institution letterhead. Orders will be billed at individual rate until proof of status is received. Foreign air speed delivery is included in all *Clinics* subscription prices. All prices are subject to change without notice. **POSTMASTER:** Send address changes to *Radiologic Clinics of North America*, Elsevier Health Sciences Division, Subscription Customer Service, 3251 Riverport Lane, Maryland Heights, MO63043. **Customer Service: Telephone: 1-800-654-2452** (U.S. and Canada); **1-314-447-8871** (outside U.S. and Canada). **Fax: 1-314-447-8029. E-mail: journalscustomerservice-usa@ elsevier.com (for print support); journalsonlinesupport-usa@elsevier.com (for online support)**.

Reprints. For copies of 100 or more of articles in this publication, please contact the Commercial Reprints Department, Elsevier Inc., 360 Park Avenue South, New York, New York 10010-1710. Tel.: +1-212-633-3874; Fax: +1-212-633-3820; E-mail: reprints@elsevier.com.

Radiologic Clinics of North America also published in Greek Paschalidis Medical Publications, Athens, Greece.

Radiologic Clinics of North America is covered in *MEDLINE/PubMed (Index Medicus), EMBASE/Excerpta Medica, Current Contents/Life Sciences, Current Contents/Clinical Medicine, RSNA Index to Imaging Literature, BIOSIS, Science Citation Index,* and *ISI/BIOMED*.

Contributors

CONSULTING EDITOR

FRANK H. MILLER, MD, FACR
Lee F. Rogers MD Professor of Medical
Education, Chief, Body Imaging Section and
Fellowship Program, Medical Director, MRI,
Department of Radiology, Northwestern
Memorial Hospital, Northwestern University
Feinberg School of Medicine, Chicago, Illinois,
USA

EDITOR

JASON M. WAGNER, MD
Associate Professor and Vice Chair,
Department of Radiological Sciences,
University of Oklahoma Health Sciences
Center, College of Medicine, Oklahoma City,
Oklahoma, USA

AUTHORS

ANTHONY M. ALLEMAN, MD, MPH
Professor, Chair, Department of Radiological
Sciences, University of Oklahoma Health
Sciences Center, College of Medicine,
Oklahoma City, Oklahoma, USA

RICHARD G. BARR, MD, PhD, FACR, FSRU, FAIUM
Professor of Radiology, Northeastern Ohio
Medical University, Editor-in-Chief, *Journal of
Ultrasound in Medicine*, Southwoods Imaging,
Youngstown, Ohio, USA

CONSTANTINE M. BURGAN, MD
Assistant Professor, Department of Radiology,
University of Alabama at Birmingham,
Birmingham, Alabama, USA

NIRVIKAR DAHIYA, MD
Associate Professor, Department of Radiology,
Mayo Clinic, Phoenix, Arizona, USA

ADRIAN A. DAWKINS, MD
Associate Professor, Chief of Abdominal
Radiology, Medical Director of Ultrasonography,
Department of Radiology, University of
Kentucky, Lexington, Kentucky, USA

AARON D. FAIN, MD
Assistant Professor, Division of
Musculoskeletal Radiology, Department of
Radiology, University of Kentucky, Lexington,
Kentucky, USA

DAVID T. FETZER, MD
Assistant Professor, Medical Director of
Ultrasound, Department of Radiology, The
University of Texas Southwestern Medical
Center, Dallas, Texas, USA

HELENA GABRIEL, MD
Associate Professor, Department of Radiology,
Northwestern University Feinberg School of
Medicine, Chicago, Illinois, USA

GOWTHAMAN GUNABUSHANAM, MD
Associate Professor, Department of Radiology and Biomedical Imaging, Yale School of Medicine, New Haven, Connecticut, USA

MINDY M. HORROW, MD, FACR
Department of Radiology, Einstein Medical Center, Philadelphia, Pennsylvania, USA

GAYATRI JOSHI, MD
Assistant Professor, Department of Radiology and Imaging Sciences, Emory University Hospital Midtown, Emory University School of Medicine, Atlanta, Georgia, USA

AYA KAMAYA, MD
Associate Professor, Director of Body Imaging Fellowship, Director of Ultrasound, Department of Radiology, Stanford University Medical Center, Stanford, California, USA

LAUREN KUMMANT, MD
Radiologist, Department of Radiology, Northwell Health, Valley Stream, New York, USA

JILL E. LANGER, MD
Professor of Radiology, Perelman School of Medicine, University of Pennsylvania, Hospital of the University of Pennsylvania, Philadelphia, Pennsylvania, USA

MARK E. LOCKHART, MD
Professor, Department of Radiology, University of Alabama at Birmingham, Birmingham, Alabama, USA

WILLIAM MIDDLETON, MD
Professor, Mallinckrodt Institute of Radiology, Washington University School of Medicine, St Louis, Missouri, USA

DANIEL C. OPPENHEIMER, MD
Assistant Professor, Department of Imaging Sciences, University of Rochester Medical Center, Rochester, New York, USA

MAITRAY D. PATEL, MD
Professor, Department of Radiology, Mayo Clinic, Phoenix, Arizona, USA

KRISTIN REBIK, DO
Assistant Professor, Department of Radiological Sciences, University of Oklahoma Health Sciences Center, Oklahoma City, Oklahoma, USA

SHUCHI K. RODGERS, MD
Clinical Associate Professor, Section Chief, Abdominal Radiology, Director of Ultrasound, Department of Radiology, Sidney Kimmel Medical College at Thomas Jefferson University, Einstein Medical Center, Philadelphia, Pennsylvania, USA

DEBORAH J. RUBENS, MD
Professor, Associate Chair, Department of Imaging Sciences, University of Rochester Medical Center, Rochester, New York, USA

RUPAN SANYAL, MD
Associate Professor, Department of Radiology, University of Alabama at Birmingham, Birmingham, Alabama, USA

LESLIE M. SCOUTT, MD
Professor of Radiology, Surgery and Cardiology, Vice Chair of Education, Department of Radiology and Biomedical Imaging, Medical Director, Non-Invasive Vascular Laboratory, Yale School of Medicine, New Haven, Connecticut, USA

JAMES H. SEOW, MBBS, FRANZCR
Department of Radiology, Royal Perth Hospital, Perth, Western Australia, Australia

STEVEN B. SOLIMAN, DO, RMSK
Assistant Professor, Division of Musculoskeletal Radiology, Department of Radiology, Henry Ford Hospital, Detroit, Michigan, USA

PAUL J. SPICER, MD
Divisions of Musculoskeletal Radiology and Breast Imaging, Assistant Professor, Department of Radiology, University of Kentucky, Lexington, Kentucky, USA

JASON M. WAGNER, MD
Associate Professor and Vice Chair, Department of Radiological Sciences, University of Oklahoma Health Sciences Center, College of Medicine, Oklahoma City, Oklahoma, USA

PETER S. WANG, MD
Department of Radiology, Einstein Medical Center, Philadelphia, Pennsylvania, USA

SCOTT W. YOUNG, MD
Assistant Professor, Department of Radiology, Mayo Clinic, Phoenix, Arizona, USA

Contents

Nodular thyroid disease is very common, and the vast majority of nodules are benign. Sonography serves as an effective diagnostic tool in identifying nodular features that are concerning for malignancy and those with a benign appearance. The American College of Radiology has developed a risk-stratification system called the Thyroid Imaging Reporting and Data System, which uses the sonographic appearance of nodules combined with nodule size to determine the need for fine-needle aspiration or sonographic surveillance to diagnose malignancy. Familiarity with the sonographic appearance of diffuse thyroid disease allows differentiation of these conditions from nodular thyroid disease.

 Video content accompanies this article at http://www.radiologic.theclinics.com.

Ultrasonography is an excellent method for imaging evaluation of cervical lymph nodes. This article provides an image-rich review of the sonographic manifestations of diseases involving the cervical lymph nodes, with an emphasis on the expected anatomic distribution of diseases.

Doppler ultrasound (US) is the primary noninvasive imaging modality for detecting, grading, and monitoring extracranial internal carotid artery (ICA) stenosis, which is a well-established surrogate marker for stroke risk. In addition, Doppler US is the primary imaging modality for surveillance of patients following carotid intervention with endarterectomy or stent placement. This article reviews the pathophysiology and epidemiology of stroke, technique for performing a carotid US examination, normal findings, and diagnostic US criteria for evaluating carotid plaque, grading stenosis in the native ICA and following intervention, as well as waveform analysis of the carotid arteries.

There is renewed interest in ultrasound imaging of the vertebral artery due to the increasing use of stent placement for treating vertebral artery stenosis. Changes in vertebral artery waveforms are helpful in detecting pathologic processes involving the proximal and distal neurovascular circulation. We review the normal anatomy, scanning technique, normal gray scale, and color Doppler ultrasound appearance and differential diagnosis of spectral Doppler waveform changes in the extracranial vertebral artery. We review the ultrasound criteria for diagnosing vertebral artery stenosis, and the imaging appearance of non-atherosclerotic pathology that may affect the vertebral artery, including dissection, pseudoaneurysm, and arteriovenous fistula.

infiltrating endometriosis), endometriomas, adenomyosis, pelvic congestion syndrome, and malpositioned intrauterine contraceptive devices. Sonographic observations regarding a number of non-gynecologic causes of pelvic pain are also described.

 Video content accompanies this article at http://www.radiologic.theclinics.com.

Ultrasound is the imaging study of choice for detection and full characterization of early pregnancies based on its accuracy, low cost, safety profile, and abundant availability. This article reviews the goals and utility of first-trimester ultrasound in gestation localization, viability determination, and abnormal pregnancies, including ectopic implantation, retained products, and molar pregnancy.

Ultrasound is the imaging modality of choice to evaluate the scrotum because of its high resolution, Doppler capabilities, availability, and lack of ionizing radiation. Acute urologic emergencies diagnosed with ultrasound include testicular torsion, testicular rupture, and Fournier gangrene. The radiologist's knowledge of sonographic features of vascular, infectious, traumatic, and benign and malignant processes that occur in the scrotum coupled with the patient's presenting symptoms, age, and physical examination allows for the correct diagnosis of a wide spectrum of scrotal pathology.

This article focuses on common sports-related injuries that are amenable to diagnosis by diagnostic ultrasonography. These injuries include rotator cuff-tears, lateral epicondylitis, distal biceps tendon tears, and anterior talofibular ligament injuries. The anatomy, scanning techniques, mechanism of injury, and sonographic appearance of each injury are discussed.

 Video content accompanies this article at http://www.radiologic.theclinics.com.

Soft tissue masses and fluid collections are frequently encountered in sonographic practice, either as principal indication for diagnostic examination or as an incidental finding during an examination performed for other indications. Sonography is a good first-line imaging modality for evaluation of superficial masses and fluid collections, but requires meticulous attention to technique to avoid diagnostic pitfalls. Although many superficial masses are diagnosed with ultrasound, there are several potential diagnostic challenges, including differentiating hematomas from sarcomas. This article provides an image-rich review of the sonographic features of common soft tissue masses, with emphasis on practical tips to accurately recognize important pathology.

RADIOLOGIC CLINICS OF NORTH AMERICA

FORTHCOMING ISSUES

July 2019
Trauma and Emergency Radiology
Stephan Anderson, *Editor*

September 2019
Imaging of the Upper Limb
Giuseppe Guglielmi and Alberto Bazzocchi, *Editors*

November 2019
Neuroradiology
Jacqueline A. Bello and Shira E. Slasky, *Editors*

RECENT ISSUES

March 2019
Topics in Spine Imaging
Lubdha M. Shah, *Editor*

January 2019
Cardiac CT Imaging
Suhny Abbara and Prabhakar Rajiah, *Editors*

November 2018
Imaging of the Pelvis and Lower Extremity
Kurt F. Scherer and Laura W. Bancroft, *Editors*

RELATED SERIES

Magnetic Resonance Imaging Clinics
Neuroimaging Clinics
PET Clinics

THE CLINICS ARE AVAILABLE ONLINE!
Access your subscription at:
www.theclinics.com

PROGRAM OBJECTIVE
The objective of the *Radiologic Clinics of North America* is to keep practicing radiologists and radiology residents up to date with current clinical practice in radiology by providing timely articles reviewing the state of the art in patient care.

TARGET AUDIENCE
Practicing radiologists, radiology residents, and other healthcare professionals who provide patient care utilizing radiologic findings.

LEARNING OBJECTIVES
Upon completion of this activity, participants will be able to:
1. Review ultrasound imaging and diagnostic criteria in the evaluation of carotid and vertebral arteries.
2. Discuss sonographic screening for hepatocellular carcinoma in patients with chronic liver disease.
3. Recognize sonographic manifestations of diseases involving the cervical lymph nodes.

ACCREDITATION
The Elsevier Office of Continuing Medical Education (EOCME) is accredited by the Accreditation Council for Continuing Medical Education (ACCME) to provide continuing medical education for physicians.

The EOCME designates this enduring material for a maximum of 15 *AMA PRA Category 1 Credit*(s)™. Physicians should claim only the credit commensurate with the extent of their participation in the activity.

All other healthcare professionals requesting continuing education credit for this enduring material will be issued a certificate of participation.

DISCLOSURE OF CONFLICTS OF INTEREST
The EOCME assesses conflict of interest with its instructors, faculty, planners, and other individuals who are in a position to control the content of CME activities. All relevant conflicts of interest that are identified are thoroughly vetted by EOCME for fair balance, scientific objectivity, and patient care recommendations. EOCME is committed to providing its learners with CME activities that promote improvements or quality in healthcare and not a specific proprietary business or a commercial interest.

The planning committee, staff, authors and editors listed below have identified no financial relationships or relationships to products or devices they or their spouse/life partner have with commercial interest related to the content of this CME activity:
Anthony M. Alleman, MD, MPH; Constantine M. Burgan, MD; Nirvikar Dahiya, MD; Adrian A. Dawkins, MD; Aaron D. Fain, MD; Helena Gabriel, MD; Gowthaman Gunabushanam, MD; Gayatri Joshi, MD; Alison Kemp; Lauren Kummant, MD; Pradeep Kuttysankaran; Jill E. Langer, MD; William Middleton, MD; Frank H. Miller, MD, FACR; Daniel C. Oppenheimer, MD; Maitray D. Patel, MD, Kristin Rebik, DO; Shuchi K. Rodgers, MD; Deborah J. Rubens, MD; Rupan Sanyal, MD; James H. Seow, MBBS, FRANZCR; Steven B. Soliman, DO, RMSK; Paul J. Spicer, MD; John Vassallo; Jason M. Wagner, MD; Peter S. Wang, MD; Scott W. Young, MD.

The planning committee, staff, authors and editors listed below have identified financial relationships or relationships to products or devices they or their spouse/life partner have with commercial interest related to the content of this CME activity:
Richard G. Barr, MD, PhD, FACR, FSRU, FAIUM: receives research support from Supersonic Imagine, BK Medical Holding Company, Inc., and General Electric Company; participates in a speakers' bureau for Mindray DS USA, Inc. and Canon Medical Systems USA; receives royalties from Thieme Medical Publishers, Inc.; participates in speakers bureau and receives research support from Siemens Medical Solutions USA, Inc. and Koninklijke Philips N.V.
David T. Fetzer, MD: participates in speakers bureau and receives research support from Koninklijke Philips N.V. and Siemens Medical Solutions USA, Inc.
Mindy M. Horrow, MD, FACR: partner is employed by Merck & Co., Inc.
Aya Kamaya, MD: receives royalties from Elsevier BV.
Mark E. Lockhart, MD: receives royalties from Oxford University Press and has an employment affiliation with John Wiley & Sons, Inc.
Leslie M. Scoutt, MD: is a consultant/advisor for Koninklijke Philips N.V.

UNAPPROVED/OFF-LABEL USE DISCLOSURE
The EOCME requires CME faculty to disclose to the participants:
1. When products or procedures being discussed are off-label, unlabelled, experimental, and/or investigational (not US Food and Drug Administration [FDA] approved); and
2. Any limitations on the information presented, such as data that are preliminary or that represent ongoing research, interim analyses, and/or unsupported opinions. Faculty may discuss information about pharmaceutical agents that is outside of FDA-approved labelling. This information is intended solely for CME and is not intended to promote off-label use of these medications. If you have any questions, contact the medical affairs department of the manufacturer for the most recent prescribing information.

TO ENROLL

To enroll in the *Radiologic Clinics of North America* Continuing Medical Education program, call customer service at 1-800-654-2452 or sign up online at http://www.theclinics.com/home/cme. The CME program is available to subscribers for an additional annual fee of USD 327.60.

METHOD OF PARTICIPATION

In order to claim credit, participants must complete the following:

1. Complete enrolment as indicated above.
2. Read the activity.
3. Complete the CME Test and Evaluation. Participants must achieve a score of 70% on the test. All CME Tests and Evaluations must be completed online.

CME INQUIRIES/SPECIAL NEEDS

For all CME inquiries or special needs, please contact elsevierCME@elsevier.com.

Preface
Ultrasound

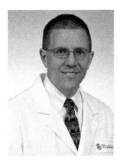

Jason M. Wagner, MD
Editor

Ultrasound remains a vibrant imaging modality, invaluable in patient evaluation and management. The advantages of ultrasound include its safety, portability, availability, and relatively low cost. Doppler interrogation of blood flow remains a unique and highly valuable advantage of ultrasound, noninvasively providing detailed physiologic information. This issue contains articles describing state-of-the-art evaluation of the carotid and vertebral arteries.

Recently, the field of ultrasound has been invigorated by the increasing use of elastography and intravenous contrast. The articles in this issue describe the evaluation of diffuse liver disease, sonographic screening for hepatocellular carcinoma in patients with chronic liver disease, and the use of contrast-enhanced ultrasound in the evaluation of focal observations in the liver. These topics represent some of the most important opportunities for high-quality ultrasound to make a difference in the lives of patients, detecting potentially lethal disease at an earlier stage. In addition, the role of ultrasound in the Liver Imaging Reporting and Data System (LI-RADS), is described by authors involved in the development of LI-RADS.

The evaluation and management of thyroid nodules remain a clinical challenge. An article describes the use of the American College of Radiology Thyroid Imaging Reporting and Data System to potentially reduce the workup of benign thyroid nodules. Evaluation of cervical lymph nodes is described from the perspective of the expected anatomic distribution of common diseases. In an article on pelvic pain in nonpregnant women, the authors challenge us to "up our game" in the detailed assessment of endometriosis. Additional articles cover common clinical indications of ultrasound, including right upper quadrant pain, renal masses, first-trimester pregnancy, scrotal pathologic condition, sports medicine, and superficial lumps and bumps.

I am grateful for the contributions of the authors, all experts in the field. They are all passionate about the use of ultrasound in patient care, and their passion is reflected in their work. It is humbling to work with such a distinguished group. On a personal note, I would like specifically thank Anthony Alleman, Mindy Horrow, Bill Middleton, Deb Rubens, and Leslie Scoutt for their teaching, mentorship, encouragement, and guidance. We are all indebted to the skilled sonographers, our partners in patient care, who produce such amazing images. Finally, I am thankful for the readers of this issue. I hope that it provides practical ways to use ultrasound to benefit your patients.

Jason M. Wagner, MD
Department of Radiological Sciences
University of Oklahoma Health Sciences Center
College of Medicine, P.O. Box 2690
Garrison Tower, Suite 4G4250
Oklahoma City, OK 73126, USA

E-mail address:
jason-wagner@ouhsc.edu

Radiol Clin N Am 57 (2019) xi
https://doi.org/10.1016/j.rcl.2019.02.011
0033-8389/19/© 2019 Published by Elsevier Inc.

Sonography of the Thyroid

Jill E. Langer, MD

KEYWORDS

- Thyroid nodules • Thyroid cancer • Fine-needle aspiration
- Thyroid imaging reporting and data system • Diffuse thyroid disease • Thyroiditis

KEY POINTS

- Nodular features that have a high correlation with thyroid malignancy are marked hypoechogenicity, infiltrative and/or lobulated margins, microcalcifications, and a taller-than-wide shape.
- Nearly entirely cystic and spongiform nodules are highly likely to be benign.
- Because the vast majority of thyroid nodules are benign lesions or nonaggressive neoplasms, fine-needle aspiration recommendations should be tailored to detect biologically significant malignancy while exposing the fewest number of patients to invasive and costly procedures.
- The American College of Radiology has developed a risk-stratification system called the Thyroid Imaging Reporting and Data System, which is able to classify thyroid nodule malignancy risk based on sonographic appearance.
- Recognition of the various patterns of diffuse thyroid disease is essential in distinguishing between these conditions and nodular thyroid disease.

INTRODUCTION

The proximity of the thyroid gland to the skin surface allows sonography to provide high-resolution imaging for evaluation of the thyroid parenchyma and thyroid lesions. Sonography of the thyroid is the imaging method of choice for the evaluation of thyroid nodules to determine their risk of malignancy and the need for fine-needle aspiration (FNA). Diffuse thyroid disease is commonly encountered both clinically and during sonographic evaluation of the thyroid. Recognition of the various patterns of diffuse thyroid disease may aid in diagnosis and distinguish these conditions from nodular thyroid disease.

NORMAL ANATOMY

The thyroid gland is a butterfly-shaped organ located in the central compartment of the neck, just below the thyroid cartilage and anterior to the trachea. It consists of 2 lateral conically shaped lobes and the isthmus, a narrow band of midline tissue (Fig. 1). The normal thyroid has relatively homogeneous, bright parenchymal echogenicity due to its relatively reflective follicular composition with a smooth overlying capsule, best seen anteriorly.[1,2] In most patients the lobes are similar in size; however, rarely there will be hypoplasia or agenesis of one or both lobes, most commonly the left, with or without isthmic agenesis (Fig. 2). The dimensions of the adult thyroid gland vary with body habitus, but they generally are 40 to 60 mm in length, 20 to 30 mm in width, and 15 to 20 mm in anteroposterior diameter; the anteroposterior diameter of the isthmus is usually less than 6 mm.

The thyroid also has a pyramidal lobe, a superior extension of thyroid tissue of variable length, which is a vestigial remnant of the thyroglossal tract that arises from the isthmus and ascends toward the hyoid bone.[1,2] The normal pyramidal lobe is quite small and often not well seen by sonography, but when hypertrophied, for example, in the setting of Graves disease, can be imaged by sonography (Fig. 3).

The Perelman School of Medicine at the University of Pennsylvania, Hospital of the University of Pennsylvania, 3400 Spruce Street, Philadelphia, PA 19104, USA
E-mail address: jill.langer@uphs.upenn.edu

Radiol Clin N Am 57 (2019) 469–483
https://doi.org/10.1016/j.rcl.2019.01.001

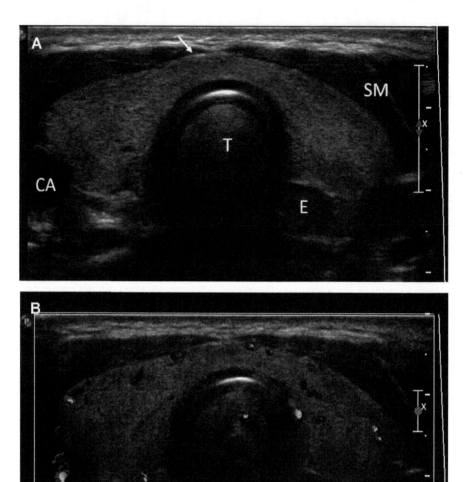

Fig. 1. Normal thyroid. (*A*) Transverse image of the neck shows that the thyroid lies anterior to the trachea (T) and is bordered laterally by the carotid artery (CA) and anteriorly by the strap muscles (SM). The normal parenchyma has homogeneous bright echogenicity due to the reflective follicular composition. A thin white line (*arrow*) representing the normal capsule is seen along the surface of the thyroid. The esophagus (E) is visible posteriorly, deep to the left lobe. (*B*) On color Doppler imaging, the parenchyma of each lobe should have a moderate amount of flow that is evenly distributed.

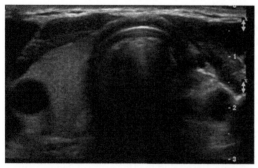

Fig. 2. Hemiagenesis of the thyroid. Transverse view of the thyroid shows a normal right lobe but absence of the isthmus and left lobe. This congenital variant has no clinical significance.

EXAMINATION TECHNIQUE

A high-frequency (10 MHz or higher) linear probe is preferred for head and neck ultrasound, because it provides optimal resolution.[2,3] Lower-frequency probes with deeper sound penetration but less spatial resolution may be needed in the setting of a large patient body habitus or to evaluate large thyroid glands. The patient should be positioned in maximal tolerated neck extension. This is achieved by pointing their chin upwards and by placing a rolled pillow under the upper back. The examination should document the 3-dimensional size of the gland and the size, number, and features of any significant focal lesions within the thyroid as well as diffuse abnormalities (**Box 1**). It is

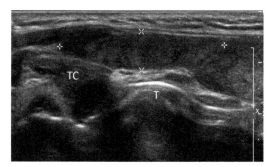

Fig. 3. Pyramidal lobe. A parasagittal image shows an enlarged and hypoechoic pyramidal lobe (partially outlined by calipers) extending cephalad over the trachea (T) and thyroid cartilage (TC) in this patient with Graves disease.

important to extend the ultrasound scanning beyond the thyroid borders, especially into the lateral neck compartment to evaluate the cervical lymph nodes as well as above the isthmus to evaluate the pyramidal lobe.[3]

FOCAL LESIONS

When a focal abnormality is noted in the thyroid parenchyma on sonography, it is called a nodule. Screening studies have shown that thyroid nodules are extremely common, especially those less than 1 cm, and they are more prevalent in women than men, and occur with increasing frequency with advancing age. As many as 67% of senior adults in the United States have focal lesions when evaluated by sonography.[4,5] The vast majority of focal nodules in the thyroid are hyperplastic regions containing nonneoplastic cells in which the orderly follicular architecture is disrupted by regions of larger and irregularly shaped follicles (Fig. 4).[5]

Follicular adenomas are the most commonly encountered thyroid neoplasms. This benign thyroid tumor is not considered to pose a risk of malignancy but a small percentage may become hyperfunctioning and lead to hyperthyroidism.[1,5] Approximately 7% to 20% of all focal nodules that are selected for biopsy are a thyroid malignancy. The incidence of cancer among detected nodules within a specific population will vary depending on patient age, the level of iodine insufficiency, the method of nodule detection, and the various selection biases in determining which nodules undergo histologic analysis.[5,6]

Most thyroid cancers are well-differentiated tumors and have an excellent prognosis.[5] Papillary thyroid cancer (PTC) is the most common thyroid cancer and has 2 subtypes, classic and follicular variant, with follicular cancer (FC) the second

most common. Medullary thyroid carcinomas (MTC) arise from the parafollicular or C cells of the thyroid and account for approximately 5% of all thyroid cancer; approximately 80% occur sporadically and 20% in patients with multiple endocrine neoplasia (MEN) type 2. The more aggressive thyroid malignances, poorly differentiated PTC and anaplastic cancers, are uncommon, are usually diagnosed at an advanced stage, and carry a poor prognosis.[7,8] Other less common focal lesions in the thyroid include a focal region of thyroiditis, an intrathryoidal parathyroid adenoma, and metastatic disease (Box 2).

Box 1
Recommended thyroid ultrasound imaging protocol and documentation

Transverse images of the superior, mid, and inferior of both lobes

Longitudinal images of the medial, mid, and lateral portions of both lobes

Measurements of lobe recorded in 3 dimensions (anteroposterior, transverse, and longitudinal planes)

At least one transverse image of the isthmus

The thickness (anteroposterior measurement) of the isthmus on the transverse view

The pyramidal lobe in 2 planes (when visible)

The location and size in 3 dimensions of all significant[a] nodules

Sufficient imaging of focal lesions to be able to characterize a nodule in terms of echogenicity, composition, margins, presence and types of echogenic foci and calcifications, effect on the thyroid capsule, and/or extension beyond the capsule.[b]

The presence, size, and anatomic location of abnormal lymph nodes in the lateral and central compartments of the neck

Color or power Doppler image of either diffuse abnormalities of the thyroid

[a] Significant is best understood to mean a nodule with imaging findings of concern for malignancy.

[b] Many nodule features are best assessed during real-time examination. Recording of cine loops of focal lesions may improve interpretation of nodule features and strongly encourages both the purposes of primary review as well as later comparison.

Adapted from the AIUM Practice Parameter for the performance of thyroid and parathyroid ultrasound examination; with permission.

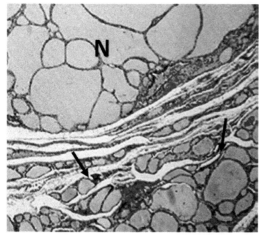

Fig. 4. Hyperplastic nodule. A photomicrograph of the thyroid with hematoxylin and eosin stain viewed at low power demonstrates the normal parenchyma (*arrows*) to be composed of follicles or roughly similar size, each composed of a circular distribution of epithelial (follicular) cells surrounding small pools of colloid, which appears light pink. The hyperplastic nodule (N) demonstrates larger and more irregularly shaped follicles that have much more central colloid, which appears as cystic regions on imaging. This type of nonneoplastic architectural distortion is the most commonly encountered nodule.

SONOGRAPHIC NODULE FEATURES

If extension of a lesion beyond the thyroid capsule or metastatic cervical lymphadenopathy is identified on imaging, a thyroid malignancy can be confidently diagnosed[7,9] (**Fig. 5**). In the absence of these findings, sonographic assessment of nodular features has emerged as the primary

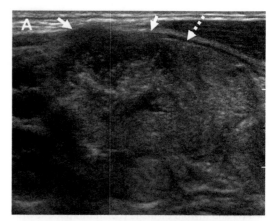

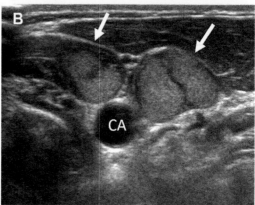

Fig. 5. Papillary thyroid cancer with extrathyroidal extension and metastatic cervical lymphadenopathy. (*A*) A sagittal image of the left lobe of the thyroid shows a 3.5 cm solid, hypoechoic, and calcified nodule. Along the inferior aspect of the lesion, the overlying normal thyroid capsule (*dashed arrow*) is intact, but along the superior aspect the lesion has grown through the capsule (*arrows*) extending into the overlying soft tissues, indicating a malignancy. (*B*) A transverse image of the left neck shows metastatic lymphadenopathy (*arrows*) adjacent to the carotid artery (CA).

imaging means to assess the likelihood of malignancy of thyroid nodules[9] (**Box 3**).

Echogenicity

The echogenicity of a thyroid nodule refers to the brightness of the solid component relative to the normal thyroid parenchyma and is classified as (1) hypoechoic, meaning darker; (2) hyperechoic, meaning brighter; or (3) isoechoic, meaning equal in echogenicity (**Fig. 6**). Marked hypoechogenicity refers to nodules that are darker than the strap muscles.[9,10] Nodules with regions of varying echogenicity may be described by the dominant echogenicity or as heterogeneous.[10] The classic type of PTC and MTC are very densely cellular and

Box 2
Focal thyroid lesions
Hyperplastic nodule (at least 75%)
Benign adenoma (5%–10%)
Thyroid carcinoma (7%–20%)
Papillary thyroid carcinoma (80%[a])
Follicular thyroid carcinoma (5–10%[a])
Medullary thyroid carcinoma (5%[a])
Anaplastic carcinoma (<1%[a])
Focal area of thyroiditis (1%–5%)
Metastatic disease (<1%)
Intrathyroidal parathyroid gland (<1%)
[a] Percentage of thyroid carcinomas in the United States.

Nodule features associated with malignancy

Capsular invasion

Coexisting metastatic lymphadenopathy

Markedly hypoechoic echogenicity

Entirely or nearly entirely solid composition[a]

Taller-than-wide shape

Infiltrative or lobulated margin

Punctate echogenic foci[b]

Irregular   or   interrupted   peripheral calcifications

[a] Especially if associated with marked hypoechogenicity and/or with calcifications.

[b] Especially when present in solid and/or hypoechoic solid regions of a nodule.

therefore usually appear as hypoechoic, often markedly hypoechoic solid nodules.[10,11] However, some benign nodules will also appear hypoechoic when compared with normal parenchyma due to regions of nonmalignant cellular proliferation. Hypoechogenicity, as a unique characteristic, is therefore only a moderately sensitive (80%) finding for malignancy,[5,6] whereas marked hypoechogenicity is less sensitive (41%), but much more specific (more than 90%).[5,6,12–14] Follicular neoplasms, including benign adenoma, follicular carcinoma, and follicular variant of papillary cancer, typically appear as solid or nearly entirely solid nodules and tend to appear isoechoic or hyperechoic because they are composed of small microfollicles that produce acoustic reflections similar to normal parenchymal echogenicity[15,16] (see **Fig. 6**).

Composition

Nodule composition is described as (1) solid or nearly entirely solid, (2) mixed cystic and solid, or (c) nearly entirely cystic.[9,10] Benign nodules account for the overwhelmingly majority of mixed cystic and solid-appearing nodules, because colloid appears cystic on sonography[5,6,9,10] (**Fig. 7**). Thyroid cancers are most commonly solid or nearly entirely solid, but some benign nodules

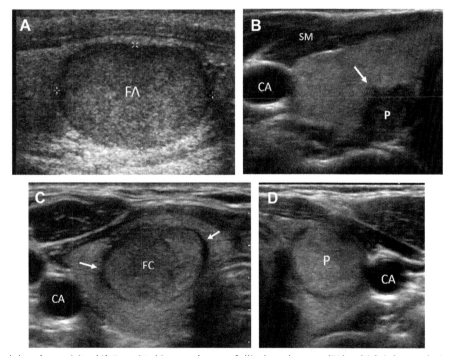

Fig. 6. Nodule echogenicity. (A) A sagittal image shows a follicular adenoma (FA), which is hypoechoic or slightly darker than the parenchyma and solid in consistency with a smooth margin. (B) A transverse image of the right lobe shows a papillary carcinoma (P), which is markedly hypoechoic, darker than the strap muscles (SM) and has a lobulated margin (*arrow*). Both of these features have a high correlation with malignancy. (C) A transverse image of the right lobe shows a follicular carcinoma (FC), which demonstrates different regions of echogenicity, appearing hypoechoic laterally and isoechoic medially. Note that there is a dark rim or halo around this nodule, which histologically represents a fibrous capsule, a finding that can also be seen in benign nodules. (D) A transverse image of the left lobe shows a follicular variant of papillary carcinoma (P), which is hyperechoic and solid. CA, carotid artery.

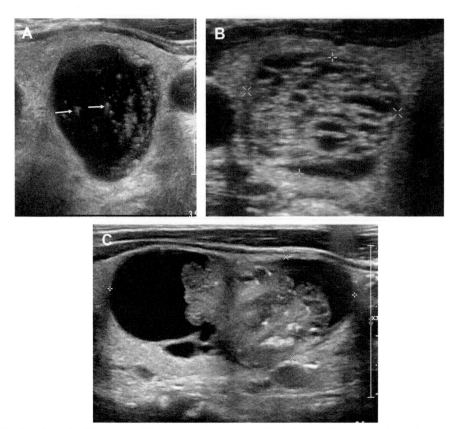

Fig. 7. Mixed cystic and solid nodules. (*A*) A transverse image of the left lobe shows a nearly entirely cystic nodule containing several echogenic foci that have large comet tail reverberation artifacts (*arrows*) caused by colloid, a finding that is highly correlated with benignity. (*B*) A transverse image of the right lobe shows a hyperplastic, mixed cystic and solid, nodule (outlined by calipers). The solid component demonstrates a spongiform appearance, defined as multiple microcytic areas that occupy more than 50% of the nodule volume. This appearance is highly likely to be benign. (*C*) A sagittal image shows a cystic papillary thyroid carcinoma (outlined by calipers). Note that the solid component appears as a frondlike, projection into the lumen of the nodule and has both calcifications and irregular borders.

will seem entirely solid, especially adenomas, such that solid consistency as a unique feature is neither specific nor sensitive for malignancy.[11–14] Thyroid neoplasms may undergo degeneration or necrosis causing cystic-appearing regions to develop.[17,18] A partially cystic nodule is considered suspicious for malignancy if the solid component is hypoechoic, has an irregular border and/or contains calcifications, and projects into the nodule with an acute angle.[17,18] Approximately 6% of all PTC will have a predominately cystic composition.[18] Conversely, if the solid component is isoechoic, smoothly marginated, and has a concentric distribution, the nodule is much more likely benign.[17] Purely cystic nodules are considered benign and nodules with a spongiform appearance, generally described as multiple microcytic areas that occupy more than 50% of the nodule volume, and have a very low risk of malignancy[5,6,9,15,19] (**Box 4**).

Shape

A taller-than-wide shape is defined as a ratio of greater than 1:1 when comparing the anteroposterior with the horizontal diameter as measured in the transverse plane and is considered an aggressive growth pattern (**Fig. 8**). This finding is not sensitive for malignancy but has specificity ranging from 82% to 93% and is most commonly noted in smaller cancers, under 1 cm.[10,20–22]

Calcifications and Echogenic Foci

Nodules may contain calcifications that are described as either macrocalcifications or microcalcifications.[10] Macrocalcifications are those calcifications large enough to cause deep acoustic shadowing on sonography and occur in both benign and malignant nodules, deposited in areas of fibrosis and tissue degeneration[5] (**Fig. 9**). Large and coarse calcifications are most worrisome for

---

Box 4
Nodule features with a very low risk of malignancy

Entirely cystic composition

Spongiform appearance

Mixed cystic and solid nodules with concentric solid portions

Large comet tail reverberation artifact

---

malignancy when seen in a solid and/or hypoechoic nodule.[23,24] Calcifications along the periphery of a nodule can be thin and regular, often called "egg-shell" calcification, and are usually benign,[25,26] whereas irregular or interrupted peripheral calcifications are more concerning for malignancy (**Fig. 10**).[24,25]

Microcalcifications appear as less than 1 mm, punctate nonshadowing echogenic foci and represent the aggregates of psammoma bodies that are found in about 40% of PTCs.[5,9] True microcalcifications almost always occur in nodules with other sonographic features of PTC, such as entirely solid consistency, hypoechogenicity (often marked), and infiltrative margins[24] (**Fig. 11**). Many nodules, particularly benign hyperplastic nodules contain echogenic foci that are not microcalcifications but instead are due to colloid or reflections from back walls of small cystic spaces.[9,19,27] Echogenic

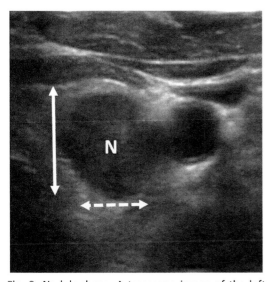

Fig. 8. Nodule shape. A transverse image of the left lobe shows a hypoechoic and solid nodule that is larger in the anteroposterior dimension (*solid arrow*) than in width (*dashed arrow*). This shape highly predicts a malignancy but tends to be seen only in small cancers, such as this 1.3 cm papillary thyroid cancer.

foci associated with large comet tail reverberation artifact, which appears as an inverted triangle measuring over 1 mm in length, are a reliable indicator of a colloid-containing nodule, the vast majority of which are benign[27] (see **Fig. 7A**). Other types of echogenic foci, such as those with a short (under 1 mm) comet tail reverberation artifact or no artifact, are nonspecific but should not be assumed to be microcalcifications, especially when not associated with other features concerning for malignancy.

Nodule Margin

The margin of a nodule refers to the border or interface between the nodule and the adjacent parenchyma.[7,10] A smooth margin is an uninterrupted, well-defined, curvilinear margin and is common in benign nodules, but up to one-third of malignancies may have a smooth border (see **Fig. 6A, C**). An irregular or infiltrating border has jagged or spiculated soft tissue protrusions extending into the parenchyma (see **Fig. 11A**). Focal, rounded soft tissue protrusions that extend into the adjacent parenchyma constitute a lobulated margin. Lobulated and infiltrative margins are considered to represent an aggressive growth pattern and carry relatively high specificity for thyroid malignancy but relatively low sensitivity (see **Fig. 6B**). An ill-defined thyroid nodule border is a common finding in benign hyperplastic nodules and is not concerning for malignancy. A halo refers to a dark rim around the periphery of the nodule and can be due to either compressed thyroid vessels displaced by the nodule, more common in benign nodules, or a fibrous capsule that is found in both benign nodules and malignant neoplasms[7] (see **Fig. 6C**).

Vascularity

Many papillary cancers lack vascularity, and increased intranodular vascularity can be seen in both benign and malignant nodules.[5,6,28] Therefore, intranodular vascularity as an individual finding does not predict malignancy, especially in nodules that lack other features of PTC. Intranodular vascularity is more commonly associated with follicular cancers that are uncommon in the United States but have a higher prevalence in Europe and iodine insufficient regions.[5,29]

INDICATIONS FOR FINE-NEEDLE ASPIRATION

Currently, the most effective diagnostic test to determine whether a nodule is neoplastic and requires surgical pathologic analysis to determine if it is a malignancy is FNA biopsy. Many

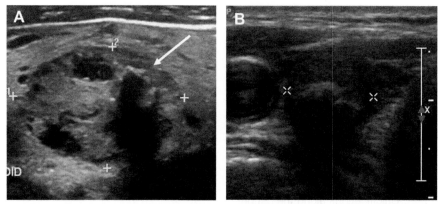

Fig. 9. Macrocalcifications. (*A*) A sagittal image shows a central macrocalcification (*arrow*), producing distal acoustic shadowing present in this benign mixed and cystic, hyperplastic nodule (outlined by calipers). (*B*) A transverse image shows a large, central dystrophic calcification in this hypoechoic and solid-appearing medullary carcinoma (outlined by calipers).

patient-related factors may influence the need for thyroid FNA, including age at the time of diagnosis, overall health, risk factors for thyroid malignancy such as a head and neck irradiation as child or a known predisposing genetic syndrome, and symptoms such as rapid growth of a solid nodule or new hoarseness.[5] However, because most thyroid lesions are benign, and even malignant nodules, particularly ones smaller than 1 cm, frequently exhibit indolent or nonaggressive behavior it is generally agreed that not all detected nodules require FNA or surgical removal.[30–33]

Several risk-stratification systems that classify thyroid nodule malignancy risk based on sonographic appearance have been introduced in the last decade.[10,34–38] All share a goal of detecting biologically significant cancers while exposing the fewest number of patients to invasive and costly medical evaluations, especially for nodules detected incidentally and/or in low-risk patients. In addition, nearly all rely on the presence of multiple suspicious features to determine the risk of malignancy rather than on individual features.

Recognizing that none of the classifications systems had been widely adopted by the radiology community in the United States, as well as the inability of the systems to classify all nodules, the American College of Radiology (ACR) developed the Thyroid Imaging Reporting and Data System (TI-RADS).[10,39] The initial step was the development of a standard set of terms (called a lexicon), which both defined and illustrated the sonographic features that can be

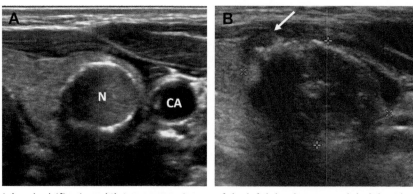

Fig. 10. Peripheral calcifications. (*A*) A transverse image of the left lobe shows a nodule (N) with smooth, peripheral or "egg shell" calcifications, a type of calcification much more common in benign nodules; FNA was performed but was nondiagnostic due to insufficient material. The nodule has remained stable in size on follow-up examinations. (*B*) A sagittal image shows a nodule (outlined by calipers) that has a region of discontinuous or interrupted calcifications through which there is a projection of hypoechoic soft tissue. Biopsy yielded PTC. CA, carotid artery.

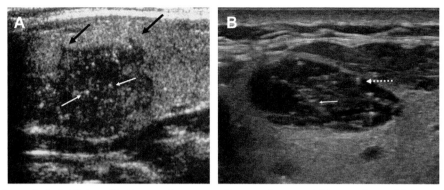

Fig. 11. Echogenic foci. (A) A sagittal image shows a papillary carcinoma, which contains multiple punctate echogenic foci (*white arrows*) due to microcalcifications. Note that the nodule is solid, markedly hypoechoic, and has infiltrating margins (*black arrows*), all features highly associated with malignancy. (B) A transverse image of the right lobe shows a mixed cystic and solid, benign hyperplastic nodule that contains many echogenic foci, some of which have large comet tail reverberation artifact (*dashed arrow*) likely related to colloid and others are linear rather than punctate (*solid arrow*) from back wall reflections from cystic spaces. These types of echogenic foci are unlikely to be microcalcifications.

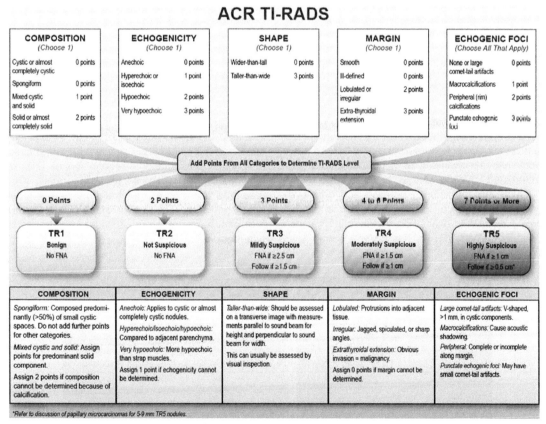

Fig. 12. ACR TI-RADS chart. The 5 nodule features of composition, echogenicity, shape, margin, and calcifications/echogenic foci are analyzed and assigned points ranging from 0 to 3 in each category. The point total determines a level of suspicion for malignancy, which ranges from TR1 (benign) to TR 5 (highly suspicious). Within each level, the size of the nodule determines if FNA of follow-up is recommended. (*From* Tessler FN, Middleton WD, Grant EG, et al. Thyroid imaging, reporting and data system (TI-RADS): white paper of the ACR TI-RADS committee. J Am Coll Radiol 2017;14(5):587–95; with permission.)

Box 5
Causes of diffuse thyroid disease
Chronic lymphocytic (Hashimoto) thyroiditis
Graves disease
Subacute granulomatous (de Quervain) thyroiditis
Drug-induced thyroiditis
Silent (subacute lymphocytic) thyroiditis
Postpartum thyroiditis

used to describe every thyroid nodule. The 5 ultrasound features of composition, echogenicity, shape, margin, and the presence of echogenic foci/calcifications of each nodule are then used to assign point values based on the relative relationship of that feature with the estimated risk of malignancy. More suspicious features are awarded higher points, and less concerning features are awarded less or no points.

The point total is summed to determine a risk assessment category of "Benign," "Minimally suspicious," "Moderately suspicious," or "Highly suspicious" for malignancy (**Fig. 12**). Within each risk category, the size of the lesion determines if FNA, sonographic follow-up, or no further evaluation is recommended. The ACR TI-RADS offers the advantage of being able to classify every nodule. For example, there are provisions to assign points to nonassessable features such as when consistency and echogenicity of a nodule cannot be determined due to dense calcifications. ACR TI-RADS also provides a detailed and definitive 5-year sonographic follow-up recommendation versus no further evaluation for nodules that do meet FNA criteria.

ACR TI-RADS is consistent with most other guidelines in recommending FNA for highly suspicious nodules only if 1 cm or larger. ACR TI-RADS differs in that it recommends higher FNA size thresholds for nodules with an intermediate level of suspicion and does not recommend either biopsy or follow-up for nodules that have a high likelihood of being benign, such as spongiform nodules of any size. The overall effect is a significant reduction in the number of biopsies performed and less follow-up of benign nodules. However, less malignant nodules over 1 cm are recommended for FNA using ACR TI-RADS (83.3%) as compared with other guidelines (93%–96%).[40] However, most of the malignant nodules that are not initially recommended for FNA by ACR TI-RADS are recommended for follow-up, allowing future opportunity for detection if growth is noted.

DIFFUSE THYROID DISEASE

Diffuse thyroid disease (DTD) refers to a group of conditions that are most commonly related to an underlying inflammatory process and typically cause thyroid enlargement, alterations in parenchymal echogenicity, coarse echotexture, increased or decreased vascularity, and surface contour changes[41,42] (**Box 5**). Autoimmune thyroid disease is by far the most commonly encountered DTD in clinical practice. There is significant overlap in the sonographic findings of these various entities, and the diagnosis is often established based on clinical presentation. Recognition of DTD is essential in determining if a focal abnormality represents a true nodule, generally meaning a focal lesion that may require FNA biopsy, or is simply part of the inflammatory process, often called a pseudonodule.

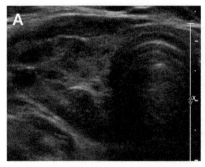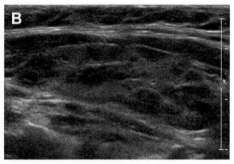

Fig. 13. Chronic lymphocytic thyroiditis. Transverse (*A*) and sagittal (*B*) views show geometrically shaped, hypoechoic patchy regions throughout the thyroid, interspersed with more normal-appearing regions. The hypoechoic regions are due to lymphocytic infiltration, and the scattered linear bright lines and irregular capsule of the thyroid occur due to fibrosis, a prominent feature of this autoimmune thyroid disease. This pattern should be recognized and described as a diffuse process rather than as a multinodular gland.

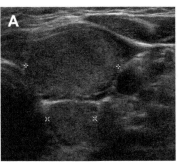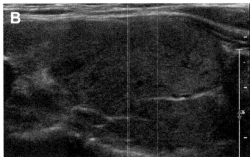

Fig. 14. Pseudonodules in chronic lymphocytic thyroiditis. Transverse (A) view shows that cursors have been placed within the left lobe around 2 nodular-appearing areas. However, on the sagittal image (B) these prove to be part of the overall heterogeneity of the parenchyma due to the thyroiditis and do not truly represent focal lesions.

Chronic Lymphocytic (Hashimoto) Thyroiditis

Chronic lymphocytic thyroiditis (CLT) is an autoimmune disease in which antibodies are directed against the thyroid leading to chronic inflammation. It is the most common cause of hypothyroidism and affects roughly 10% of the US population. It tends to run in families and most commonly affects middle-aged women but can occur at any age.[41] The hallmark histologic changes are lymphocytic infiltration, follicle destruction, and fibrosis.[42] The sonographic appearance of CLT is quite variable.[43–46] The lymphocytic infiltrates produce patchy regions of hypoechogenicity, which range from subcentimeter in size, to larger infiltrative and/or more nodular appearing, to entirely replacing the gland (Fig. 13). The degree of hypoechogenicity is relatively predictive of the severity of hypothyroidism. Later in the progression of thyroid inflammation, fibrosis develops and appears as hyperechoic linear and curvilinear bands and causes nodular surface changes. The gland may be normal in size, enlarged or small, if end stage and atrophic. Both the patchy hypoechoic regions and the parenchymal distortions caused by fibrosis may simulate nodules but are best considered to be "pseudonodules" because these regions, when recognized to be part of a more diffuse process, would not be considered candidates for FNA (Fig. 14). It has been suggested that there is a higher prevalence of PTC in patients with CLT.[47] Malignant nodules may be more challenging to detect within the heterogeneity of CLT but should be suspected if focal dense and/or psammomatous calcifications are noted[44,45,48] (Fig. 15). In general, hyperechoic, noncalcified nodules or patchy hyperechoic regions found in CLT glands represent less affected parenchyma and are thought to be a type of pseudonodule.[19,24]

Lymph node reactivity is almost invariably present in patients with CLT, most commonly in the paratracheal and pretracheal space and less commonly in the lateral neck.[49] Pathologic changes in the nodes, such as cystic change or calcifications, should raise concern for occult PTC and be assessed by nodal FNA. Patients with long-standing CLT may develop primary thyroid lymphoma, which is often diagnosed when patients note rapid enlargement of the thyroid in a previously atrophic gland. Thyroid lymphoma appears as one or multiple hypoechoic masses in the thyroid, often with increased sound through transmission[45,50] (Fig. 16).

Graves Disease

Graves disease is an autoimmune disorder in which the body produces antibodies to the receptor for thyroid-stimulating hormone causing hyperthyroidism. There is marked epithelial hyperplasia causing the gland to enlarge and become hypoechoic. Fibrosis is unusual unless

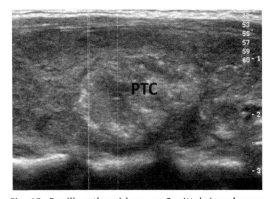

Fig. 15. Papillary thyroid cancer. Sagittal view shows a papillary thyroid cancer (PTC) occurring in a gland with chronic lymphocytic thyroiditis. The echogenicity of the nodule is similar to the background but the calcifications with the lesion facilitate its detection.

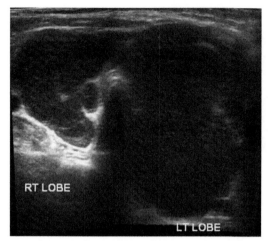

Fig. 16. Thyroid lymphoma. Transverse view of the thyroid in a patient with long-standing chronic lymphocytic thyroiditis who noted new neck swelling due to the development of primary thyroid lymphoma. The lymphomatous infiltration is asymmetrically involving the left lobe, which appears markedly enlarged, but the contour of the thyroid is preserved. Note how the involved parenchyma of both lobes is homogenously hypoechoic with good through transmission of sound. This sonographic feature highly suggests lymphoma because regions of lymphocytic thyroiditis tend to be more heterogeneously hypoechoic and attenuate sound due to underlying fibrosis.

the disease is long-standing such that the surface of the gland remains smooth and often scalloped.[42] The classic sonographic feature of Graves disease is increased Doppler flow in the gland referred to as the "thyroid inferno"[51] (**Fig. 17**). There is, however, overlap in blood flow patterns between Graves and other types of thyroiditis such that Doppler characteristics alone may not be sufficient to distinguish these 2 diagnostic entities.[52,53]

Subacute Granulomatous (de Quervain) Thyroiditis

Subacute granulomatous or de Quervain thyroiditis is a relatively uncommon condition, which is thought to be an immune response to a viral infection of the upper respiratory tract. Patients present with sudden onset of neck pain, that may last weeks or months, often with fever and other systemic symptoms. Patients may initially be hyperthyroid during the acute phase and later hypothyroid. The typical appearance is a patchy, poorly defined hypoechoic region in one or both lobes, mostly commonly with diminished flow in the affected areas[54] (**Fig. 18**). The changes will evolve over time and may take months to fully resolve.

Drug-Induced and Other Painless Thyroiditis

Patients treated with a wide variety of medications including amiodarone, interleukin-2, interferon-alpha, cytokines, tyrosine kinase inhibitors, and immunomodulating anticancer therapies may develop destructive thyroiditis without pain, although typically with clinical thyroid hormone dysfunction.[42,55] The gland may rapidly enlarge and develop diffuse changes of hypoechoic infiltrates. Silent thyroiditis is considered to be an autoimmune process and has been referred to as subacute lymphocytic thyroiditis because it may be a form of transient Hashimoto thyroiditis. It occurs primarily in women aged 30 to 50 years and tends to have lower levels of thyroid autoantibodies than seen in Hashimoto thyroiditis. Thyroiditis may also develop in the postpartum setting.[42]

In summary, nodular thyroid disease is very common, and the vast majority of nodules are benign, hyperplastic regions of the thyroid or benign adenomas, with the minority representing

A   **B**

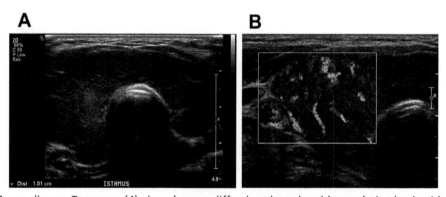

Fig. 17. Graves disease. Transverse (*A*) view shows a diffusely enlarged and hypoechoic gland, with smoothly lobulated surface. A color Doppler sagittal view (*B*) shows vascularity throughout the entire gland, a characteristic feature of Graves disease.

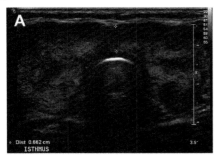 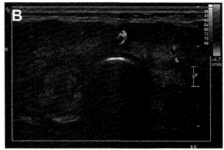

Fig. 18. Subacute granulomatous (de Quervain) thyroiditis. Transverse views in gray scale (*A*) and color Doppler (*B*) of the thyroid in a 43-year-old patient who presented with neck pain and fever show patchy hypoechoic regions in a relatively avascular gland. The patient had an elevated serum sedimentation rate and the symptoms and imaging features resolved in a few weeks.

a malignancy. Sonography serves as an effective diagnostic tool in determining the need for FNA to diagnose or exclude thyroid malignancy, especially in low-risk patients. Familiarity with the sonographic appearance of diffuse thyroid diseases allows differentiation of these conditions from nodular thyroid disease and will aid in the detection of coexisting malignancy.

REFERENCES

1. Khati N, Adamson T, Johnson KS, et al. Ultrasound of the thyroid and parathyroid glands. Ultrasound Q 2003;19:162–76.

2. Mazzaglia PJ, Muraveika L. Normal thyroid appearance and anatomic landmarks in neck ultrasound. In: Milas M, Mandel S, Langer JE, editors. Advanced thyroid and parathyroid ultrasound. Cham (Switzerland): Springer; 2017. p. 77–86.

3. AIUM practice guideline for the performance of ultrasound examinations of the head and neck. J Ultrasound Med 2014;33:366–02.

4. Mazzaferri EL. Management of a solitary thyroid nodule. N Engl J Med 1993;328(8):553–9.

5. Haugen BR, Alexander EK, Bible KC, et al. 2015 American Thyroid Association Management guidelines for adult patients with thyroid nodules and differentiated thyroid cancer: the American Thyroid Association guidelines task force on thyroid nodules and differentiated thyroid cancer. Thyroid 2016; 26(1):1–133.

6. Brito JP, Gionfriddo MR, Al Nofal A, et al. The accuracy of thyroid nodule ultrasound to predict thyroid cancer: systematic review and meta-analysis. J Clin Endocrinol Metab 2014; 99(4):1253–63.

7. Milas M, Tollison DM, Milas ZI. Feature illustration: thyroid nodule margins and extrathyroidal extention. In: Milas M, Mandel S, Langer JE, editors. Advanced thyroid and parathyroid ultrasound. Cham (Switzerland): Springer; 2017. p. 95–104.

8. Suh HJ, Moon HJ, Kwak JY, et al. Anaplastic thyroid cancer: ultrasonographic findings and the role of ultrasonography-guided fine needle aspiration. Yonsei Med J 2013;54:1400–6.

9. Frates MC, Benson CB, Charboneau JW, et al. Management of thyroid nodules detected at US: Society of Radiologists in Ultrasound consensus conference statement. Radiology 2005;237:794–800.

10. Grant EG, Tessler FN, Hoang JK, et al. Thyroid ultrasound reporting lexicon: white paper of the ACT thyroid imaging, reporting and data system (TI-RADS) committee. J Am Coll Radiol 2015;12: 1272–9.

11. Papini E, Guglielmi R, Bianchini A, et al. Risk of malignancy in nonpalpable thyroid nodules: predictive value of ultrasound and color-Doppler features. J Clin Endocrinol Metab 2002;87:1941–6.

12. Moon WJ, Jung SL, Lee JH, et al. Benign and malignant thyroid nodules: US differentiation–multicenter retrospective study. Radiology 2008;247:762–70.

13. Kim EK, Park CS, Chung WY, et al. New sonographic criteria for recommending fine-needle aspiration biopsy of nonpalpable solid nodules of the thyroid. AJR Am J Roentgenol 2002;178:687–91.

14. Ahn SS, Kim EK, Kang DR, et al. Biopsy of thyroid nodules: Comparison of three sets of guidelines. AJR Am J Roentgenol 2010;194:31–7.

15. Jeh SK, Jung SL, Kim BS, et al. Evaluating the degree of conformity of papillary carcinoma and follicular carcinoma to the reported ultrasonographic findings of malignant thyroid tumor. Korean J Radiol 2007;8:192–7.

16. Kim DS, Kim JH, Na DG, et al. Sonographic features of follicular variant papillary thyroid carcinomas in comparison with conventional papillary thyroid carcinomas. J Ultrasound Med 2009;28:1685–92.

17. Kim DW, Lee EJ, In HS, et al. Sonographic differentiation of partially cystic thyroid nodules: a prospective study. AJNR Am J Neuroradiol 2010;31:1961–6.

18. Henrichsen TL, Reading CC, Charboneau JW, et al. Cystic change in thyroid carcinoma: prevalence

and estimated volume in 360 carcinomas. J Clin Ul-trasound 2010;38:361–6.

19. Bonavita JA, Mayo J, Babb J, et al. Pattern recognition of benign nodules at ultrasound of the thyroid: which nodules can be left alone? AJR Am J Roentgenol 2009;193:207–13.

20. Moon HJ, Kwak JY, Kim EK, et al. A taller-than-wide shape in thyroid nodules in transverse and longitudinal ultrasonographic planes and the prediction of malignancy. Thyroid 2011;21:1249–53.

21. Chen SP, Hu YP, Chen B. Taller-than-wide sign for predicting thyroid microcarcinoma: Comparison and combination of two ultrasonographic planes. Ultrasound Med Biol 2014;40:2004–11.

22. Ren J, Liu B, Zhang LL, et al. A taller-than-wide shape is a good predictor of papillary thyroid carcinoma in small solid nodules. J Ultra Med 2015;34: 19–26.

23. Frates MC, Benson CB, Doubilet PM, et al. Prevalence and distribution of carcinoma in patients with solitary and multiple thyroid nodules on sonography. J Clin Endocrinol Metab 2006;91(9):3411–7.

24. Reading CC, Charboneau JW, Hay ID, et al. Sonography of thyroid nodules: a "classic pattern" diagnostic approach. Ultrasound Q 2005;21(3):157–65.

25. Taki S, Terahata S, Yamashita R, et al. Thyroid calcifications: Sonographic patterns and incidence of cancer. Clin Imaging 2004;28(5):368–71.

26. Park YJ, Kim JA, Son EJ, et al. Thyroid nodules with macrocalcification: sonographic findings predictive of malignancy. Yonsei Med J 2014;55:339–44.

27. Malhi H, Beland MD, Cen SY, et al. Echogenic foci in thyroid nodules: significance of posterior acoustic artifacts. AJR Am J Roentgenol 2014;203(6):1310–6.

28. Moon HJ, Kwak JY, Kim MJ, et al. Can vascularity at power Doppler US help predict thyroid malignancy? Radiology 2010;255(1):260–9.

29. Remonti LR, Kramer CK, Leitao CB, et al. Thyroid ultrasound features and risk of carcinoma: a systematic review and meta-analysis of observational studies. Thyroid 2015;25(5):538–50.

30. Welch HG, Black WC. Overdiagnosis in cancer. J Natl Cancer Inst 2010;102(9):605–13.

31. Hoang JK, Langer JE, Middleton WD, et al. Managing incidental thyroid nodules detected on imaging: white paper of the ACR Incidental Thyroid Findings Committee. J Am Coll Radiol 2015;12:143–50.

32. Ito Y, Miyauchi A, Inoue H, et al. An observational trial for papillary thyroid microcarcinoma in Japanese patients. World J Surg 2010;34:28–35.

33. Miyauchi A. Clinical trials of active surveillance of papillary microcarcinoma of the thyroid. World J Surg 2016;40(3):516–22.

34. Horvath E, Majlis S, Rossi R, et al. An ultrasonogram reporting system for thyroid nodules stratifying cancer risk for clinical management. J Clin Endocrinol Metab 2009;94:1748–51.

35. Park JY, Lee HJ, Jang HW, et al. A proposal for a thyroid imaging reporting and data system for ultrasound features of thyroid carcinoma. Thyroid 2009; 19(11):1257–64.

36. Kwak JY, Han KH, Yoon JH, et al. Thyroid imaging reporting and data system for US features of nodules: a step in establishing better stratification of cancer risk. Radiology 2011;260:892–9.

37. Russ G, Royer B, Bigorgne C, et al. Prospective evaluation of thyroid imaging reporting and data system on 4550 nodules with and without elastography. Eur J Endocrinol 2013;168(5):649–55.

38. Shin JH, Baek JH, Chung J, et al. Ultrasonography diagnosis and imaging-based management of thyroid nodules: revised Korean Society of Thyroid radiology consensus statement and recommendations. Korean J Radiol 2016;17:370–95.

39. Tessler FN, Middleton WD, Grant EG, et al. Thyroid imaging, reporting and data system (TI-RADS): white paper of the ACR TI-RADS committee. J Am Coll Radiol 2017;14(5):587–95.

40. Hoang JK, Middleton WD, Farjat AE, et al. Reduction in thyroid nodule biopsies and improved accuracy with American College of Radiology Thyroid Imaging and Reporting Data System. Radiology 2018;287: 185–93.

41. Pearce E, Farwell A, Braverman L. Current concepts: thyroiditis. N Engl J Med 2003;384(26): 2646–55.

42. Livolsi VA. The pathology of autoimmune thyroid disease: a review. Thyroid 1994;4(3):333–9.

43. Ahn HS, Kim DW, Lee YJ, et al. Diagnostic accuracy of real-time sonography in differinetiating diffuse thyroid disease from normal thyroid parenchyma: a multicenter study. AJR Am J Roentgenol 2018;211: 1–6.

44. Anderson L, Middleton WD, Teefey SA, et al. Hashimoto thyroiditis: part 1, sonographic analysis of the nodular form of Hashimoto thyroiditis. AJR Am J Roentgenol 2010;195:208–15.

45. Anderson L, Middleton W, Teefey SA, et al. Hashimoto thyroiditis: part 2, sonographic analysis of benign and malignant nodules in patients with diffuse hashimoto thyroiditis. AJR Am J Roentgenol 2010;195:216–22.

46. Yeh H, Futterweit W, Gilbert P. Micronodulation: ultrasonographic sign of Hashimoto thyroiditis. J Ultrasound Med 1996;15:813–9.

47. Gul K, Dirikoc A, Kiyak G, et al. The association between thyroid carcinoma and Hashimoto's thyroiditis: The ultrasonographic and histopathologic characteristics of malignant nodules. Thyroid 2010; 20:873–8.

48. Durfee SM, Benson CB, Arthaud DM, et al. Sonographic appearance of thyroid cancer in patients with Hashimoto thyroiditis. J Ultrasound Med 2015; 34(4):697–704.

49. Brancato D, Citarrella R, Richiusa P, et al. Neck lymph nodes in chronic autoimmune thyroiditis: the sonographic pattern. Thyroid 2013;23(2):173–7.

50. Ma B, Jia Y, Wang Q, et al. Ultrasound of primary non-Hodgkin's lymphoma. Clin Imaging 2014;38: 621–6.

51. Ralls PW, Mayekawa DS, Lee KP, et al. Color-flow Doppler sonography in Graves' disease: "Thyroid Inferno". AJR Am J Roentgenol 1988;150(4):781–4.

52. Sipos JA, Kahaly GJ. Imaging of thyrotoxicosis. Am J Med 2012;125(9):S1–20.

53. Alzahrani AS, Ceresini G, Aldasouqi SA. Role of ultrasonography in the differential diagnosis of thyrotoxicosis: a noninvasive, cost-effective, and widely available but underutilized diagnostic tool. Endocr Pract 2012;18(4):567–78.

54. Frates MC, Marqusee E, Benson CB, et al. Subacute granulomatous (deQuervain's) thyroiditis. J Ultrasound Med 2013;32:505–11.

55. Hamnvik OR, Larsen PR, Marqusee E. Thyroid dysfunction from antineoplastic agents. J Natl Cancer Inst 2011;103:1572–87.

Ultrasonography of Cervical Lymph Nodes

Jason M. Wagner, MD*, Anthony M. Alleman, MD, MPH

KEYWORDS

- Ultrasound • Cervical lymph nodes • Neck mass • Squamous cell carcinoma
- Papillary thyroid cancer

KEY POINTS

- Important considerations in the evaluation of cervical lymph nodes include patient history, node location, nodal morphology, and node size—in that order.
- Nodal metastatic disease in the neck generally follows a predictable pattern of spread in an untreated neck.
- Level 2/3 nodal metastatic disease may displace the carotid arteries medial and posterior. Paragangliomas and other deep masses displace the carotid lateral and anterior.
- A cystic lateral neck mass in an adult should be regarded as metastatic squamous cell carcinoma until proved otherwise.
- In the postoperative neck, particular attention must be paid to the margins of prior node dissection.

 Video content accompanies this article at http://www.radiologic.theclinics.com.

INTRODUCTION

The head and neck contain 40% of the estimated 800 lymph nodes in the body.[1,2] Cervical lymph nodes are commonly involved by a variety of benign and malignant conditions, for which accurate assessment of nodal involvement is crucial to patient management. Sonography is an excellent modality for imaging cervical lymph nodes because of its high spatial resolution, portability, low cost, lack of ionizing radiation, ability to assess tissue blood flow, and ability to guide needle biopsy. Sonography of the cervical lymph nodes is most valuable when correlated with the patient's clinical presentation, surgical history, pathology of any prior biopsy or resection, and prior imaging.

ANATOMY

The anatomic location of cervical lymph nodes is classified based on a system endorsed by the American Head and Neck Society and American Academy of Otolaryngology—Head and Neck Surgery (Fig. 1).[3,4]

- Level I lymph nodes are located superior to the hyoid and inferior to the mandible. Level IA (submental) nodes are located medial to the anterior belly of the digastric muscle. Level IB (submandibular) nodes are located between the anterior belly of the digastric and the lateral border of the submandibular gland.
- Level II lymph nodes are located above the level of the hyoid bone and between the lateral

---

Disclosure: None.
Department of Radiological Sciences, University of Oklahoma Health Sciences Center, College of Medicine, P.O. Box 2690, Garrison Tower, Suite 4G4250, Oklahoma City, OK 73126, USA
* Corresponding author.
E-mail address: jason-wagner@ouhsc.edu

Radiol Clin N Am 57 (2019) 485–500
https://doi.org/10.1016/j.rcl.2019.01.005

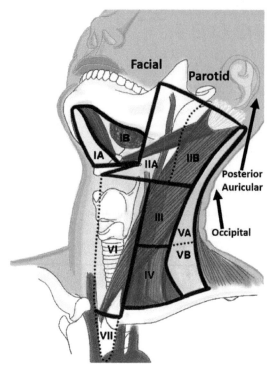

Fig. 1. Anatomic classification of cervical lymph nodes. The occipital nodes are in the posterior neck. The retropharyngeal lymph nodes are not depicted and are usually poorly visualized with transcutaneous ultrasound.

bone and the manubrium and to regard the upper half as above the cricoid (level III) and the lower half as below the cricoid (level IV).

- Level V (posterior triangle) lymph nodes are located posterior to the posterior border of the sternocleidomastoid muscle (except in the inferior neck where the anterior border is the posterolateral margin of the anterior scalene muscle) and anterior to the trapezius muscle.
- Level VI (central compartment) lymph nodes are medial to the common carotid arteries and between the hyoid bone and the manubrium.

It is important to apply this nodal classification system with the patient's neck in neutral position, as turning the head can sometimes alter the relationship of lymph nodes with anatomic landmarks (**Fig. 2** and Video 1). The supraclavicular lymph nodes can be defined as those lateral to the medial border of the common carotid and at or below the level of the clavicle on axial computed tomography (CT) images, which includes the inferior portions of levels IV and V.

There are several nodal locations that are not included in this system, including the intraparotid, facial, posterior auricular, and occipital lymph nodes. The retropharyngeal lymph nodes are not included in the system and are occasionally a site of metastasis for thyroid, nasopharyngeal, and posterior wall pharyngeal tumors.[4] An important limitation of ultrasonography is the inability to visualize most retropharyngeal lymph nodes.

HEAD AND NECK SQUAMOUS CELL CANCER

Evaluation of cervical lymph nodes requires an understanding of the frequently encountered diseases. Squamous cell carcinoma of the upper aerodigestive tract is the most common cause of nodal metastasis in the neck.[5] Early detection of nodal disease is critical because the presence

border of the submandibular gland and the posterior border of the sternocleidomastoid. Lymph nodes in level II may abut the lateral border of the submandibular gland.

- Level III and IV lymph nodes are below the level of the hyoid bone and lateral to the medial border of the common carotid artery. Level III is above the level of inferior margin of the cricoid and level IV below this level. The cricoid is the one border-forming structure in this system that is not easily visualized with ultrasound. A simple approximation is to consider the distance between the hyoid

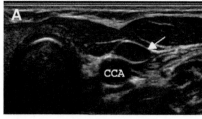
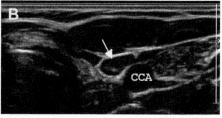

Fig. 2. (A) Left level IV lymph node (arrow) is located lateral to the common carotid artery (CCA) with the head in neutral position. (B) When the head is turned to the right, the same node appears to be medial to the carotid and could be incorrectly interpreted as level VI.

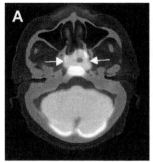 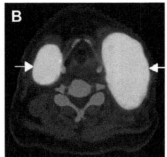 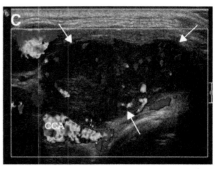

Fig. 3. Nasopharyngeal carcinoma. (A) FDG-PET/CT shows a hypermetabolic mass in the nasopharynx (arrows). (B) FDG-PET/CT shows bilateral hypermetabolic level II/III nodal metastases (arrows). (C) Transverse ultrasound scan of the right level II/III metastasis (arrows). Note that the common carotid artery (CCA) is displaced posteriorly and medially.

of nodal disease significantly affects survival and may alter treatment strategies. Head and neck squamous cell cancer should not be regarded as one disease, but as a group of diseases with variable biology, treatment, and prognosis depending on the location of the primary tumor.

(nonkeratinizing) type of nasopharyngeal carcinoma is strongly associated with Epstein-Barr virus and is most common in Asian men.[6] Nasopharyngeal carcinoma frequently produces bilateral nodal metastasis to the retropharyngeal and level II nodes (Fig. 3).[6,7]

Nasopharyngeal Carcinoma

Although nasopharyngeal carcinoma is the most common malignancy of the nasopharynx, it is rare in the Western world. The most common

Oropharyngeal Carcinoma

Oropharyngeal squamous cell carcinoma frequently arises in the posterior one-third of the tongue or the tonsils and accounts for 15%

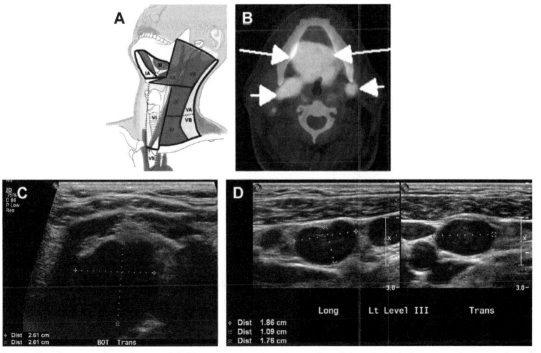

Fig. 4. Oropharyngeal carcinoma. (A) Most common locations of nodal metastasis from oropharyngeal carcinoma. (B) FDG-PET/CT showing a primary tumor in the base of the tongue (long arrows) and bilateral level II nodal metastasis (short arrows). (C) Transverse ultrasound image of this base-of-tongue tumor (calipers) obtained from a submental approach. (D) Left level III nodal metastasis (calipers) in the same patient.

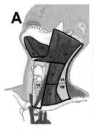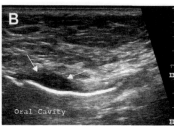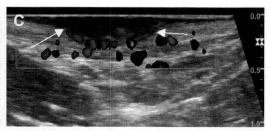

Fig. 5. Oral cavity cancer. (*A*) Most common locations of nodal metastatic disease in oral cavity cancer. (*B*) Squamous cell carcinoma of the buccal mucosa (*arrows*) imaged from a transcutaneous approach with puffed cheeks to fill the oral cavity with air. (*C*) The same tumor (*arrows*) imaged from a direct transmucosal approach, to evaluate the relationship of the tumor with the underlying buccinator muscle for operative planning.

to 30% of all head and neck tumors.[8] Oropharyngeal tumors commonly present with bilateral level II to IV metastasis and are a common location of "occult" primaries in patients presenting with lateral neck metastases. Tumors at the base of the tongue can frequently be visualized with transcutaneous ultrasound using a submental approach (**Fig. 4** and Video 2) and ultrasound-guided needle biopsy of base-of-tongue tumors is feasible, although uncommonly indicated.[9,10] Most oropharyngeal cancers are treated nonoperatively, with definitive chemoradiotherapy.

Many oropharyngeal carcinomas are associated with human papilloma virus (HPV) infection, particularly in younger patients. HPV-positive tumors have a significantly improved survival in comparison with HPV-negative tumors, particularly in patients without a history of smoking. The impact of HPV is so significant that there now are separate staging systems for HPV-positive and HPV-negative oropharyngeal carcinoma.[11]

Oral Cavity Cancer

Oral cavity carcinoma frequently involves the anterior two-thirds of the tongue, the floor of the mouth, or the buccal mucosa. Although most oral cavity cancers can be evaluated with direct inspection, there is a role for transmucosal ultrasound to determine tumor thickness, which can affect management (**Fig. 5**).[12] Oral cavity cancer most commonly spreads to the ipsilateral level I and II nodes, and the presence of nodal metastasis is the most important prognostic factor.[13] The primary therapy for oral cavity cancer is surgery, so accurate identification of nodal metastasis is necessary to guide neck dissection. The role of HPV in oral cavity cancer remains unclear.[14]

Laryngeal Carcinoma

Laryngeal carcinoma is highly associated with smoking and drinking alcohol.[15] Laryngeal carcinoma most commonly spreads to lymph nodes in levels II, III, and IV. Less commonly, advanced laryngeal carcinoma will involve the anterior level

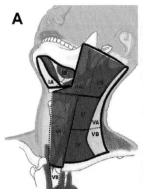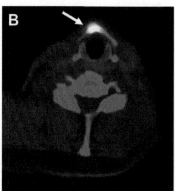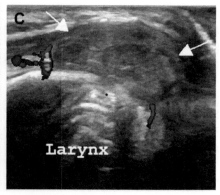

Fig. 6. Laryngeal cancer with involvement of the Delphian node. (*A*) Common locations for nodal metastasis from laryngeal cancer. (*B*) FDG-PET/CT shows hypermetabolism in the anterior midline near the larynx (*arrow*). (*C*) Transverse ultrasound scan of this location, followed by biopsy, confirmed nodal recurrence of cancer (*arrows*).

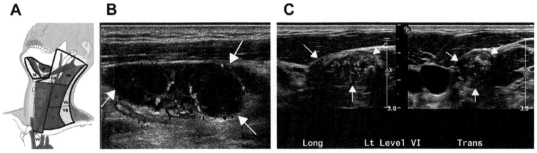

Fig. 7. Papillary thyroid cancer. (A) Most common locations of nodal metastatic disease of thyroid cancer. Lymph nodes (*arrows*) with cystic changes (B) and calcifications (C) characteristic of metastatic papillary thyroid cancer.

VI (Delphian) node, which is a negative prognostic sign (**Fig. 6**). Treatment of laryngeal cancer may involve surgery, radiation, and/or chemotherapy depending on stage.

THYROID CANCER

The most common thyroid malignancy is papillary thyroid cancer. The most common locations for the spread of papillary thyroid carcinoma are levels VI, III, and IV. Levels II and V may also be involved, but usually only when levels III and IV are involved. Involvement of level I is rare.[16,17] Metastatic papillary thyroid cancer in cervical lymph nodes frequently produces intranodal cystic changes, calcifications, and increased echogenicity (**Fig. 7**; Videos 3 and 4).[18] The significance of cervical nodal metastasis in differentiated thyroid cancer remains controversial.[19] Cervical nodal metastasis from differentiated thyroid cancer is treated surgically, and accurate preoperative mapping of disease extent using ultrasound is critical for patient management.[20,21]

METASTASIS FROM OTHER SITES

Cutaneous malignancies of the head and neck, including melanoma and aggressive squamous cell carcinoma, can metastasize to adjacent lymph node levels, but show a propensity to metastasize to the parotid gland (**Fig. 8**).[22,23] Metastatic disease

to the neck from distant primary sites, such as the lung, breast, abdomen, or pelvis, most commonly presents as supraclavicular adenopathy (**Fig. 9**).[24] Metastatic disease from a distant primary presenting as only upper neck adenopathy without supraclavicular adenopathy does occur but is uncommon. Thus, even in patients with a history of a distant primary malignancy, the finding of isolated upper neck adenopathy should raise suspicion for a head or neck primary (**Fig. 10**; see Video 4).

LYMPHOMA

Lymphoma can involve any cervical nodal level. Just as the term lymphoma encompasses a heterogeneous group of diseases, the sonographic appearance of lymphoma is highly variable. Lymph nodes involved with lymphoma can have a reticular echotexture or can be intensely hypoechoic, simulating a cystic lymph node (**Figs. 11** and **12**).[1,25] Low-grade lymphoma can present as a cluster of mildly enlarged lymph nodes with otherwise normal morphology, and simulate reactive adenopathy. High-grade lymphoma can present as ill-defined infiltrative masses (**Fig. 13** and Video 5).

NONMALIGNANT CAUSES OF ADENOPATHY

In addition to malignancy, there are many infectious and noninfectious causes of cervical adenopathy. Diffuse bilateral cervical adenopathy can be caused

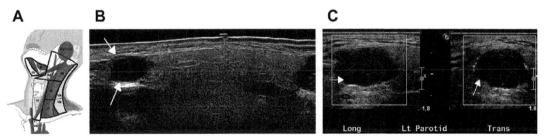

Fig. 8. Metastatic skin cancer. (A) Cutaneous malignancies of the head and neck have a propensity to metastasize to intraparotid lymph nodes. (B) Longitudinal image demonstrates metastatic melanoma (*arrows*) at the superior aspect of the parotid. (C) Metastatic cutaneous squamous cell carcinoma to the parotid with areas of necrosis (*arrows*).

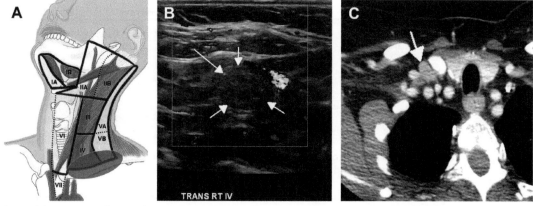

Fig. 9. (*A*) Metastases from a distant primary most commonly involve the supraclavicular lymph nodes. (*B*) Transverse ultrasound scan of the inferior right neck demonstrates metastatic ovarian cancer in a supraclavicular lymph node (*short arrows*), containing a small calcification (*long arrow*). (*C*) Corresponding CT demonstrates the same node (*arrow*).

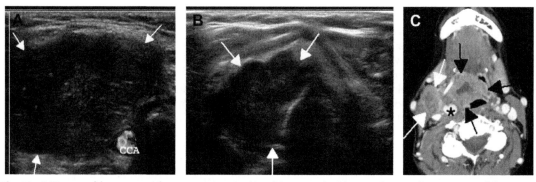

Fig. 10. A 71-year-old woman with an extensive smoking history and a history of treated squamous cell lung cancer who presented with a right neck mass. (*A*) Initial transverse ultrasound scan of the mass showed a level III nodal mass (*arrows*) consistent with metastasis, which was biopsied showing squamous cell carcinoma. The distal common carotid artery (CCA) is displaced medial and posterior. (*B*) As there was no supraclavicular adenopathy, a search was made for a primary malignancy, and a supraglottic laryngeal tumor (*arrows*) was identified (see Video 4). (*C*) Subsequent CT confirmed the supraglottic tumor (*black arrows*) and the nodal metastasis (*white arrow*). The asterisk marks the distal common carotid.

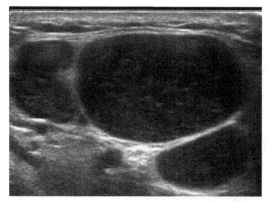

Fig. 11. Lymphoma. Three adjacent level IV lymph nodes with a reticular echotexture typical of lymphoma.

by viral or fungal infection (**Figs. 14** and **15**).[26] Unilateral or regional adenopathy can be caused by acute bacterial or mycobacterial infection (**Fig. 16**). Other causes of cervical adenopathy include sarcoidosis, amyloidosis, Kikuchi-Fujimoto disease, and Castleman disease (**Fig. 17**).[26]

EVALUATION OF CERVICAL LYMPH NODES

Patient history and node location are paramount in the evaluation of cervical lymph nodes. In an untreated neck, metastatic disease to the cervical lymph nodes tends to follow a predictable pattern based on the primary malignancy (**Table 1**). For instance, in a patient presenting for staging of an oral cavity cancer, a borderline

A

B

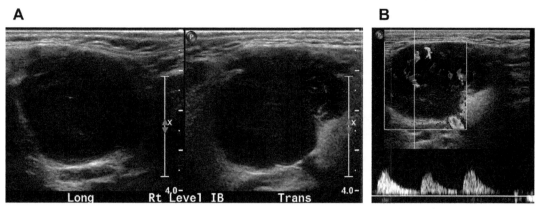

Fig. 12. Lymphoma (A) Hypoechoic level I mass could be confused for a fluid collection with internal debris; however, Doppler evaluation (B) shows internal blood flow.

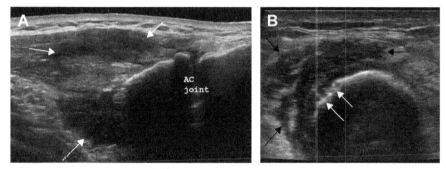

Fig. 13. High-grade lymphoma. (A) Ill-defined mass (arrows) infiltrating the shoulder musculature near the acromiclavicular joint (AC joint). (B) Image taken perpendicular to the shaft of the clavicle in the same patient demonstrates an ill-defined mass (black arrows) involving the clavicle with permeative destruction of the cortex (white arrows, see Video 5).

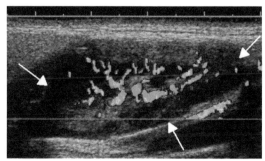

Fig. 14. Enlarged level II lymph node (arrows) in a 16-year-old boy with Epstein-Barr virus infection.

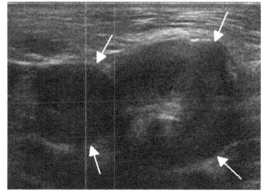

Fig. 15. Level II adenopathy (arrows) caused by coccidioidomycosis in a patient with AIDS.

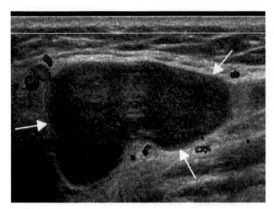

Fig. 16. Enlarged cervical lymph node (*arrows*) caused by mycobacterial infection.

abnormal ipsilateral level IB lymph would be regarded with a high level of suspicion and likely warrant a biopsy.

In a treated neck, however, the expected location of metastasis should be altered based on the treatment rendered. Although isolated metastasis of thyroid cancer to level II is uncommon at presentation, the authors have seen several cases of "isolated" metastasis to level II following ipsilateral level III/IV neck dissection. Similarly, isolated metastasis of oral cavity cancer to level IV is unusual, but the authors have seen cases of "isolated" metastasis to level IV following ipsilateral level II/III neck dissection.

Lymph Node Morphology

The high spatial resolution of ultrasound allows detailed evaluation of nodal morphology. Normal

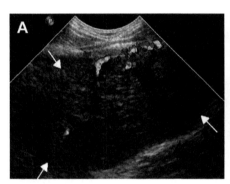
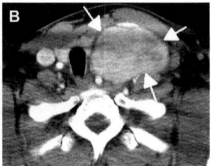

Fig. 17. (*A*) Castleman disease presenting in a 24-year-old man presenting as a massively enlarged level IV lymph node (*arrows*). (*B*) Avid enhancement on CT is typical of Castleman disease.

Table 1
Expected distribution of nodal metastatic disease in an untreated neck

Primary Malignancy	Most Common	Reasonably Common	Uncommon	Rare
Nasopharyngeal	Retropharyngeal	II, V, III, IV	I, intraparotid	VI
Oropharyngeal	II (often bilateral)	III, IV, retropharyngeal	I, V, VI	
Oral cavity	I, II	III, IV	VI	V (except in diffuse disease)
Laryngeal	II, III, IV	VI (Delphian node)	V, I	
Thyroid	VI, III, IV	II, V (when III/IV are involved)	II, V (when III/IV are not involved)	I
Skin cancer	Intraparotid	Any level depending on location of primary		
Chest/abdominal/ pelvic primary	Supraclavicular (inferior IV and V)	II, III (when supraclavicular nodes are involved)	II, III (when supraclavicular nodes are not involved)	I (except in diffuse disease)

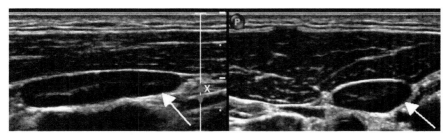

Fig. 18. Longitudinal and transverse images of a normal cervical lymph node (*arrows*).

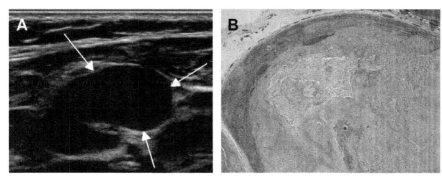

Fig. 19. (*A*) Level II lymph node with asymmetric enlargement of the anterior portion (*arrows*, see Video 6). This node was found on a staging sonogram for oral cavity carcinoma. Needle biopsy and subsequent resection confirmed metastatic squamous cell carcinoma. (*B*) 2× hematoxylin-eosin stain of the resected node shows metastatic carcinoma (pink tissue) surrounded by a rind of lymphoid tissue (purple tissue).

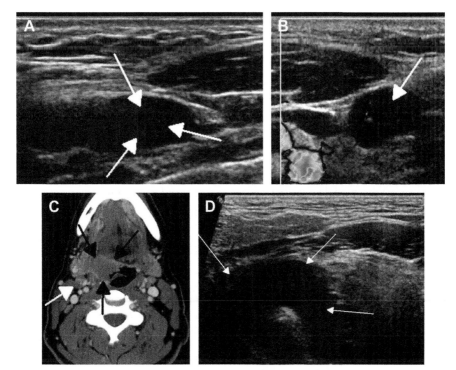

Fig. 20. Longitudinal (*A*) and transverse with color Doppler (*B*) images of a right level II lymph node with focal involvement (*white arrows*) from metastatic oropharyngeal carcinoma. Transverse CT (*C*) shows the focal abnormality in the node (*white arrow*) and the primary malignancy (*black arrows*). (*D*) Transverse submandibular ultrasound scan of the primary malignancy in the right tonsil (*arrows*).

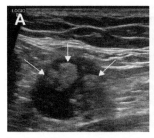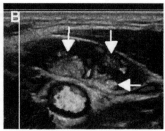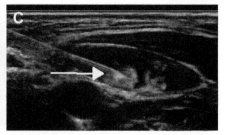

Fig. 21. (*A*) Hyperechoic foci of metastatic oral cavity cancer (*arrows,* see Video 7) in a level I node. (*B*) Hyperechoic foci of metastatic papillary thyroid cancer (*arrows*) in a level III node. (*C*) Ultrasound-guided fine-needle aspiration targeting a hyperechoic focus (*arrow*).

cervical lymph nodes are typically oval and elongated in the craniocaudal (longitudinal) plane, with a central echogenic hilum (**Fig. 18**). Normal level I nodes often have a more spherical shape. Patterns of malignant nodal involvement include diffuse enlargement, asymmetric enlargement, focal involvement, and loss of the echogenic hilum (**Figs. 19–21**; Videos 6 and 7). Fatty change in lymph nodes, which can be diffuse or, less commonly, focal, can mimic metastatic involvement (**Figs. 22 and 23**).

Cystic Changes

Cystic-appearing changes in cervical lymph nodes are generally pathologic and can be due to infection, malignancy-associated necrosis, or neoplastic cyst formation (see **Fig. 7**; **Figs. 24 and 25**). An interesting clinical challenge is an adult presenting with a lateral cystic neck mass. Although a branchial cleft cyst is a leading diagnosis for a cystic lateral neck mass in a child or young adult, it is an uncommon diagnosis in a middle-aged or older adult (**Fig. 26**). Metastatic papillary thyroid carcinoma can produce large cystic lateral neck masses, but metastatic nodes are usually multiple and a suspicious thyroid nodule is usually detectable (**Fig. 27** and Video 8).

Cystic lateral neck masses presenting in middle-aged or older adults should be regarded as metastatic squamous cell carcinoma unless proved otherwise (**Fig. 28**). Many of these are metastatic HPV-positive oropharyngeal carcinoma and the appropriate workup is needle biopsy of the cystic mass, fluorodeoxyglucose (FDG)-PET/CT, and panendoscopy to locate the primary tumor. In some cases, a primary lesion will not be found.[27]

Lymph Node Calcifications

Intranodal calcifications are seen in a variety of metastatic malignancies including papillary thyroid cancer, medullary thyroid cancer, metastatic adenocarcinoma, and head and neck squamous cell carcinoma (**Fig. 29**). Although prior granulomatous disease can produce calcified cervical lymph nodes (which are usually densely calcified), this is far less common than in the mediastinum. Enlarged cervical lymph nodes containing calcifications are likely malignant. Treated nodal metastases may be calcified, but should be stable or shrink over time.

Extranodal Spread

Nodal metastatic disease can spread into adjacent tissues, occasionally presenting as invasion of the sternocleidomastoid muscle or carotid arteries. Extranodal spread of tumor in squamous cell carcinoma doubles the risk of local recurrence and distant metastasis, and significantly decreases overall survival.[28] Ultrasonography performs as well as MRI in diagnosing extranodal spread of tumor.[29] Findings of extranodal spread include a shaggy nodal margin, a vanishing nodal margin, and extension of tumor into adjacent structures (**Fig. 30**; Videos 9 and 10).[29] Infectious causes of adenopathy, including tuberculosis, may have findings that mimic extranodal spread of tumor.[30]

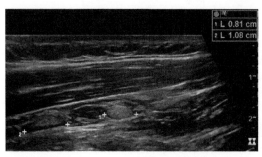

Fig. 22. Level IV nodes (*calipers*), which appear hyperechoic because of near complete fatty replacement. Notice the thin rim of hypoechoic cortical tissue.

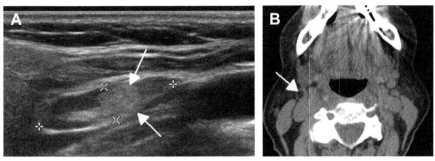

Fig. 23. (A) Longitudinal image of a level II lymph node (*calipers*) with a hyperechoic focus (*arrows*). (B) Corresponding axial noncontrast CT shows focal fatty change in the lymph node (*arrow*). This patient had no history of cancer and the finding was unchanged on an ultrasound scan performed 1 year later. In a patient with known or suspected cancer, a hyperechoic focus such as this would generally warrant biopsy, unless proved to be focal fatty change with CT or MRI.

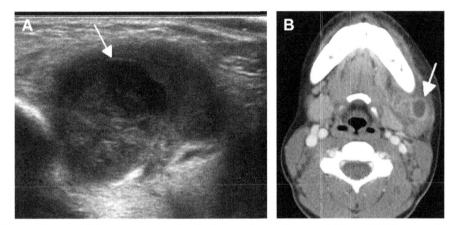

Fig. 24. Suppurative level IB lymph node in a febrile 6-year-old on ultrasound (A) and CT (B) scan, with an area of internal liquefaction (*arrows*).

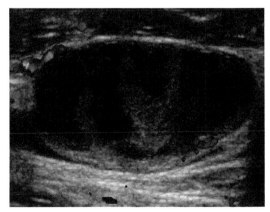

Fig. 25. Nodal metastasis from tongue cancer with extensive central necrosis and deep acoustic enhancement.

Doppler

One of the strengths of ultrasonography is the assessment of blood flow using Doppler. Although metastatic papillary thyroid cancer tends to be hypervascular, metastatic nodes can range from hypervascular to avascular. Normal and reactive lymph nodes have an organized hilar pattern of blood flow (see **Fig. 14**). A disorganized pattern of nonhilar blood flow is a specific but insensitive sign of metastatic disease (**Fig. 31**).[18]

Lymph Node Size

As clinicians we love to measure things with ultrasound and commonly measure structures in 3 orthogonal planes. Cervical nodal measurements by CT are commonly reported as only the short axis (smallest measurement) in the axial plane.

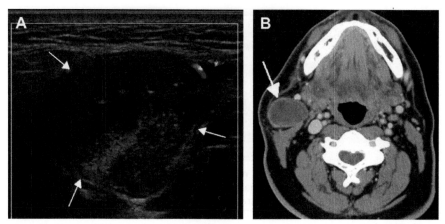

Fig. 26. (*A, B*) Unusual case of a benign branchial cleft cyst (*arrows*) presenting in a 44-year-old man. Following a negative needle biopsy and negative panendoscopy, this was resected, confirming a benign cyst.

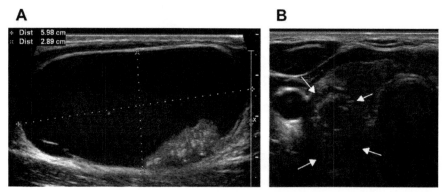

Fig. 27. (*A*) Papillary thyroid cancer with a large level IV cystic nodal metastasis. See Video 8 for additional cystic nodes. (*B*) The primary thyroid cancer in the same patient (*arrows*).

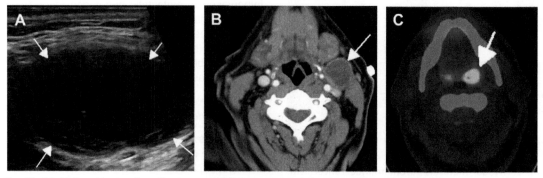

Fig. 28. (*A, B*) Squamous cell carcinoma presenting as cystic left level II neck mass (*arrows*) in a 61-year-old man. (*C*) FDG-PET/CT demonstrates an occult left tonsillar cancer (*arrow*), which was confirmed surgically.

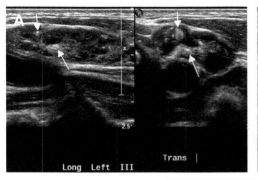
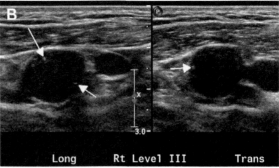
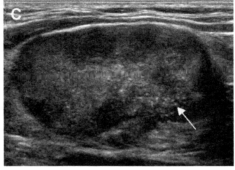

Fig. 29. Intranodal calcifications (*arrows*) caused by metastatic papillary thyroid cancer (*A*), metastatic tongue cancer (*B*), and metastatic colon cancer (*C*).

Most cervical lymph nodes (except some level I nodes) are longest in the craniocaudal (longitudinal) plane. In fact, many normal nodes are well over 2 cm in craniocaudal dimension. Thus, the "CT short axis" dimension is generally the smallest dimension obtained by 3-plane ultrasound measurements. As size criteria for cervical lymph nodes are frequently based on the axial short axis, reporting the longitudinal measurement

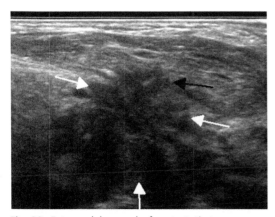

Fig. 30. Extranodal spread of metastatic tongue cancer. The level II nodal metastasis (*white arrows*) has an irregular border and focal extension into the sternocleidomastoid muscle (*black arrow*). See Videos 9 and 10.

obtained with ultrasound can create confusion (and inappropriately upstage disease) because the longitudinal dimension of many normal nodes would be "abnormal" if interpreted using criteria based on short-axis measurements.

Even when appropriate short-axis measurements are used, cervical nodal size is a not a reliable marker of malignancy.[4] There is no uniform agreement on size cutoffs for cervical lymph nodes. A suggested criterion for abnormality using the minimum axial diameter is greater than 11 mm for level II and greater than 10 mm for other levels.[5] Other criteria regard a level II lymph node as abnormal at greater than 15 mm. A multicenter study of neck dissections for head and neck squamous cell cancer found that 46% of metastatic nodes were less than 10 mm.[31]

CONDITIONS THAT MIMIC ADENOPATHY

Not all solid lateral neck masses are adenopathy. A potential mimic of adenopathy is a paraganglioma (Fig. 32). When evaluating a lateral neck mass of unknown cause, it is helpful to determine the relationship of the mass to the carotid artery. Paragangliomas tend to displace the carotid anterior and lateral, whereas adenopathy tends to displace the carotid medial and posterior (Fig. 33). Carotid body tumors are located at

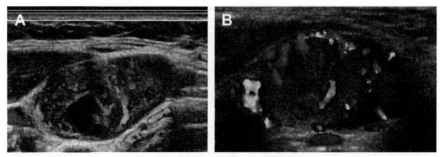

Fig. 31. (*A*, *B*) Disordered nonhilar blood flow in metastatic papillary thyroid cancer.

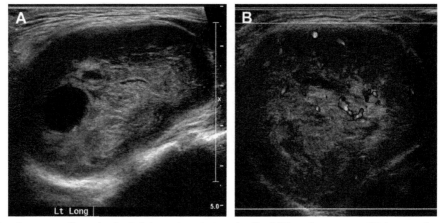

Fig. 32. Vagal paraganglioma in the left lateral neck. Longitudinal (*A*) and transverse (*B*) images demonstrate a mostly solid mass with smooth margins.

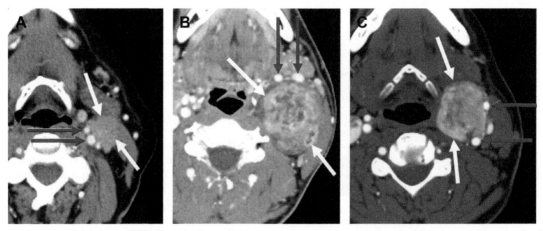

Fig. 33. The relationship of lateral neck masses (*white arrows*) with the internal and external carotid arteries (*red arrows*). (*A*) Nodal metastatic disease displaces the carotids medial and posterior. (*B*) Vagal paraganglioma displaces the carotids anterior and lateral. (*C*) Carotid body tumor splays the carotid arteries.

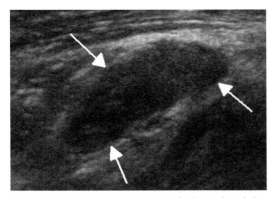

Fig. 34. Posttraumatic neuroma in the lateral neck (*arrows*), 12 years after neck dissection for melanoma.

the carotid bifurcation and will splay the internal and external carotid. Another potential mimic of adenopathy is a posttraumatic neuroma, which tends to occur in an operative bed years after surgery (**Fig. 34**).[32]

SUMMARY

Ultrasonography is an excellent imaging method for cervical lymph nodes, allowing detailed assessment of nodal architecture and blood flow as well as providing guidance for needle biopsy of suspicious lymph nodes. Many diseases involving the cervical lymph nodes have a predictable anatomic distribution and typical sonographic findings. Ultrasound of the cervical lymph nodes is most successful when knowledge of these patterns is applied to the sonographic findings and clinical history.

ACKNOWLEDGMENTS

The authors would like to acknowledge Marjorie Somerville, professional artist, for her drawing of the cervical lymph node stations.

SUPPLEMENTARY DATA

Supplementary videos related to this article can be found at https://doi.org/10.1016/j.rcl.2019.01.005.

REFERENCES

1. Prativadi R, Dahiya N, Kamaya A, et al. Chapter 5. Ultrasound characteristics of benign vs malignant cervical lymph nodes. Semin Ultrasound CT MR 2017;38(5):506–15.
2. Kulzer MH, Branstetter BF. Chapter 1. Neck anatomy, imaging-based level nodal classification and impact of primary tumor site on patterns of nodal metastasis. Semin Ultrasound CT MR 2017;38(5):454–65.
3. Som P, Curtin H, Mancuso AA. An imaging-based classification for the cervical nodes designed as an adjunct to recent clinically based nodal classifications. Arch Otolaryngol Head Neck Surg 1999;125:388–96.
4. Hoang JK, Vanka J, Ludwig BJ, et al. Evaluation of cervical lymph nodes in head and neck cancer with CT and MRI: tips, traps, and a systematic approach. AJR Am J Roentgenol 2013;200(1):W17–25.
5. Kelly HR, Curtin HD. Chapter 2. Squamous cell carcinoma of the head and neck-imaging evaluation of regional lymph nodes and implications for management. Semin Ultrasound CT MR 2017;38(5):466–78.
6. Glastonbury CM, Salzman KL. Pitfalls in the staging of cancer of nasopharyngeal carcinoma. Neuroimaging Clin N Am 2013;23(1):9–25.
7. Ho FC, Tham IW, Earnest A, et al. Patterns of regional lymph node metastasis of nasopharyngeal carcinoma: a meta-analysis of clinical evidence. BMC Cancer 2012;12:98.
8. Corey A. Pitfalls in the staging of cancer of the oropharyngeal squamous cell carcinoma. Neuroimaging Clin N Am 2013;23(1):47–66.
9. Blanco RG, Califano J, Messing B, et al. Transcervical ultrasonography is feasible to visualize and evaluate base of tongue cancers. PLoS One 2014;9(1):e87565.
10. Wagner JM, Conrad RD, Cannon TY, et al. Ultrasound-guided transcutaneous needle biopsy of the base of the tongue and floor of the mouth from a submental approach. J Ultrasound Med 2016;35(5):1009–13.
11. Porceddu SV. A TNM classification for HPV+ oropharyngeal cancer. Lancet Oncol 2016;17(4):403–4.
12. Mark Taylor S, Drover C, Maceachern R, et al. Is preoperative ultrasonography accurate in measuring tumor thickness and predicting the incidence of cervical metastasis in oral cancer? Oral Oncol 2010;46(1):38–41.
13. Brennan PA, Subramaniam S, Tsioryannis C, et al. An update on the latest evidence for managing the clinically negative neck (cN0) in oral squamous cell carcinoma. Oral Dis 2017;23(3):287–91.
14. Hubbers CU, Akgul B. HPV and cancer of the oral cavity. Virulence 2015;6(3):244–8.
15. Baugnon KL, Beitler JJ. Pitfalls in the staging of cancer of the laryngeal squamous cell carcinoma. Neuroimaging Clin N Am 2013;23(1):81–105.
16. Onoda N, Ishikawa T, Kawajiri H, et al. Pattern of initial metastasis in the cervical lymph node from papillary thyroid carcinoma. Surg Today 2013;43(2):178–84.
17. Kupferman ME, Patterson M, Mandel SJ, et al. Patterns of lateral neck metastasis in papillary thyroid

carcinoma. Arch Otolaryngol Head Neck Surg 2004; 130(7):857–60.

18. Kim DW, Choo HJ, Lee YJ, et al. Sonographic features of cervical lymph nodes after thyroidectomy for papillary thyroid carcinoma. J Ultrasound Med 2013;32(7):1173–80.

19. Wang LY, Ganly I. Nodal metastases in thyroid cancer: prognostic implications and management. Future Oncol 2016;12(7):981–94.

20. Sturgeon C, Yang A, Elaraj D. Surgical management of lymph node compartments in papillary thyroid cancer. Surg Oncol Clin N Am 2016;25(1):17–40.

21. Wang LY, Palmer FL, Thomas D, et al. Preoperative neck ultrasound in clinical node-negative differentiated thyroid cancer. J Clin Endocrinol Metab 2014; 99(10):3686–93.

22. Barzilai G, Greenberg E, Cohen-Kerem R, et al. Pattern of regional metastases from cutaneous squamous cell carcinoma of the head and neck. Otolaryngol Head Neck Surg 2005;132(6):852–6.

23. Pathak I, O'Brien CJ, Petersen-Schaeffer K, et al. Do nodal metastases from cutaneous melanoma of the head and neck follow a clinically predictable pattern? Head Neck 2001;23(9):785–90.

24. Lopez F, Rodrigo JP, Silver CE, et al. Cervical lymph node metastases from remote primary tumor sites. Head Neck 2016;38(Suppl 1):E2374–85.

25. Wagner JM, Lamprich BK. Ultrasonography of lumps and bumps. Ultrasound Clin 2014;9(3): 373–90.

26. Agarwal M, Nabavizadeh SA, Mohan S. Chapter 6. Non-squamous cell causes of cervical lymphadenopathy. Semin Ultrasound CT MR 2017;38(5): 516–30.

27. Miller FR, Karnad AB, Eng T, et al. Management of the unknown primary carcinoma: long-term follow-up on a negative PET scan and negative panendoscopy. Head Neck 2008;30(1):28–34.

28. Shaw RJ, Lowe D, Woolgar JA, et al. Extracapsular spread in oral squamous cell carcinoma. Head Neck 2010;32(6):714–22.

29. Katayama I, Sasaki M, Kimura Y, et al. Comparison between ultrasonography and MR imaging for discriminating squamous cell carcinoma nodes with extranodal spread in the neck. Eur J Radiol 2012;81(11):3326–31.

30. Moon IS, Kim DW, Baek HJ. Ultrasound-based diagnosis for the cervical lymph nodes in a tuberculosis-endemic area. Laryngoscope 2015;125(5):1113–7.

31. Saindane AM. Pitfalls in the staging of cervical lymph node metastasis. Neuroimaging Clin N Am 2013;23(1):147–66.

32. Kwak JY, Kim EK, Kim MJ, et al. Sonographic features of traumatic neuromas after neck dissection. J Clin Ultrasound 2009;37(4):189–93.

Carotid Ultrasound

Leslie M. Scoutt, MD*, Gowthaman Gunabushanam, MD

KEYWORDS

- Carotid ultrasound • Spectral Doppler • Internal carotid artery stenosis • Carotid plaque
- Intimal medial thickening

KEY POINTS

- Most strokes are ischemic and caused by thromboemboli rather than by a flow-reducing lesion (watershed infarct).
- Carotid ultrasound (US) is the primary noninvasive imaging modality for diagnosis and follow-up of internal carotid artery stenosis.
- The carotid US examination should assess plaque, degree of stenosis, and carotid waveforms.
- Peak systolic velocities of 125 to 230 cm/s and greater than 230 cm/s are the primary Doppler US criteria for diagnosing 50% to 69% and ≥70% internal carotid artery stenosis, respectively. However, in certain scenarios, peak systolic velocity ratio and end diastolic velocity may be more accurate.
- Spectral Doppler criteria may be selected to maximize sensitivity or specificity and should always be correlated with gray-scale and color Doppler findings as well as waveform patterns.
- Changes in the carotid waveforms may help diagnose more proximal and distal cardiovascular disease as well as nonatherosclerotic pathologic conditions.

INTRODUCTION

Cerebrovascular disease is a significant cause of disability and mortality, and the yearly direct and indirect costs of stroke in the United States have been estimated to exceed 40 billion dollars.[1] An oft quoted sobering statistic is that a stroke occurs every 40 seconds in the United States at an estimated incidence of 795,000 strokes per year, although the incidence and mortality have declined in the past few decades.[1–3] Risk factors for stroke include older age, hypertension, diabetes mellitus, elevated cholesterol and lipid levels, smoking, inactivity, chronic renal disease, and genetic predisposition.[1] In addition, atrial fibrillation increases the risk of stroke by a factor of 5.[1] A Mediterranean-style diet containing nuts and extra virgin olive oil has been recently reported to reduce stroke risk.[4]

Most strokes are ischemic, and most ischemic strokes occur secondary to emboli, of which approximately 15% likely originate from vulnerable plaque at the carotid bifurcation.[5] Other sources of emboli include the heart, origins of the carotid and vertebral arteries, distal cerebrovascular circulation, venous thromboembolism (in the setting of a right to left shunt), or percutaneous arterial intervention. Ischemic watershed infarcts due to a flow-reducing lesion are much less common. Hypoperfusion and increased intracranial pressure/edema are uncommon causes of ischemic stroke. Approximately 10% of strokes are hemorrhagic, most commonly from hypertension and more rarely caused by tumors, arteriovenous malformations, or trauma.

Extracranial internal carotid artery (ICA) stenosis, most commonly occurring at the carotid

---

Disclosures: Dr L.M. Scoutt is an educational consultant for Philips Healthcare. Dr G. Gunabushanam has no disclosures.
Department of Radiology and Biomedical Imaging, Yale School of Medicine, 333 Cedar Street, PO Box 208042, New Haven, CT 06520-8042, USA
* Corresponding author.
E-mail address: leslie.scoutt@yale.edu

Radiol Clin N Am 57 (2019) 501–518
https://doi.org/10.1016/j.rcl.2019.01.008

bifurcation, is a well-established surrogate marker for stroke risk. Doppler ultrasound (US) has emerged as the primary noninvasive imaging modality for detecting, grading, and monitoring ICA stenosis due to its high sensitivity and specificity, relatively low cost, lack of ionizing radiation, and avoidance of iodinated and gadolinium-based intravenous contrast. There are 3 major components of the carotid Doppler US examination: plaque characterization, grading ICA stenosis using Doppler velocity criteria, and waveform analysis.

SCAN TECHNIQUE

Carotid Doppler US examination is optimally performed with the patient in a supine position with the neck slightly hyperextended and turned toward the contralateral side. A high-resolution 5-MHz or greater linear array transducer should be used.[6] However, if the vessels are deep, scanning with a 3- to 5-MHz curved array transducer may be necessary. Occasionally, a small footprint transducer is useful to angle under the mandible to better visualize a high carotid bifurcation or under the sternal notch to evaluate the origins of the carotid arteries. Either an anterior or a posterior approach may be used, although the sternocleidomastoid muscle generally provides a good acoustic window.

The cervical carotid arteries should be assessed in the sagittal and transverse planes using gray-scale and color Doppler, documenting the proximal and distal common carotid arteries (CCAs), the carotid bifurcation; origin, mid, and distal ICAs; origins of the external carotid arteries (ECAs); and mid vertebral arteries (VAs). Additional images are recorded of any abnormal area or pathology. Gray-scale and color Doppler cine clips of the carotid bifurcation in the sagittal and transverse planes are often valuable in roughly quantifying the extent of plaque.

On gray-scale imaging, the focal zone is placed at the posterior margin of the vessel, and the gain is set such that the normal 3 layers of the CCA wall are clearly depicted. For color Doppler imaging, the color gain is increased until color speckles are observed in the surrounding soft tissues, and then the color gain is decreased until color signal remains only in the vessel lumen. The color Doppler scale is set such that color fills the vessel lumen but does not overwrite the vessel wall. If no flow is seen, increasing the color Doppler gain, decreasing the color scale, decreasing the wall filter, using a small straight color box and/or using power Doppler imaging will help increase sensitivity for the detection of flow.

Spectral Doppler waveforms are obtained on sagittal images in the proximal and distal CCA; bifurcation; proximal, mid, and distal ICA; proximal ECA; and mid VA as well as at any area of plaque, significant narrowing, or focal color aliasing. The Doppler angle is kept between 45° and 60°.[6] It is best not to vary the incident Doppler angle by more than 5° between vessel segments or on follow-up examinations because peak systolic velocity (PSV) measurements are less reliable at higher angles. Peak systolic velocity ratio (PSVR) is calculated by dividing the maximal PSV at or just distal to the ICA stenosis by the PSV in the distal CCA. Three measurements at each vessel segment should be obtained with the highest PSV, PSVR, and end diastolic velocity (EDV) recorded. PSV in the distal CCA should be routinely measured 2 to 3 cm below the carotid bulb to avoid obtaining an artificially low PSV where the bulb widens, because that may result in false positive elevation of the PSVR. Most laboratories measure the Doppler angle in the plane of the residual lumen rather than aligned to the vessel wall if the 2 planes are not parallel. The sample gate is kept between 1.5 and 2.5 mm in width and placed centrally in the vessel lumen. The spectral Doppler scale or pulse repetition frequency should be set low enough such that the waveform fills the available space without aliasing.

NORMAL FINDINGS

The carotid arteries supply the anterior circulation of the brain. In most patients, the right CCA arises from the brachiocephalic artery and the left CCA arises directly from the aorta. The CCA dilates slightly to form the carotid bulb just before or at the carotid bifurcation. This dilatation extends variably into the origins of the ICA and/or ECA. The ICA is typically larger and posterolateral to the ECA. However, the most reliable way of differentiating the ICA from the ECA is by the identification of branches arising from the ECA rather than by arterial size, location, or waveform pattern (Fig. 1).

The CCA, ICA, and ECA each have characteristic waveform patterns, which largely reflect peripheral vascular resistance and oxygen consumption of the distal vascular bed. All the carotid arteries should demonstrate a sharp systolic upstroke and narrow spectral envelope outlining a spectral window, and waveforms should be symmetric right to left in all 3 vessels. The normal ICA waveform is characterized by a relatively thicker spectral envelope and continuous forward

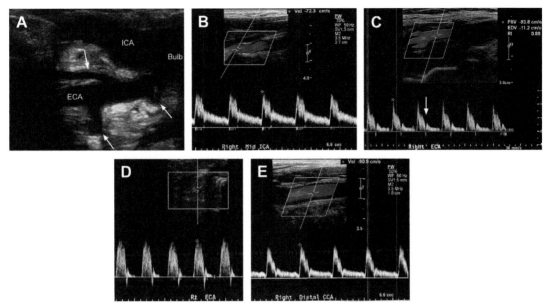

Fig. 1. Normal carotid Doppler examination. (A) Sagittal gray-scale image demonstrating multiple branches (arrows) arising from the ECA; ICA; bulb (Bulb). (B) Spectral Doppler tracing of the normal ICA demonstrating a sharp systolic upstroke, thin spectral envelope, and continuous forward diastolic flow. (C) Spectral Doppler tracing of the normal ECA demonstrating a sharp systolic upstroke, thin spectral envelope with early diastolic notch (arrow), and relatively little diastolic flow. Note 2 distal branches arising from the ECA. (D) Spectral Doppler tracing of the normal ECA from a different patient demonstrates no end diastolic flow. Although the amount of diastolic flow in the normal ECA may be variable, in a given patient it should always be symmetric right to left and less than the amount of diastolic flow in the ICA. (E) Spectral Doppler tracing of the normal CCA demonstrating sharp systolic upstroke and thin spectral envelope with an intermediate amount of diastolic flow and less prominent early diastolic notch.

diastolic flow due to low peripheral vascular resistance and relatively higher oxygen consumption (see **Fig. 1**). The ECA supplies blood to the muscles of the head and neck, which are not as metabolically active as the brain parenchyma and, therefore, the normal ECA waveform characteristically has less diastolic flow and a thinner spectral envelope. An early diastolic notch is often observed (see **Fig. 1**). The exact amount of diastolic flow in the ECA is variable but should be symmetric right to left and less than in the ICA in a given patient. The CCA, which supplies blood to both the ICA and the ECA, has an intermediate shaped waveform with continuous forward diastolic flow, but less than the ICA (see **Fig. 1**). PSV in the CCA normally ranges from 60 to 100 cm/s and decreases slightly distally.

PLAQUE CHARACTERIZATION

Plaque characterization is extremely important because risk of embolization is directly related to plaque composition and morphology, but only indirectly related to degree of stenosis. Intraplaque neovascularity/hemorrhage, inflammation, necrosis, high lipid content, and thinning of the fibrous cap are thought to predispose to plaque rupture, exposing the necrotic core to the circulating blood and resulting in the formation of unstable thrombus on the plaque surface. This unstable thrombus or plaque debris may then be dislodged by the high-velocity jet of blood coursing through the narrowed lumen, resulting in distal embolus or stroke (**Fig. 2**).[7–9] Irregularly surfaced or ulcerated plaque also predisposes to formation of unstable thrombus on plaque surfaces due to either stagnant flow or exposure of the central necrotic core.[10] Conversely, thrombus is less likely to form on smoothly surfaced hyalinized, fibrous, or calcified plaque, which has a reduced risk of distal embolization and rupture (see **Fig. 2**).

Gray-scale and color Doppler assessment of plaque should focus on evaluating plaque burden, echogenicity, and surface characteristics. Echogenicity is described as hypoechoic versus echogenic and heterogeneous versus homogeneous (**Fig. 3**). Hemorrhagic and lipid-laden plaque is more likely to be hypoechoic and is most

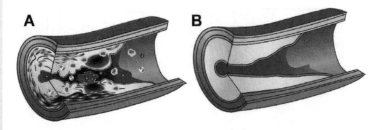

Fig. 2. Plaque schematics. (A) Vulnerable plaque is characterized by neovascularity, inflammation, central necrosis, and thinning of the fibrous cap. Hemorrhage from plaque neovascularity and inflammatory cell death due to cholesterol and lipid toxicity result in central necrosis, swelling, and ultimately plaque rupture, exposing the thrombogenic necrotic core to circulating blood. Thrombus forming on the surface of the ruptured plaque or plaque debris is then at risk for distal embolization. (B) Hyalinized, fibrous, or calcified plaque has less inflammation and neovascularity and is less likely to undergo central necrosis and rupture. Thus, unless the surface is irregular resulting in stagnant flow, thrombus is unlikely to form on the surface of the plaque.

concerning if greater than 50% of the plaque is hypoechoic.[11,12] Numerous studies have shown that hypoechoic plaque is more likely to be symptomatic.[13,14] However, plaque hypoechogenicity is a nonspecific finding, and fibrous or hyalinized plaque may also be hypoechoic.[11,12] Echogenic plaque with or without shadowing is unlikely to be vulnerable plaque (see **Fig. 3**). Irregularly surfaced,

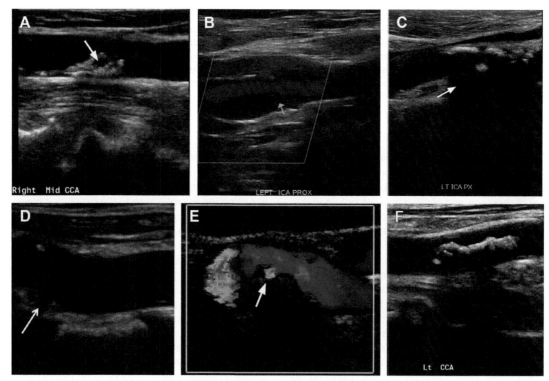

Fig. 3. Variable appearance of plaque. (A) Focal area of hypoechoic plaque (arrow). Such areas are concerning for hemorrhage, inflammation, or necrosis, especially if comprising greater than 50% of plaque volume. The surface is slightly irregular. (B) Homogeneously hypoechoic plaque (arrow) with a smooth surface contour. This is a nonspecific appearance and can be seen with fibrous, fatty, or hyalinized plaque in addition to hemorrhagic plaque. (C) Echogenic plaque. Posterior acoustic shadowing (arrow) is noted, likely indicating calcification. Echogenic plaque is less likely to be vulnerable. (D) Gray-scale image demonstrating an ulcer (arrow) that fills in (arrow) with color Doppler imaging (E). Plaque with an irregular surface (F) carries a poor prognosis as stagnant flow in the indentations or crevices may lead to platelet aggregation and thrombus formation on the surface of the plaque.

fissured, or undermined plaque should be differentiated from smooth surfaced plaque. A surface defect deeper than 2 mm in 2 orthogonal imaging planes is described as an ulcer (see **Fig. 3**). The plaque should also be quantified on gray-scale and color Doppler imaging as large plaques, especially if rapidly progressing, are more likely to be hemorrhagic and symptomatic.

Plaque evaluation requires meticulous scanning with both gray-scale and color Doppler imaging in sagittal and transverse planes. Spatial compounding and harmonic imaging may improve resolution. If the gray-scale gain is set too low, plaque may appear falsely hypoechoic, mimicking vulnerable plaque. Conversely, increasing the gain may create artifactual echoes in hypoechoic plaque, resulting in a false negative examination. Extremely hypoechoic plaque or thrombus may not be visible on gray-scale imaging and may only be recognized as a color void. However, one should not rely on color Doppler alone to evaluate plaque, because color Doppler may overwrite or obscure plaque, particularly if the color gain is set too high. Surface characteristics of plaque are often best visualized on color/power Doppler imaging or contrast-enhanced ultrasound (CEUS).[15] Recently, 3dimensional imaging has been reported to be highly accurate in assessing plaque burden and progression,[16] with large plaque volume associated with elevated coronary artery calcium score[17] and increased risk of cardiovascular events.[18] In addition, estimation of degree of stenosis on gray-scale and color Doppler provides contemporaneous quality assurance (QA) of spectral Doppler measurements because these findings should be concordant. If a large amount of plaque is found without associated increased PSV or vice versa, an explanation and/or correlative imaging should be sought.

Feinstein[15] reported that early-phase CEUS could identify plaque neovascularity. Other investigators have reported a similar association of early-phase US contrast enhancement of hypoechoic plaque with both plaque neovascularity and acute symptoms.[19,20] Feinstein also reported that early-phase CEUS provided better depiction of irregularly surfaced plaque and ulcerations than gray-scale or color Doppler.[15] Furthermore, Owen and colleagues[21] reported that late-phase (20-minute delay) contrast enhancement of plaque in symptomatic patients was associated with inflammatory plaque and that such areas were also hypoechoic on gray-scale imaging.

Increased intima-media thickness (IMT) of the CCA and ICA has long been proposed as an independent risk factor for cardiovascular disease and a predictor of myocardial infarction, sudden death, and stroke.[22–25] In a large meta-analysis, Lorenz and colleagues[26] reported that a 0.1-mm increase in IMT increased stroke risk by 13% to 18% and the risk of myocardial infarction by 10% to 15%. However, more recent large epidemiologic studies suggest that carotid IMT measurement does not improve risk stratification for future cardiovascular events[27,28] or provides such a small improvement in risk prediction that it is unlikely to be of clinical significance.[29,30] It has been suggested that the CCA IMT is more closely associated with stroke risk than IMT measurement of the ICA, which has a stronger association with myocardial infarction.[31]

In addition, controversy exists regarding both the technique and the reporting parameters for carotid IMT measurement, which vary widely between studies. In 2008, the American Society of Echocardiography issued a consensus statement recommending that the IMT be measured bilaterally on magnified images along the posterior wall of the mid CCA 1 cm below the bulb separate

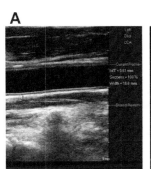 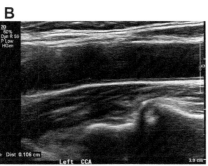

Fig. 4. Measurement of IMT. (*A*) Sagittal gray-scale image demonstrating the 3 layers of the normal CCA wall resulting in a characteristic "tram track" appearance of 2 parallel echogenic lines. The IMT is measured between the interface of the hypoechoic middle layer, the media, with the outer echogenic adventitia, and the interface of the echogenic intima with the anechoic vessel lumen. The adventitial layer is not included in the measurement. This computer-generated measurement of 0.61 mm is normal. (*B*) In a different patient, the IMT has been measured with hand-placed calipers (+) and is abnormal at 1.1 mm.

from any area of plaque (defined as vessel wall thickness >1.5 mm) using a high-frequency linear array transducer with the CCA oriented perpendicular to the insonating US beam (parallel to the transducer face) (**Fig. 4**).[32] The IMT varies with age, gender, and race and is reportedly thickest in older African American men and thinnest in younger Asian women.[32] An IMT measurement less than 0.7 to 0.8 mm is considered normal.[32]

GRADING INTERNAL CAROTID ARTERY STENOSIS

In 1991, the North American Symptomatic Carotid Endarterectomy Trial (NASCET) reported that symptomatic patients with a ≥70% ICA stenosis who underwent carotid endarterectomy (CEA) had an absolute ipsilateral stroke risk reduction of 17% when compared with treatment with then state-of-the-art medical management.[33] Multiple subsequent trials have reported clinically significant, but relatively lower benefit in asymptomatic individuals and in patients with moderate (50%–69%) ICA stenosis.[34,35] More recent trials have demonstrated an equivalent decrease in the incidence of ipsilateral stroke following carotid artery stent (CAS) placement.[36,37] In order to reduce interobserver and intraobserver variability in the NASCET study, percent ICA stenosis was calculated by dividing the smallest residual ICA luminal diameter by the luminal diameter of the distal normal ICA, because both of these can be precisely measured angiographically (**Fig. 5**). Therefore, a 70% ICA stenosis as calculated by the NASCET method is tighter than a 70% ICA stenosis as calculated by the previous method, which compared the diameter of the residual lumen with an estimate of the width of the ICA from outer wall to outer wall at the site of stenosis. Although plaque burden can be significantly underestimated by the NASCET method, it remains widely accepted as the preferred method of grading an ICA stenosis.[38]

In 2002, the Society of Radiologists in Ultrasound (SRU) consensus panel recommended using PSV as the primary Doppler criterion for grading ICA stenosis (**Figs. 6** and **7**, **Table 1**), with PSVR and EDV as potential additional parameters.[39] In addition, the panel emphasized that the stenosis grade estimated using PSV criteria should be correlated with the gray-scale and color Doppler findings.[39] Although the SRU consensus criteria are the most commonly used criteria for grading ICA stenosis in the United States,[40] other charts may be equally effective, and vascular laboratories are strongly encouraged to routinely perform QA to validate their chosen criteria.

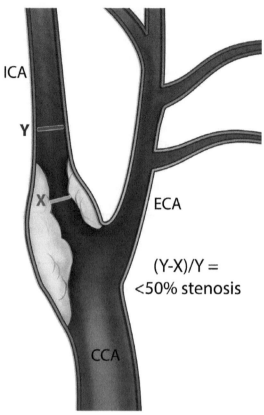

Fig. 5. Schematic image demonstrating calculation of ICA stenosis according to the NASCET method. According to the NASCET study design, percent ICA stenosis is calculated by comparing the diameter of the residual lumen (X) to the diameter of the distal normal ICA (Y). In this schematic image, there is less than 50% ICA stenosis despite the presence of a large amount of plaque. Although the NASCET method reduces interobserver and intraobserver variability, it may significantly underestimate plaque burden.

PITFALLS IN GRADING AN INTERNAL CAROTID ARTERY STENOSIS

Although PSV is generally considered the single most reliable Doppler criterion for grading an ICA stenosis, there are scenarios where PSVR or EDV may provide a more accurate gauge of an ICA stenosis, or when all Doppler criteria may be inaccurate. Correlation with gray-scale and color Doppler estimation of plaque burden as well as attention to the individual patient's hemodynamics will help avoid such interpretative pitfalls. If there is significant discordance between spectral Doppler and gray-scale/color Doppler findings, or between spectral Doppler criteria, an explanation should be sought. If no explanation can be found, additional imaging using CT angiography may be needed.

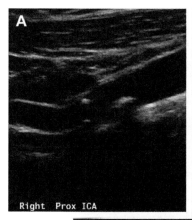

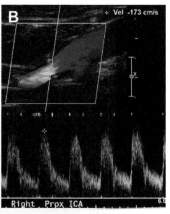

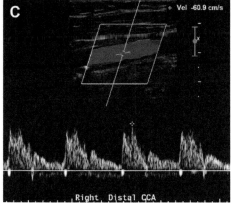

Fig. 6. Fifty percent to 69% ICA stenosis. (*A*) Echogenic plaque on gray-scale image reduces the arterial lumen by slightly more than 50%. (*B*) PSV in the ICA is 173 cm/s and PSV in the distal CCA (*C*) is 61 cm/s for a PSVR of less than 3. By the SRU criteria, these findings would correspond to a 50% to 69% ICA stenosis.

Increased Peak Systolic Velocity Without Significant Stenosis

Absolute PSV is less reliable in diagnosing ICA stenosis in patients with increased or decreased cardiac output (Table 2), and PSVR may be a more reliable Doppler criterion. In patients with high output states, CCA PSV is often greater than 100 cm/s, and using the standard PSV criterion of greater than 230 cm/s to diagnose a ≥70% ICA stenosis will result in overestimation of ICA stenosis and false positive diagnosis. Conversely, in patients with low cardiac output, CCA PSV is often less than 60 cm/s, and reliance on the PSV alone will underestimate ICA stenosis resulting in false negative results.

Causes of elevated PSV in the absence of significant plaque include vessel tortuosity and contralateral high-grade carotid stenosis or occlusion. PSV does increase in a tortuous artery. In addition, it is difficult to correctly orient the Doppler angle given the rapidly changing direction of blood flow around a curve, which may lead to overestimation of PSV. Increased compensatory flow due to a contralateral high-grade ICA/CCA stenosis or occlusion increases PSV in both the ICA and the CCA if these arteries provide collateral flow.[41,42] Hence, reliance on PSV as the sole diagnostic Doppler US criterion will result in overestimation of ICA stenosis; in these cases, PSVR is a better Doppler criterion even though it may not fully correct because the amount of compensatory flow may differ in the ICA and CCA.[41] Correlation with gray-scale and color Doppler findings is key in these scenarios.

Significant Stenosis with Normal Peak Systolic Velocity Values

If a large amount of ICA plaque is visualized without the expected increase in PSV, one should consider the possibility of tandem lesions, a long segment stenosis, or a high-grade nearly occlusive lesion. When tandem stenoses are present, PSV in the more distal lesion will not be as elevated as expected for the degree of stenosis. PSV will also not be as high as expected in a long segment stenosis (>2 cm) (Fig. 8) likely because of inflow resistance. Finally, PSV will decrease in a nearly occlusive lesion, as predicted by the Spencer and Reid diagram.[43] Careful correlation with the gray-scale

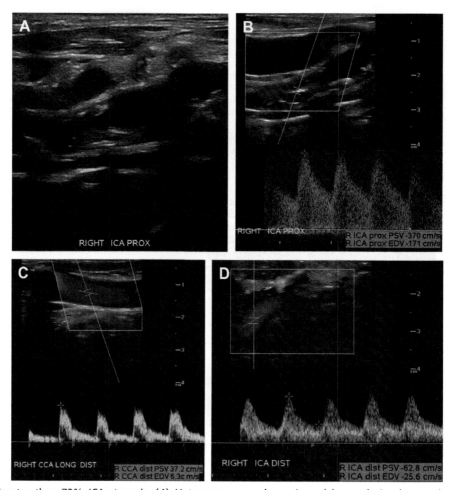

Fig. 7. Greater than 70% ICA stenosis. (A) Heterogeneous echogenic and hypoechoic plaque on gray-scale sagittal image reduces the arterial lumen by more than 70%. (B) PSV in the ICA is 370 cm/s with an EDV of 171 cm/s. An EDV greater than 100 cm/s is a highly specific criterion for a lesion that should be treated. PSV in the distal CCA (C) is 37 cm/s for a PSVR of 10. By the SRU criteria, these findings would correspond to a ≥70% ICA stenosis. (D) Note tardus parvus waveforms in distal ICA.

Table 1
Society of Radiologists in Ultrasound consensus conference guidelines for grading an internal carotid artery stenosis

| % Stenosis | Primary Criteria | | Additional Criteria | |
	ICA PSV	Plaque Estimate (%)[a]	PSVR	EDV
<50%	<125 cm/s	<50%	<2.0	<40 cm/s
50%–69%	125–230 cm/s	≥50%	2.0–4.0	40–100 cm/s
≥70%, near occlusion	>230 cm/s	≥50%	>4.0	>100 cm/s
Near occlusion	Variable (high, low, or undetectable)	>95%	Variable	Variable

[a] Plaque estimate (diameter reduction) with gray-scale and color Doppler US.

From Grant EG, Benson CB, Moneta GL, et al. Carotid artery stenosis: gray-scale and Doppler US diagnosis–Society of Radiologists in Ultrasound consensus conference. Radiology 2003;229(2):344; with permission.

Table 2	
Common causes of changes in cardiac output	
Causes	
Increased cardiac output	Hyperdynamic heart (young athlete)
	Hypertension
	Thyrotoxicosis
	AR
Decreased cardiac output	Hypotension
	Cardiomyopathy
	Left ventricular aneurysm
	Left ventricular dysfunction
	Aortic valve stenosis
	Pericardial effusion

and color Doppler images and waveform assessment of the proximal and distal arteries may provide additional clues to the presence of a high-grade stenosis (**Fig. 9**).

WAVEFORM ANALYSIS OF THE CAROTID ARTERIES

The tardus parvus (TP) waveform pattern, characterized by a slow rate of systolic upstroke, rounding of the systolic peak, and decreased PSV, is often observed distal to a high-grade stenosis[44] and becomes more pronounced the tighter the

proximal stenosis and the farther downstream from the stenosis that the artery is sampled. The distribution of the TP waveform in the cervical vessels will help to pinpoint the location of the proximal stenosis. For example, a TP waveform in the distal ICA but a sharp systolic upstroke in the distal CCA indicates that the stenosis is in the proximal ICA (see **Fig. 9**), whereas TP waveforms in the ipsilateral internal and common carotid arteries but sharp systolic upstrokes in the contralateral carotid arteries suggest the stenosis is at the origin of the ipsilateral CCA or brachiocephalic artery. TP waveforms in all the cervical vessels including the VAs suggest that the stenosis is proximal to all the great vessels of the neck, most likely at the level of the aortic valve (**Fig. 10**). Stenoses, including aortic valve stenosis, generally must be moderate to severe to cause a distal TP waveform.[45-47]

The "knocking," "staccato," or thump waveform pattern characterized by decreased PSV, decreased, absent, or even reversed diastolic flow and a sharp systolic upstroke is observed proximal to a high-grade stenosis or occlusion and becomes more pronounced the closer one samples to the obstructing lesion.[45] A knocking waveform in the CCA suggests a high-grade stenosis/occlusion in the ipsilateral ICA (**Fig. 11**). High-resistance waveforms in the ipsilateral CCA and ICA with a normally patent ICA on color Doppler suggest occlusion of the ipsilateral

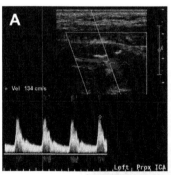
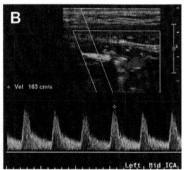
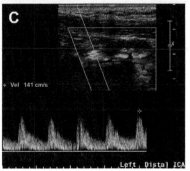

Fig. 8. Long segment ICA stenosis. Longitudinal spectral and color Doppler images of the proximal (A), mid (B), and distal (C) ICA demonstrate a long segment narrowing of the proximal and mid ICA with diffuse heterogeneous hypoechoic and echogenic plaque. There is mild poststenotic dilatation (C). Color Doppler findings suggest a high-grade stenosis, much greater than 70%. However, the highest PSV obtained was 163 cm/s, well below the the SRU threshold criterion of 230 cm/s for a ≥70% stenosis. PSV will be less than expected in a long segment stenosis due to inflow resistance.

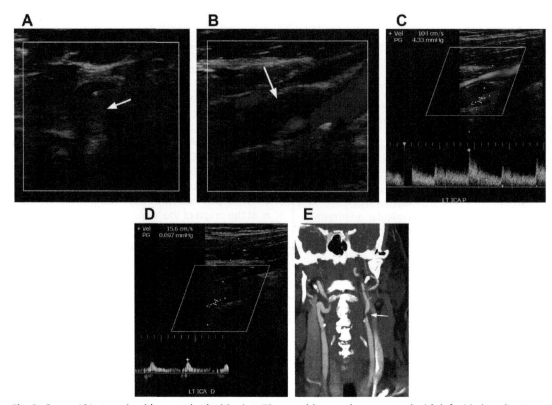

Fig. 9. Severe ICA stenosis with normal velocities in a 53-year-old man who presented with left-sided stroke. Transverse (A) and longitudinal color Doppler (B) images show a large amount of homogeneously hypoechoic plaque (*arrows* in A, B) causing a tight stenosis of the left proximal ICA. (C) Spectral Doppler image of the left proximal ICA demonstrates a PSV of 104 cm/s, consistent with a < 50% stenosis. (D) Tardus parvus waveforms with a PSV of 16 cm/s are noted in the left distal ICA. These findings are concerning for a high-grade stenosis of the left proximal ICA, which was confirmed on a coronal maximum intensity projection CT angiography image (E, *arrow*).

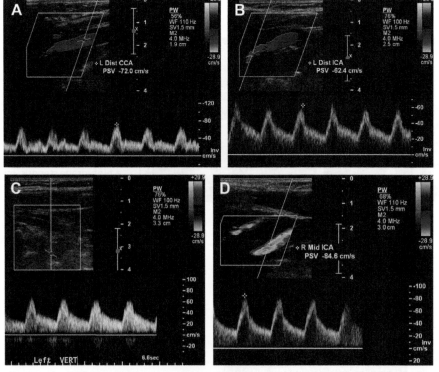

Fig. 10. Aortic stenosis. A 73-year-old woman with severe aortic valve stenosis. Spectral Doppler images of the left CCA (A), left ICA (B), left VA (C), and right ICA (D) show TP waveforms throughout.

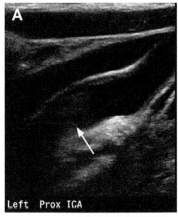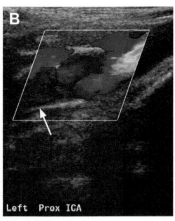

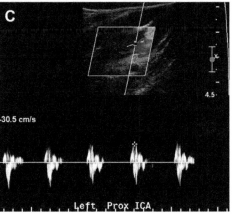

Fig. 11. Staccato waveform. Sagittal gray-scale (A) and color Doppler (B) images demonstrating hypoechoic plaque and/or thrombus (arrow) completely occluding the left ICA. Spectral Doppler waveform of the proximal ICA (C) demonstrating diminished PSV, sharp systolic up-stroke, and no diastolic flow. This waveform has been termed a "knocking" or "staccato" waveform and is seen proximal to a high-grade stenosis or occlusion.

intracranial ICA or middle cerebral artery. More rarely, a unilateral knocking ICA waveform may be seen in patients with distal dissection, arteritis, or vasospasm. Bilateral CCA, ICA, and VA knocking waveforms suggest increased intracranial pressure and/or increased peripheral vascular resistance, commonly caused by a mass lesion, hematoma, edema, and/or vasospasm.[45,48] Diastolic flow reversal with normal to increased PSV in all the cervical great vessels suggests aortic regurgitation (AR).[45,48] AR must be moderately severe to cause this abnormal waveform pattern, which is more pronounced closer to the regurgitant valve in the proximal CCAs and normalizes more distally in the ICAs.[45,48]

Patients with intra-aortic balloon pumps (IABPs) will have a characteristic waveform pattern in all the great vessels of the neck with 2 closely approximated forward peaks and reversal of flow in end diastole (Fig. 12). The first peak corresponds to systole, and the second peak of forward flow occurs at the onset of diastole when the balloon is inflated. PSV may be increased or decreased following IABP

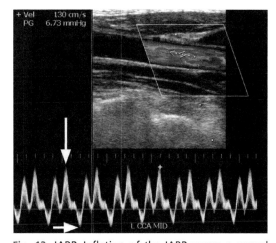

Fig. 12. IABP. Inflation of the IABP causes a second peak of forward flow during early diastole (long arrow), increasing blood flow to the coronary arteries in this patient with unstable angina. Deflation of the balloon at end diastole causes transient flow reversal (short arrow). This waveform will be noted in all the vessels in the neck including the bilateral ICAs, ECAs, and VAs (not shown).

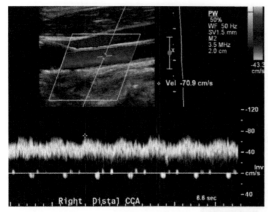

Fig. 13. LVAD. In this patient with refractory congestive heart failure, an LVAD was placed as a bridge to cardiac transplantation. The spectral Doppler waveform of the right CCA has a markedly TP configuration. Similar arterial waveforms will be visualized throughout the body. In some patients with LVADs, the systolic peak may be extremely attenuated or even undetectable, mimicking a venous waveform.

placement, and the 2 peaks may vary in height. Therefore, PSVR, gray-scale, and color Doppler findings are of increased importance.[48,49] Placement of a left ventricular assist device (LVAD) most commonly results in a monophasic waveform pattern with a marked TP morphology and low PSV (**Fig. 13**). Sometimes a systolic peak cannot be clearly visualized, mimicking a venous waveform.[49,50]

NONATHEROSCLEROTIC PATHOLOGIC CONDITIONS

Pseudoaneurysms (PSAs) most often occur following penetrating trauma, such as inadvertent needle puncture or surgical intervention, but may also develop as a complication of arteritis, radiation therapy, carotid dissection, or invasion of the carotid artery by malignancy. On gray-scale imaging, an outpouching arising from the carotid artery will be noted. Color Doppler will demonstrate slowly swirling blood flow in a "yin-yang" pattern and a color void if intraluminal thrombus is present. If the neck is thin, a characteristic "to-and-fro" waveform with flow heading toward the PSA during systole and reversed flow during diastole will be observed (**Fig. 14**).

Arteriovenous fistulas most often occur in the setting of penetrating trauma or surgery but may be congenital in origin. A tract may be seen connecting the artery and vein with markedly elevated PSV and EDV on the spectral Doppler tracing (**Fig. 15**). Pulsatile high-velocity flow is present in the draining vein. Vibration of the adjacent soft tissues may create a soft tissue color bruit.

Trauma is the most common cause of carotid artery dissections, which may also arise spontaneously or as an extension of thoracic aortic dissections. Predisposing risk factors include hypertension and conditions that weaken the vessel wall, such as Marfan syndrome, Ehlers-Danlos syndrome, fibromuscular dysplasia (FMD), and cystic medial necrosis.[51,52] CCA dissections are

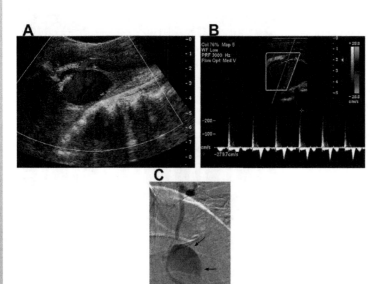

Fig. 14. PSA. A 59-year-old man with head and neck cancer, who underwent surgery and radiation therapy, and subsequently developed a pulsatile neck mass. (A) Color Doppler image shows a 3-cm structure arising from the right ICA, which fills with color with a "yin-yang" appearance. (B) Spectral Doppler image shows "to-and-fro" flow in the neck of the PSA. (C) Angiogram shows a contrast-filled outpouching (*arrows*) arising from the right ICA.

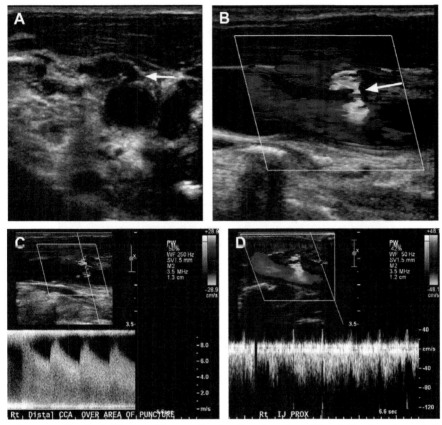

Fig. 15. Arteriovenous fistula. A 63-year-old man who developed neck swelling following attempted central line placement. Transverse gray-scale (*A*) and longitudinal color Doppler (*B*) images show a communication (*arrows*) between the CCA and internal jugular vein. Note the color Doppler aliasing on (*B*). (*C*) Spectral Doppler image shows a low-resistance waveform with spectral broadening and PSV >800 cm/s within the fistula. (*D*) Spectral Doppler image demonstrating a pulsatile waveform with increased velocity approximating 80 cm/s within the right internal jugular vein consistent with an arteriovenous fistula.

readily diagnosed on US by identification of an echogenic intraluminal flap (**Fig. 16**). The true lumen typically has a normal Doppler waveform, although PSV may be elevated secondary to compression by the false lumen, which often has a more atypical waveform pattern.[48] Rarely, a CCA dissection may present with a homogeneously hypoechoic mural hematoma spiraling around the vessel lumen. ICA dissections are more common in younger patients, who typically present with headache, stroke, Horner syndrome, or following trauma. Most ICA dissections begin at the skull base and dissect down toward the carotid bifurcation. Visualization of a dissection flap is rare, and the most common US finding is a high-resistance waveform pattern in the proximal ICA due to distal ICA occlusion/stenosis. Thrombosis of the false lumen or mural hematoma may result in homogeneous hypoechoic thickening of the ICA wall with a flame-shaped lumen smoothly tapering toward the head. Absence of calcified atherosclerotic plaque in the proximal ICA and a high index of clinical suspicion given the patient's age and presentation are helpful in making the diagnosis, which can readily be confirmed on MR imaging.

The ICA is the second most common artery to be affected by FMD. A beaded configuration of the ICA will be observed in the middle to distal ICA on gray-scale or color/power Doppler. Spectral Doppler criteria are unreliable for grading ICA stenosis in patients with FMD due to the presence of multiple tandem lesions. Takayasu arteritis causes diffuse wall thickening at the origins of the great vessels arising from the aorta, and when the CCA is involved, rarely extends into or beyond the carotid bulb. Significant narrowing of the vessel lumen may cause increased PSV in the CCA and TP waveforms in the ICA and ECA. Radiation arteritis, a form of accelerated inflammatory

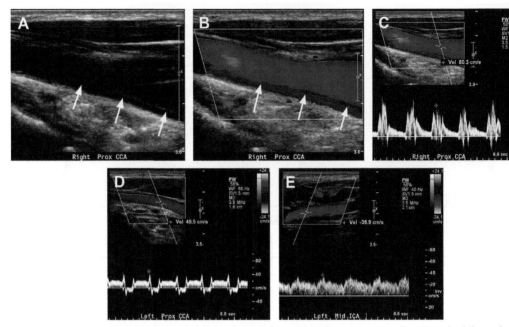

Fig. 16. Dissection. A young woman with known ascending aortic dissection extending into the bilateral common carotid arteries. Longitudinal gray-scale (*A*) and color Doppler (*B*) images show a thin, linear echogenic dissection flap (*arrows*) in the right CCA. Note that due to dynamic obstruction, a variety of waveforms can be observed in carotid dissections, including an irregular waveform with multiple peaks as seen here in the right proximal CCA (*C*), a presteal waveform as observed in the left proximal CCA (*D*), or a TP waveform as noted in this patient's left mid ICA (*E*).

atherosclerosis, may occur 10 to 15 years following high-dose cervical radiation therapy and will cause diffuse wall thickening in the mid-CCA.

IMAGING OF THE CAROTID ARTERIES AFTER INTERVENTION

Both CEA and CAS placement have been demonstrated to be effective treatments for patients with carotid stenosis. The risk of periprocedural mortality, myocardial infarction, and cranial nerve palsy is higher following CEA, but the periprocedural stroke risk is higher in patients following CAS placement, particularly in symptomatic patients with tortuous vessels, high-grade stenoses, and vulnerable plaque.[37] The long-term risks of stroke and restenosis are similar for both procedures, and surveillance US at 6- to 12-month intervals is recommended. Note that the SRU consensus criteria should not be applied for the

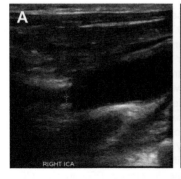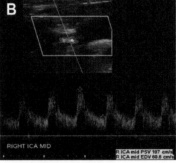

Fig. 17. Restenosis post-CEA. This patient presented with transient ischemic attacks several years following CEA. (*A*) Gray-scale image demonstrates significant narrowing (calipers) of the residual lumen from plaque in the mid ICA above the dilated endarterectomy site. However, PSV is only 197 cm/s (*B*), well below what one would expect for this degree of stenosis. Following CEA, the diameter of the carotid bulb increases secondary to placement of the patch, resulting in a decrease in PSV. Therefore, PSV for a given percent stenosis will be lower than in the native vessel, and gray-scale findings and PSVR are likely more accurate predictors of degree of stenosis.

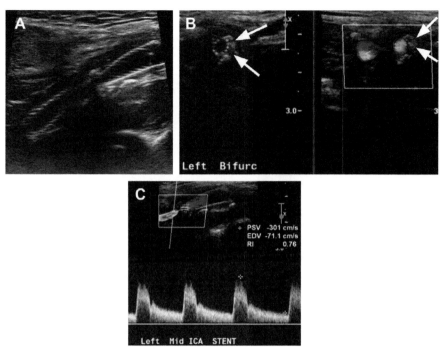

Fig. 18. Normal findings after carotid stent placement. Sagittal gray-scale (A) and (B) transverse split screen gray-scale and color Doppler images of left ICA stent demonstrating compression and narrowing of the stent by excluded echogenic plaque (arrows, B). Spectral Doppler tracing (C) obtained from the narrowed portion of the stent reveals increased PSV of 301 cm/s. However, no intraluminal echoes are noted. Therefore, the elevated PSV is likely due to narrowing of the stent by the excluded plaque rather than a true in-stent restenosis, and no further imaging (other than continued surveillance) or intervention is required.

diagnosis of restenosis following intervention. Placement of a patch in the carotid bulb during CEA increases the luminal diameter and, thus, decreases PSV, and also changes vessel wall compliance. Hence, the PSV threshold for diagnosing a ≥70% stenosis following CEA is likely lower than for the native artery, although no specific PSV threshold number is universally accepted. Therefore, PSVR, gray-scale, and color Doppler findings as well as change over time are likely more reliable criteria for grading an ICA stenosis following CEA (Fig. 17). CAS placement also changes vessel hemodynamics: compliance is decreased; partial occlusion of the ECA will shunt blood into the ICA; narrowing of the stent may persist either due to lack of expansion (termed "waisting") or from compression by excluded calcified plaque (Fig. 18). All these factors will increase PSV. Virtually all reported studies have shown that PSV and PSVR criteria for a ≥70% ICA stenosis are higher following CAS than for the native vessel. Although there is no consensus on a specific threshold number, PSV greater than 300 to 325 cm/s may be indicative of a ≥70% stenosis.[53,54] In addition, increase in PSV and PSVR over time and concordance with gray-scale and color Doppler findings are extremely helpful in diagnosing in-stent restenosis. Additionally, one should exercise caution in making the diagnosis of in-stent restenosis unless intraluminal echoes due to neointimal hyperplasia, thrombus, or plaque are observed on gray-scale or color Doppler (Fig. 19). When US findings are equivocal, CT angiography or angiography should be considered.

SUMMARY

Doppler US is the primary noninvasive imaging modality for the diagnosis of ICA stenosis, for following mild to moderate stenoses that do not require immediate intervention, and for surveillance of patients after intervention. Although PSV is the primary Doppler US criterion for grading an ICA stenosis, in certain scenarios PSVR or EDV may provide more accurate assessment. Furthermore, there are no widely accepted Doppler criteria for grading an ICA stenosis in patients with severe contralateral disease, tandem lesions, long segment, or nearly occlusive ICA lesions, or following CEA or CAS placement. In these situations, gray-scale and color Doppler findings as

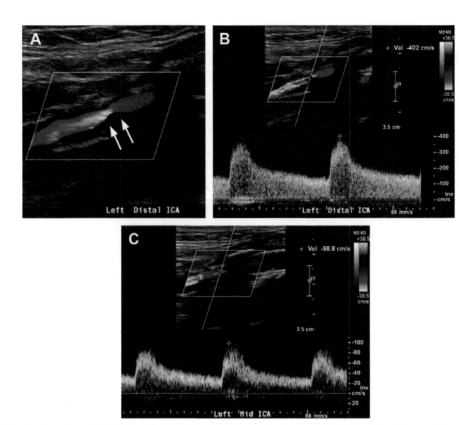

Fig. 19. In-stent restenosis. (*A*) Color Doppler sagittal image from a patient presenting for surveillance 2 years following carotid stent placement in the left ICA reveals hypoechoic material (*arrows*), likely neointimomedial thickening or thrombus narrowing the lumen of the distal stent. (*B*) Duplex Doppler sagittal image demonstrating narrowing, focal color aliasing, and increased PSV of 402 cm/s in comparison to 99 cm/s in the proximal segment of the stent (*C*) yielding a PSVR of 4.0. These findings are consistent with a greater than 70% in-stent restenosis. Because PSV is typically higher within a stent than in the native vessel, the same Doppler criteria cannot be used to grade stenoses following stent placement. PSV criteria are higher than for the native vessel, and the PSVR and gray-scale and color Doppler findings have increased importance. One should be cautious in diagnosing an in-stent restenosis in the absence of intraluminal echoes narrowing the residual lumen.

well as change over time become critically important. In addition, waveform analysis may provide important clues regarding the severity of an ICA stenosis as well as the presence of proximal or distal cardiovascular disease and nonatherosclerotic carotid pathology.

At the time of the SRU consensus conference in 2002, available data indicated that intervention in symptomatic patients with a ≥70% ICA stenosis resulted in substantial stroke risk reduction, with a more modest stroke risk reduction in patients with a 50% to 69% ICA stenosis. Hence, the Doppler criteria for diagnosing a ≥70% ICA stenosis were chosen to emphasize sensitivity rather than specificity as the consequence of missing a ≥70% ICA stenosis (false negative examination) was deemed far worse than the consequence of misclassifying a 50% to 69% ICA stenosis as a ≥70% stenosis (false positive examination).[55] However, improvements in medical management

with statins as well as more aggressive antiplatelet therapy have resulted in a significant decline in the incidence of stroke. Therefore, these assumptions may no longer be valid, and spectral Doppler criteria may need to be revised upwards to provide more specificity because medical management may now be more appropriate for patients with moderate ICA stenosis.[56]

REFERENCES

1. Benjamin EJ, Virani SS, Callaway CW, et al. Heart disease and stroke statistics - 2018 update: a report from the American Heart Association. Circulation 2018;137:e67–492.

2. Kleindorfer DO, Khoury J, Moomaw CJ, et al. Stroke incidence is decreasing in whites but not in blacks: a population-based estimate of temporal trends in stroke incidence from the Greater Cincinnati/Northern Kentucky Stroke Study. Stroke 2010;41:1326–31.

3. Carandang R, Seshadri S, Beiser A, et al. Trends in incidence, lifetime risk, severity, and 30-day mortality of stroke over the past 50 years. JAMA 2006;296: 2939–46.

4. Estruch R, Ros E, Salas-Salvado J, et al. Retraction and republication: primary prevention of cardiovascular disease in a Mediterranean diet supplemented with extra-virgin olive oil or nuts. N Engl J Med 2018; 378:2441–2. e34(1)–e34(14).

5. Fairhead JF, Rothwell PM. The need for urgency in identification and treatment of symptomatic carotid stenosis is already established. Cerebrovasc Dis 2005;19:355–8.

6. AIUM practice parameter for the performance of an ultrasound examination of the extracranial cerebrovascular system. 2016. Available at: https://www.aium.org/resources/guidelines/extracranial.pdf. Accessed October 25, 2018.

7. Hansson GK. Inflammation, atherosclerosis, and coronary artery disease. N Engl J Med 2005;352: 1685–95.

8. Ross R. Atherosclerosis-an inflammatory disease. N Engl J Med 1999;340:115–26.

9. Bonati LH, Nederkoorn PJ. Clinical perspective of carotid plaque imaging. Neuroimaging Clin N Am 2016;26:175–82.

10. Fisher M, Paganini-Hill A, Martin A, et al. Carotid plaque pathology: thrombosis, ulceration and stroke pathogenesis. Stroke 2005;6(2):253–7.

11. Bluth EI, Kay D, Merritt CR, et al. Sonographic characterization of carotid plaque: detection of hemorrhage. AJR Am J Roentgenol 1986;146:1061–5.

12. Gerrit L, Sijbrands EJ, Straub D, et al. Noninvasive imaging of the vulnerable atherosclerotic plaque. Curr Probl Cardiol 2010;35:556–91.

13. Polak JF, Shemanski L, O'Leary DH, et al. Hypoechoic plaque at US of the carotid artery: an independent risk factor for incident stroke in adults aged 65 years or older. Cardiovascular Healthy Study. Radiology 1998;208(3):649–54.

14. Gupta A, Kesavabhotla K, Baradaran H, et al. Plaque echolucency and stroke risk in asymptomatic carotid stenosis: a systemic review and meta-analysis. Stroke 2015;46:91–7.

15. Feinstein SB. Contrast ultrasound imaging of the carotid artery vasa vasorum and atherosclerotic plaque neovascularization. J Am Coll Cardiol 2006;48: 236–43.

16. Schminke U, Motsch L, Griewing B, et al. Three-dimensional power-mode ultrasound for quantification of the progression of carotid artery atherosclerosis. J Neurol 2000;247:106–11.

17. Sillesen H, Muntendam P, Adourian A, et al. Carotid plaque burden as a measure of subclinical atherosclerosis: comparison with other tests for subclinical arterial disease in the High Risk Plaque BioImage study. JACC Cardiovasc Imaging 2012;5:681–9.

18. van Engelen A, Wannarong T, Parraga G, et al. Three-dimensional carotid ultrasound plaque texture predicts vascular events. Stroke 2014;45: 2695–701.

19. Coli S, Magnoni M, Sangiorgi G, et al. Contrast-enhanced ultrasound imaging of intraplaque neovascularization in carotid arteries: correlation with histology and plaque echogenicity. J Am Coll Cardiol 2008;52:223–30.

20. Giannoni MF, Vincenzini E, Citone M, et al. Contrast carotid ultrasound for the detection of unstable plaques with neoangiogenesis: a pilot study. Eur J Vasc Endovasc Surg 2009;37:722–7.

21. Owen DR, Shalhoub J, Miller S, et al. Inflammation within carotid atherosclerotic plaque: assessment with late-phase contrast-enhanced US. Radiology 2010;255(2):638–44.

22. Salonen JT, Salonen R. Ultrasonographically assessed carotid morphology and the risk of coronary heart disease. Arterioscler Thromb 1991;11: 1245–9.

23. Chambless LE, Heiss G, Folsom AR, et al. Association of coronary heart disease incidence with carotid arterial wall thickness and major risk factors: The Arteriosclerosis Risk in Communities (ARIC) Study 1993-1997. Am J Epidemiol 1997;146:483–94.

24. Bots ML, Hoes AW, Koudstaal PJ, et al. Common carotid artery intima-media thickness as a risk factor for myocardial infarction: The Rotterdam Study. Circulation 1997;96:1432–7.

25. O'Leary DH, Polak JF, Kronmal RA, et al. Carotid-artery intima and media thickness as a risk factor for myocardial infarction and stroke in older adults. Cardiovascular Health Study. N Engl J Med 1999;340: 14–22.

26. Lorenz MW, Markus HS, Bots ML, et al. Prediction of clinical cardiovascular events with carotid intima-media thickness: a systemic review and meta-analysis. Circulation 2007;115:459–67.

27. Helfand M, Buckley DI, Freeman M, et al. Emerging risk factors for coronary heart disease: a summary of systemic reviews conducted for the U.S. Preventive Services Task Force. Ann Intern Med 2009;151: 496–507.

28. Zavodni AEH, Wasserman BA, McClelland RL, et al. Carotid artery plaque morphology and composition in relation to incident cardiovascular events: The Multi-Ethnic Study of Atherosclerosis (MESA). Radiology 2014;271(2):381–9.

29. Den Ruijter HM, Peters SA, Anderson TJ, et al. Common carotid intima-media thickness measurements in cardiovascular risk prediction: a meta-analysis. JAMA 2012;308(8):796–803.

30. van den Oord SCH, Sijbrands EJG, Gerrit L, et al. Carotid intima-media thickness for cardiovascular risk assessment: systemic review and meta-analysis. Atherosclerosis 2013;228:1–11.

31. O'Leary DH, Bots ML. Imaging of atheroscleroisis: carotid intima-media thickness. Eur Heart J 2010; 31:1682–9.

32. Stein JH, Korcarz CE, Hurst RT, et al. Use of carotid ultrasound to identify subclinical disease and evaluate cardiovascular risk: a consensus statement from the American Society of Echocardiography carotid intima-media thickness task force endorsed by the Society of Vascular Medicine. J Am Soc Echocardiogr 2008;21:93–111.

33. North American Symptomatic Carotid Endarterectomy Trial Collaborators (NASCET), Barnett HJM, Taylor DW, Haynes RB, et al. Beneficial effect of carotid endarterectomy in symptomatic patients with high-grade carotid stenosis. N Engl J Med 1991; 325(7):445–53.

34. Executive Committee for the Asymptomatic Carotid Atherosclerosis Study. Endarterectomy for asymptomatic carotid artery stenosis. JAMA 1995;273: 1421–8.

35. Rothwell PM, Eliasziw M, Gutnikov SA, et al. Analysis of pooled data from the randomized controlled trials of endarterectomy for symptomatic carotid stenosis. Lancet 2003;361:107–16.

36. Yadav JS, Wholey MH, Kuntz RE, et al. Protected carotid-artery stenting versus endarterectomy in high-risk patients. N Engl J Med 2004;351: 1439–501.

37. Bangalore S, Kumar S, Wettersley J, et al. Carotid artery stenting vs. carotid Endarterectomy: Meta-analysis and diversity-adjusted trial sequential analysis of randomized trials. Arch Neurol 2011;68(2): 172–84.

38. Brott TG, Halperin JL, Abbara S, et al. 2011 ASA/ ACCF/AHA/AANN/AANS/ACR/ASNR/CNS/SAIP/ SCAI/SIR/SNIS/SVM/SVS guideline on the management of patients with extracranial carotid and vertebral artery disease. J Am Coll Cardiol 2011;57(8): 1002–44.

39. Grant EG, Benson CB, Moneta GL, et al. Carotid artery stenosis: gray-scale and Doppler US diagnosis–Society of Radiologists in Ultrasound consensus conference. Radiology 2003;229(2): 340–6.

40. IAC vascular testing white paper on carotid stenosis interpretation criteria. 2014. Available at: https:// www.intersocietal.org/vascular/forms/IACCarotid CriteriaWhitePaper1-2014.pdf. Accessed October 25, 2018.

41. AbuRama AF, Richmond BK, Robinson PA, et al. Effect of contralateral severe stenosis or carotid occlusion on duplex criteria of ipsilateral stenoses. Comparative study of various duplex parameters. J Vasc Surg 1995;22:751–62.

42. Grajo JR, Barr RG. Duplex Doppler sonography of the carotid artery. Velocity measurements in an artery with contralateral stenosis. Ultrasound Q 2007; 23:199–202.

43. Spencer MP, Reid JM. Quantitation of carotid stenosis with continuous wave (CW) Doppler ultrasound. Stroke 1979;10:326–30.

44. Kotval PS. Doppler waveform parvus and tardus. A sign of proximal flow obstruction. J Ultrasound Med 1989;8(8):435–40.

45. Rohren EM, Kliewer MA, Carroll BA, et al. A spectrum of Doppler waveforms in the carotid and vertebral arteries. AJR Am J Roentgenol 2003; 181:1695–704.

46. O'Boyle MK, Vibharak N, Chung J, et al. Duplex sonography of the carotid arteries in patients with isolated aortic stenosis: imaging findings and relation to severity of stenosis. AJR Am J Roentgenol 1996; 166:197–202.

47. Gunabushanam G, Millet JD, Stilp E, et al. Computer-assisted detection of tardus parvus waveforms on Doppler ultrasound. Ultrasound 2018; 26(2):81–92.

48. Scoutt LM, Lin FL, Kliewer M. Waveform analysis of the carotid arteries. Ultrasound Clin 2006;1:133–59.

49. Nuffer Z, Rupasov A, Bhatt S. Doppler ultrasound evaluation of circulatory support devices. Ultrasound Q 2017;33(3):193–200.

50. Cervini P, Park SJ, Shah DK, et al. Carotid Doppler ultrasound findings in patients with left ventricular assist devices. Ultrasound Q 2010;26(4):255–61.

51. Flis CM, Jager HR, Sidhu PS. Carotid and vertebral artery dissections: clinical aspects, imaging features and endovascular treatment. Eur Radiol 2007;17: 820–34.

52. Debette S, Leys D. Cervical-artery dissections: predisposing factors, diagnosis, and outcome. Lancet Neurol 2009;8(7):668–78.

53. Setacci C, Chisci E, Setacci F, et al. Grading carotid intrastent restenosis: a 6-year follow up study. Stroke 2008;39:1189–96.

54. Dai Z, Xu G. Restenosis after carotid artery stenting. Vascular 2017;25(6):576–86.

55. Heijenbrok-Kal MH, Buskens E, Nederkoorn PJ, et al. Optimal peak systolic velocity threshold at duplex US for determining the need for carotid endarterectomy: a decision analytic approach. Radiology 2005;238:480–8.

56. AbuRama AF, Srivastava M, Stone PA, et al. Critical appraisal of the carotid duplex consensus criteria in the diagnosis of carotid artery stenosis. J Vasc Surg 2011;53:53–60.

Vertebral Artery Ultrasound

Gowthaman Gunabushanam, MD[a],*, Lauren Kummant, MD[b], Leslie M. Scoutt, MD[a]

KEYWORDS

- Vertebral artery ultrasound • Spectral Doppler • Vertebral artery stenosis

KEY POINTS

- Waveform analysis of the vertebral arteries may provide useful clues regarding pathology in the subclavian, carotid, brachiocephalic, and intracranial arteries.
- Provocative maneuvers can convert a pre-steal waveform to a complete steal or deepen the mid systolic retraction of the pre-steal waveform.
- Approximately 90% of vertebral artery stenoses occur at the vertebral artery origin, which often can be imaged well on ultrasound.
- Peak systolic velocity greater than 115–140 cm/s and a peak systolic velocity ratio greater than 2.1–2.2 are suggestive of greater than 50% stenosis at the vertebral artery origin.
- Given its wide availability, relatively low cost, and lack of ionizing radiation, ultrasound is especially useful for serial monitoring of pathology involving the extracranial vertebral artery.

INTRODUCTION

The vertebral arteries (VAs) supply the posterior circulation of the central nervous system. A single waveform of the mid VA is routinely obtained as part of the carotid Doppler ultrasound examination.[1] Previously, except in the context of subclavian steal syndrome, there was limited interest in imaging the VAs, partly due to lack of readily available and widely accepted treatment options. However, in current practice, VA stenosis is increasingly being treated by stent placement. In addition, ultrasound (US) evaluation of the VAs may provide useful clues about cerebrovascular pathology proximal or distal to the field of view. In this article, we review the anatomy, scanning technique, and sonographic appearance of the normal VAs as well as VA stenosis, dissection, pseudoaneurysm (PSA), and arteriovenous fistula (AVF). Direct ultrasound assessment of the

intracranial segment of the VA using transcranial Doppler is beyond the scope of this article.

NORMAL ANATOMY AND IMAGING TECHNIQUE

The VAs are paired vessels, typically measuring 3 to 5 mm in diameter, which most commonly arise from the ipsilateral subclavian arteries (Fig. 1). The VA has been divided into 4 segments (V1 through V4). The V1 segment extends from the origin of the VA to the transverse foramen of the sixth cervical vertebra. The V2 segment travels through the transverse foramina of the sixth through second cervical vertebra. The V3 segment extends from the transverse foramen of the axis to the point of entry into the dura mater. The terminal segment of the VA, V4, is intradural and joins the contralateral VA to form the basilar artery (BA), which in turn terminates into the circle of Willis,

Disclosures: L.M. Scoutt is an educational consultant to Philips Healthcare (unrelated to this article). The other authors have no disclosures.
[a] Department of Radiology and Biomedical Imaging, Yale University School of Medicine, 333 Cedar Street, PO Box 208042, New Haven, CT 06520-8042, USA; [b] Department of Radiology, Northwell Health, 900 Franklin Avenue, Valley Stream, NY 11580, USA
* Corresponding author.
E-mail address: gowthaman.gunabushanam@yale.edu

Radiol Clin N Am 57 (2019) 519–533
https://doi.org/10.1016/j.rcl.2019.01.011

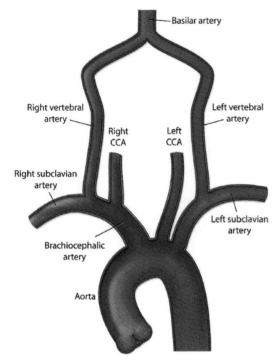

Fig. 1. Schematic image showing vertebral artery anatomy. CCA, common carotid artery.

connecting the posterior circulation to the anterior cerebral circulation supplied by the carotid arteries.[2]

The VAs give off many tiny branches in the V1 through V3 segments, including cervical muscular branches and meningeal arteries, but these are too small to be visualized on US. The posterior inferior cerebellar artery is the largest branch of the VA and arises from the V4 segment. In 3% to 5% of individuals, the VA (usually the left VA) arises directly from the aorta.[3] Less common variants include origin of the VA from the left common carotid or external carotid arteries.[3] Not uncommonly, one of the VAs is hypoplastic or terminates prematurely after the origin of the posterior inferior cerebellar artery, in which case only one VA contributes to form the BA.

The cervical VA can be evaluated by US in most patients by using a 5- to 12-MHz linear array transducer. Typically, the V2 segment of the VA is imaged first by locating the mid common carotid artery (CCA) in the sagittal plane, and then angulating the US probe posterolaterally until the VA is seen as it courses between the foramina of the transverse processes of the cervical vertebra (**Fig. 2**). Color and spectral Doppler are often helpful in distinguishing the artery from the adjacent vertebral vein (see **Fig. 2**).[3] The V1 segment, including the VA origin, can then be assessed by

following the V2 segment inferiorly (see **Fig. 2**).[4] The V3 segment of the VA is assessed by placing the US probe below the mastoid process lateral to the sternocleidomastoid muscle and angulating the probe toward the contralateral orbit.[2]

NORMAL ULTRASOUND FINDINGS

Owing to the relatively small caliber and deep location of the cervical VA, it can be difficult to visualize the arterial wall and lumen well or to characterize atherosclerotic disease on grayscale imaging. The extra-osseous portion of the V2 segment is visualized between shadowing from the transverse processes of the cervical vertebra. The normal spectral Doppler waveform of the VA has a low-resistance pattern characterized by continuous forward diastolic flow, similar to the waveform of the internal carotid artery, as the artery supplies the low-resistance posterior circulation. Vertebral artery waveforms should have a sharp systolic upstroke and well-defined systolic peak. The peak systolic velocity (PSV) typically ranges from 20 to 60 cm/s. Spectral broadening is commonly seen due to a relatively large sample volume compared with the small vessel caliber. Although waveforms are most often bilaterally symmetric, many patients have a dominant VA (usually the left), which may have a larger diameter and higher PSV than the contralateral VA.[5]

WAVEFORM ANALYSIS
High-Resistance Waveforms

High-resistance waveforms with complete loss of, reversed or decreased diastolic flow and often decreased PSV may be indicative of distal pathology causing obstruction to flow, such as distal VA stenosis, occlusion, hypoplasia, or dissection (**Table 1**). However, in a study of 79 patients with high-resistance VA waveforms, no vascular pathology was observed in approximately 19% of patients.[6] Up to 15% of all individuals have a dominant VA,[5] and the contralateral hypoplastic VA may demonstrate relatively increased vascular resistance due to a small lumen diameter, which is often less than 2 mm (**Fig. 3**).[7] Bilateral high-resistance waveforms in the VA with normal carotid artery waveforms are suggestive of pathology in the BA. High-resistance waveforms in both VAs, as well as in the carotid arteries, may be observed with increased intracranial pressure, vasospasm, and/or brain death. Reversal of diastolic flow in the vertebral and carotid arteries may also be noted in patients with severe aortic regurgitation, but PSV is usually elevated in such cases.

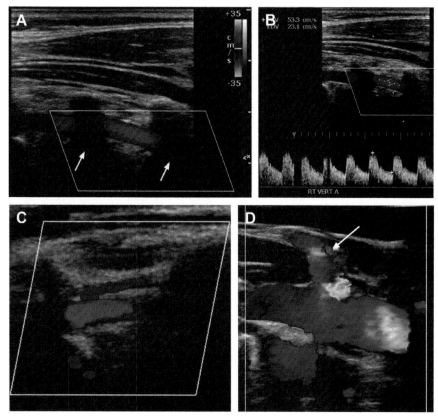

Fig. 2. (A) Sagittal color Doppler image showing the normal appearance of the vertebral artery coursing through the foramina of the transverse processes of the cervical spine. Arrows point to shadowing from the transverse processes. (B) Spectral Doppler image shows a normal low-resistance waveform with a brisk systolic upstroke and continuous forward diastolic flow. Peak systolic velocity of 53 cm/s is within the normal range of 20–60 cm/s. (C) Sagittal color Doppler image demonstrating a normal vertebral artery (*red*) with the adjacent vein (*blue*). (D) Color Doppler image shows vertebral artery origin (*arrow*) from the subclavian artery.

Increased Flow

Increased PSV along the length of the VA is usually secondary to compensatory increased flow. Causes include contralateral VA hypoplasia or congenital absence, contralateral subclavian steal, and high-grade stenosis/occlusion of the ipsilateral carotid artery (**Fig. 4**) or contralateral VA.[8]

Pre-steal and Steal Waveforms

Subclavian steal syndrome is said to occur when there is partial or complete reversal of flow within the VA with symptoms of either vertebrobasilar insufficiency, such as stroke, transient ischemic attack, syncope, dizziness, vertigo, blurred vision, and diplopia,[9] or upper extremity arterial insufficiency such as arm pain and tingling. However, most patients with VA flow reversal are asymptomatic,[10] and this finding has been termed the subclavian steal phenomenon.

Subclavian steal usually occurs because of stenosis or occlusion of the proximal subclavian artery, and is 3 times more common on the left compared with the right. Stenosis within the subclavian artery will often manifest as a "pre-steal" VA waveform before complete reversal of flow occurs. It has been postulated that, due to the Venturi effect, a transient pressure drop occurs during early to mid systole at the VA origin as the high-velocity jet caused by the subclavian artery stenosis courses under the origin of the VA.[5,11] This, combined with the normal intraluminal pressure in the contralateral VA and BA alters the net pressure gradient in the ipsilateral VA, resulting in a very narrow first systolic peak followed by a mid systolic retraction or brief reversal of flow in early to mid systole and reappearance of forward flow in late systole and diastole (**Fig. 5**). This waveform appearance has been referred to as the "vertebral bunny" or pre-steal waveform, and in

Table 1	
Differential diagnosis of qualitative changes in vertebral artery waveforms	
Imaging Findings	**Possible Causes**
Unilateral high-resistance waveform	Distal vertebral artery stenosis or occlusion
	Hypoplastic vertebral artery (normal variant)
	Normal finding (no distal abnormality)
Unilateral increased flow	Hypoplasia of contralateral vertebral artery
	Stenosis/occlusion of contralateral vertebral artery
	Stenosis/occlusion of ipsilateral carotid artery
	Subclavian steal phenomenon on contralateral side
Bilateral high-resistance vertebral artery waveforms with normal carotid artery waveforms	Basilar artery stenosis or occlusion
Bilateral high-resistance vertebral and carotid artery waveforms	Increased intracranial pressure due to any cause, including a mass, hematoma, or cerebral edema
	Diffuse vasospasm
	Brain death

general the depth of the mid systolic retraction roughly correlates with the degree of subclavian artery stenosis.[8] Another potential explanation for the pre-steal waveform pattern is that the transient reversal of flow in mid systole is simply related to changes in the arterial pressure gradient during the cardiac cycle.

Pitfalls can occur in diagnosing a pre-steal waveform. Occasionally, slow bidirectional flow within the VA can be mistaken for complete occlusion due to a very small net movement of blood within the artery.[12,13] A hypoplastic VA and proximal VA stenosis or occlusion may also result in bidirectional flow within the VA, and mimic the subclavian steal phenomenon.[14] In addition, it is important to not misdiagnose pulsatile flow within the adjacent vertebral vein as reversal of flow within the VA.

Because the right VA originates from the right subclavian artery, which in turn arises from the brachiocephalic (innominate) artery, steal and pre-steal phenomena in the right VA may be caused by narrowing or occlusion within either the right subclavian or brachiocephalic arteries. It is helpful to image the right carotid arteries in these cases, because a brachiocephalic artery stenosis will alter the waveforms in the right carotid arteries (**Fig. 6**), whereas the right carotid arterial waveforms will be normal if the stenosis/occlusion is within the subclavian artery (**Fig. 7**). In the case of a brachiocephalic artery occlusion, reversed flow in the right VA may supply blood flow not only to the right arm but also to the right carotid system, depending on the presence of intracranial collaterals. Hence, flow is often reversed in the segment of the right subclavian artery between the origin of the right VA and the right CCA (see **Fig. 6**). However, if the predominant collateral flow to the right anterior circulation is from collaterals through the circle of Willis or between the external carotid arteries, flow will be reversed in the right internal and common carotid arteries, but forward toward the hand in the right subclavian artery distal to the origin of the right CCA.

If reversed flow or a pre-steal waveform is noted in the VA, Doppler US evaluation of the proximal ipsilateral subclavian artery is recommended to search for increased PSV at the site of the stenosis or an occlusion. Other findings that support the diagnosis of subclavian steal are a greater than 20 mm Hg pressure difference between the patient's right and left arm (the stenosis/occlusion will be on the side with the decreased pressure) and tardus parvus spectral Doppler waveforms within the lateral subclavian or axillary arteries.[13]

Provocative maneuvers are useful in eliciting reversal of flow within the VA, thus aiding in the diagnosis of subclavian stenosis. These include inflating a blood pressure cuff above systolic blood pressure for 3 to 5 minutes and then releasing the cuff, or asking the patient to exercise their arm by repeatedly clenching and unclenching their fist until symptoms in the hand occur, and then immediately obtaining a waveform in the VA.[8,15] These maneuvers increase oxygen demand, decrease peripheral vascular resistance within the limb and thereby accentuate the steal phenomenon. Immediately repeating the Doppler examination will either demonstrate deepening of the mid systolic retraction or complete flow reversal in the ipsilateral VA.[12,13,16] Symptomatic patients with subclavian steal syndrome due to subclavian artery stenosis are usually treated using subclavian artery stent placement. It should be noted that if partial or complete subclavian steal is observed on

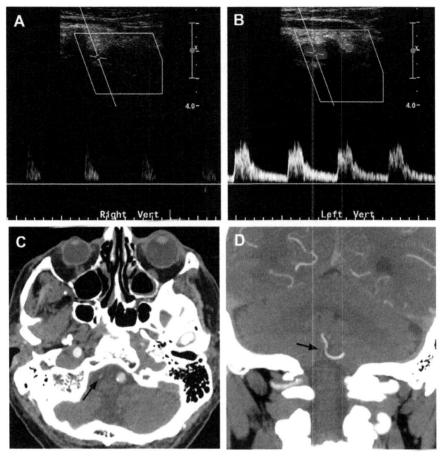

Fig. 3. An 83-year-old woman with a hypoplastic right vertebral artery. (A) A markedly high-resistance waveform is noted In the right vertebral artery with complete absence of diastolic flow. (B) Note normal-appearing low-resistance waveform in the left vertebral artery with continuous forward diastolic flow. Axial (C) and coronal re-formatted (D) CT angiogram shows the diminutive size of the right vertebral artery (arrows) compared with the left side.

imaging, and a careful history reveals the patient to be asymptomatic, no further imaging workup or treatment may be needed.[17]

SPECIFIC PATHOLOGIES
Vertebral Artery Stenosis

Approximately 25% of all strokes occur in the vertebrobasilar system, and 20% of these strokes are related to stenosis of the proximal VA.[18] In addition, the risk of recurrent stroke because of VA stenosis is reportedly much higher than the risk of recurrent stroke due to plaque/stenosis at the origin of the internal carotid artery, especially in the acute phase.[19,20] Hence, stent placement in the VA is increasingly performed to treat ≥50% VA stenoses to prevent new or recurrent stroke.[21] Ultrasound has an important role in the diagnosis and follow-up management of VA stenosis in comparison with computed tomography (CT) angiography,

MR angiography, and digital subtraction angiography (DSA) because of the advantages of low cost, wide availability, and lack of risk factors associated with intravenous contrast use, making US the ideal modality for repeat measurements and continued surveillance of the VAs. Approximately 90% of VA stenoses occur at the vessel origin, which can be well visualized with US (Fig. 8).[5,22]

The arterial lumen may appear narrowed on color Doppler and be accompanied by color Doppler aliasing due to increased PSV. However, spectral Doppler velocity criteria for diagnosing VA stenosis are not well established (Table 2). Yurdakul and Tola[4] studied 96 VAs in 48 patients. Of these, 77 VAs were included and 19 excluded from final analysis because of one of the following conditions: origin directly from the aorta rather than from the subclavian artery, hypoplastic VAs, VA occlusion, and subclavian artery occlusion. They suggested a PSV ratio of greater than 2.2 as the

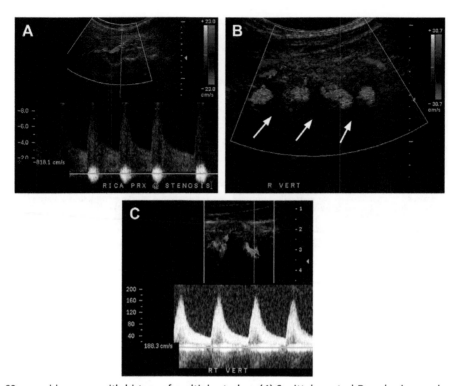

Fig. 4. A 69-year-old woman with history of multiple strokes. (*A*) Sagittal spectral Doppler image demonstrates high-grade stenosis in the right proximal internal carotid artery with a PSV of 818 cm/s. (*B*) Sagittal color Doppler image demonstrating compensatory hypertrophy of the right vertebral artery, which is quite dilated and tortuous as it courses between the cervical vertebral transverse processes. Arrows indicate shadowing from the bone. Note color aliasing indicates high velocity flow. (*C*) On spectral Doppler interrogation, PSV in the right vertebral artery is elevated at 188 cm/s.

optimal Doppler criterion for identifying a proximal VA stenosis of ≥50%. Other useful Doppler parameters were PSV greater than 108 cm/s, end diastolic velocity (EDV) >36 cm/s and EDV ratio >1.7. Koch and colleagues[23] performed a study correlating VA Doppler US findings with angiography in 218 patients (436 VAs). Of the 386 VAs that were angiographically visible, 72 (19%: 33 right and 39 left) VA origins could not be visualized on US. Vertebral artery origin in 50% to 99% stenosis was observed in 36 vessels (9%). For the detection of 50% to 99% stenosis, PSV at the VA origin of 114 cm/s had a reported sensitivity of 71% and specificity of 90%, whereas a PSV cutoff of 77 cm/s had a reported sensitivity of 80% and specificity of 71%. In a study of 62 patients, Skoda and colleagues[24] found a PSV of ≥135 cm/s and PSV ratio of ≥2.2 to be similarly accurate for the detection of 50% to 99% VA stenosis.

In a large correlative study of patients who underwent VA Doppler US as well as DSA within 2 weeks of each other, Hua and colleagues[25] reported that PSV at the VA origin of 85 to

139 cm/s (<50% stenosis), 140 to 209 cm/s (50%–69% stenosis), and ≥210 cm/s (70%–99% stenosis) had an accuracy of 94.5%, 96.2%, and 88.7%, respectively. However, it is important to note that the study by Hua and colleagues,[25] excluded patients with severe stenosis or dissection of the intracranial VAs or BA, greater than 50% stenosis of the contralateral VA, occlusion of the VA, VA hypoplasia, greater than 70% stenosis of a carotid artery or subclavian artery, and other conditions including cerebral hemorrhage detected with CT and severe heart disease with low cerebral blood flow. In fact, only 247 of 653 (37.8%) patients met all inclusion criteria, and, therefore, the real-world accuracy of VA Doppler US is likely to be significantly lower than reported in this study. Indeed, in a comparison study of Doppler US, contrast-enhanced CT and MR angiography, and DSA in 46 patients, US had a reported sensitivity of 67% (95% confidence interval: 35%–88%) and specificity of 98% (95% confidence interval: 91%–100%) for stenosis at the VA origin.[26] For VA stenosis at all locations, the specificity of US was similar at 95% (95%

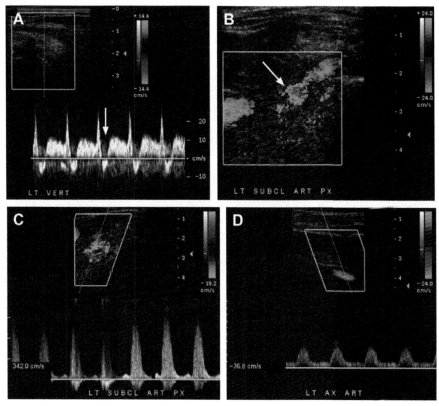

Fig. 5. A 66-year-old woman with left arm claudication. (*A*) Spectral Doppler image shows pre-steal waveforms in the left vertebral artery with a sharp but narrow early systolic peak and early to mid systolic retraction (*arrow*). (*B*) Color Doppler image demonstrating aliasing at the origin of the left subclavian artery (*arrow*) as well as a soft tissue color bruit (color pixels outside the vessel lumen). (*C*) Spectral Doppler image demonstrating increased peak systolic velocity of 342 cm/s at the origin of the left subclavian artery, consistent with severe stenosis. (*D*) Spectral Doppler tracing from the left axillary artery demonstrating a tardus parvus waveform distal to the left subclavian artery stenosis.

confidence interval: 86%–98%), but the sensitivity was lower at 44% (95% confidence interval: 23%–67%). In the same study, contrast-enhanced MR angiography had the highest reported sensitivity of 83% to 89% and specificity of 87% to 91%.

The above Doppler velocity criteria apply only to the native VAs; following stent placement, the optimal criteria in one study for detection of 50% to 69% in-stent restenosis were intra-stent PSV ≥170 cm/s, EDV ≥45 cm/s, and PSV ratio ≥2.7, and those for 70% to 99% in-stent restenosis were intra-stent PSV ≥220 cm/s, EDV ≥55 cm/s, and PSV ratio ≥4.2.[27]

Narrowing of the VA may also be due to extrinsic compression such as from an osteophyte (**Fig. 9**) or a herniated disc. In cases where the VA origin cannot be directly assessed due to tortuosity, deep location or shadowing from the clavicle, tardus parvus waveforms in the distal VA with a slow systolic upstroke and poorly defined rounded low velocity systolic peak suggests proximal

stenosis.[3] However, it is important to remember that tardus parvus waveforms are a non-specific finding, and merely indicate that there is a stenosis proximal to the imaged vessel, including subclavian artery, brachiocephalic artery, or even aortic valve stenosis. Therefore, another imaging modality such as CT or MR angiography may be necessary to localize the stenosis.

Dissection

Vertebral artery dissections although uncommon, with a reported annual incidence of 1 to 1.5 per 100,000 population,[28] account for approximately 10% to 15% of strokes in young adults. The most common cause of VA dissection is either blunt or penetrating trauma. The dissection entry point typically occurs at the atlanto-axial segment, due to increased mobility at this level.[29] Other causative factors include extension of an aortic dissection, fibromuscular dysplasia, connective tissue

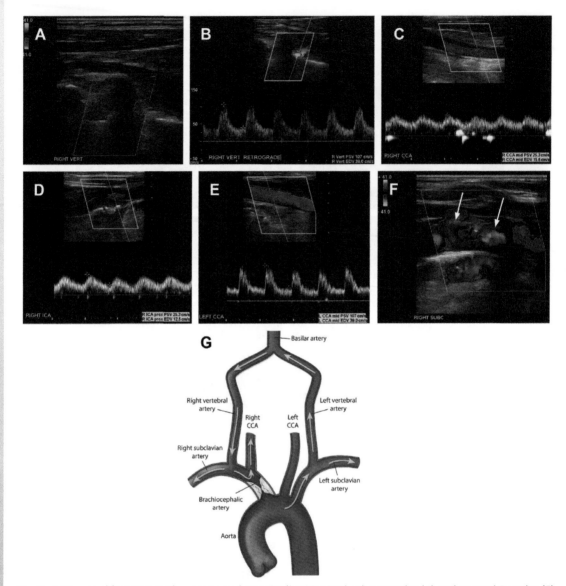

Fig. 6. A 74-year-old woman with syncope and arm tingling. Sagittal color Doppler (*A*) and spectral Doppler (*B*) images show retrograde flow within the right vertebral artery. Spectral Doppler shows tardus parvus waveforms with relatively low peak systolic velocities of approximately 25 cm/s in the right common carotid (*C*) and internal carotid arteries (*D*). (*E*) The left common carotid artery shows normal waveforms with a brisk systolic upstroke and a normal peak systolic velocity of 107 cm/s. (*F*) Color Doppler image shows reversal of flow within the very proximal segment of right subclavian artery (*white arrows*). These findings are suggestive of occlusion of the brachiocephalic artery, with reversal of flow in the right vertebral artery with retrograde filling of the right carotid system from the right vertebral artery, as depicted on the schematic image (*G*). CCA, common carotid artery.

diseases, and atherosclerosis. Patients with extracranial VA dissections often present with nonspecific symptoms such as dizziness, vertigo, amnesia, tinnitus, hemianopia, nausea and vomiting, or posterior cerebral circulation infarcts. However, many patients are completely asymptomatic.[28]

Ultrasound has a reported sensitivity ranging from 66% to 90% for the detection of VA dissection, which is low compared with CT and MR

angiography. The pathognomonic but uncommonly seen US finding is an echogenic intimal flap, with demonstration of a true and false lumen on color Doppler. However, more often, the false lumen is thrombosed resulting in homogeneous thickening of the VA wall causing a smooth-surfaced long segment stenosis or narrowing of the lumen without a detectable dissection flap (**Fig. 10**). Often, the only findings observed are

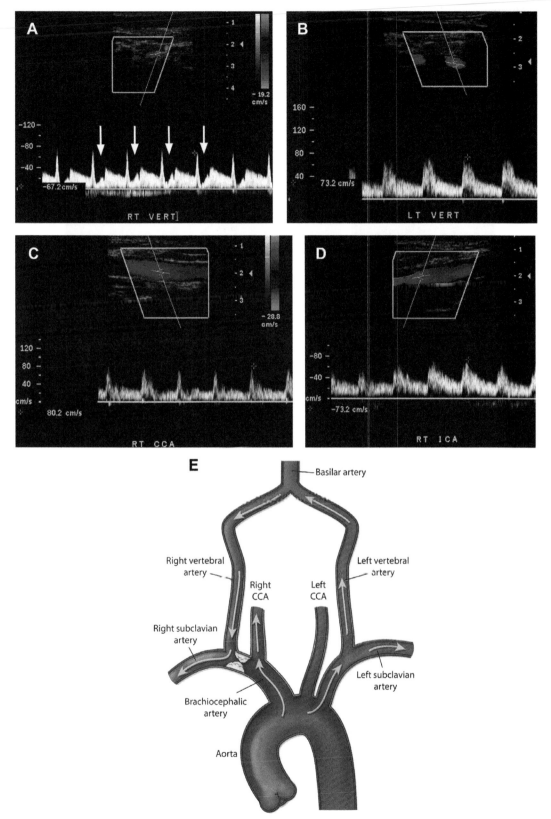

Fig. 7. A 47-year-old woman with dizziness. (*A*) Sagittal spectral Doppler image shows early-mid systolic retraction (*arrows*), consistent with a pre-steal waveform. (*B*) Compare this with the normal-appearing waveform in the left vertebral artery. Spectral Doppler images of the right common (*C*) and internal carotid arteries (*D*) demonstrate normal waveforms as well. These findings are suggestive of a high-grade stenosis in the right subclavian artery proximal to the origin of the right vertebral artery, as depicted on the schematic image (*E*). CCA, common carotid artery.

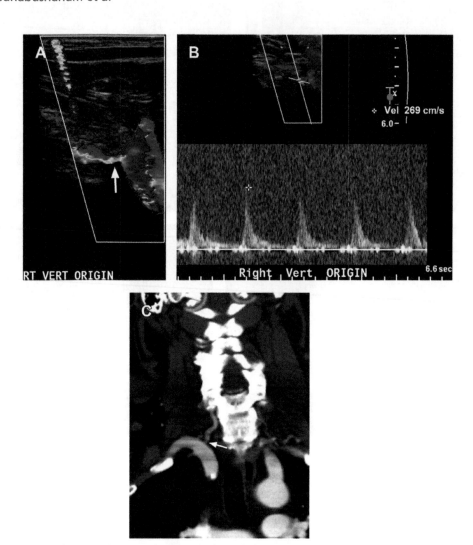

Fig. 8. A 47-year-old man with remote history of left cerebellar stroke presenting with weakness and dysarthria. (*A*) Sagittal color Doppler ultrasound image shows narrowing (*arrow*) at the origin of the right vertebral artery with color aliasing. (*B*) Peak systolic velocity is 269 cm/s on spectral Doppler image. (*C*) Coronal maximum intensity projection image of a CT angiogram confirms the high-grade stenosis at the origin of the right vertebral artery (*arrow*).

flow alterations. A high-resistance obstructive waveform pattern may be seen proximal to a VA dissection if it narrows the residual lumen enough to obstruct flow. In addition, increased PSV may be seen if the lumen is significantly narrowed. However, these patterns of flow alteration are non-specific and may be mimicked by other pathology resulting in obstruction to VA flow or narrowing of the VA lumen.

Ultrasound has been reported to overestimate the degree of luminal narrowing.[29,30] In addition, short segment VA dissections may be missed on US, especially at the skull base, where VA dissections are actually quite common, and in the V2 segment due to shadowing from the cervical transverse processes. Thus, if there is strong clinical suspicion for VA dissection and the Doppler US examination is negative, further evaluation with CT or MR angiography should be considered. T1-weighted MR imaging with fat saturation is highly sensitive and specific for the detection of VA dissection, and is particularly useful in diagnosing VA dissections at the skull base and within the transverse foramina. However, US is very useful in follow-up imaging as it can depict alterations in patency and size of the true and false lumen, PSV and direction, and screen for complications such development of a PSA.[31]

Dissections are usually managed using antiplatelet or anticoagulant therapy.[32] Endovascular therapy is used in patients who fail medical therapy; for example, due to a new ischemic event,

Table 2
Quantitative criteria for diagnosis of vertebral artery stenosis

Author	% Stenosis	Number of Patients	PSV (cm/s)	PSV Ratio	EDV (cm/s)	Other Criteria
Hua et al,[25] 2009	<50	247	85–139[a]	1.3–2.0	27–34	—
	50–69		140–209[a]	2.1–3.9	35–49	—
	70–99		≥210[a]	≥4.0	≥50	—
Koch et al,[23] 2009	50–99	218	≥114[a]	—	—	—
Yurdakul & Tola,[4] 2011	50–99	48	>108	>2.2[a]	>36	EDV ratio >1.7
Skoda et al,[24] 2014	50–99	62	≥135[a]	>2.2[a]	—	—

Abbreviations: EDV ratio, end diastolic velocity at site of stenosis/end diastolic velocity distal to stenosis at V2 segment; EDV, end diastolic velocity at site of stenosis of vertebral artery (usually the origin); PSV ratio, peak systolic velocity at site of stenosis/peak systolic velocity distal to stenosis (usually V2 segment but Skoda and colleagues[24] used distal V1); PSV, peak systolic velocity at site of stenosis of vertebral artery (usually the origin).
[a] Indicates the parameter(s) suggested by authors as most accurate.

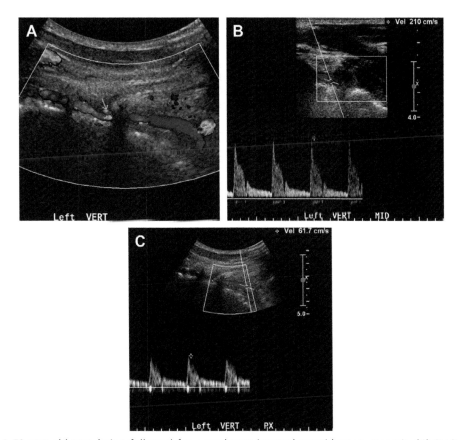

Fig. 9. A 78-year-old man being followed for a moderate internal carotid artery stenosis. (*A*) Sagittal color Doppler image shows vertebral artery narrowing immediately superior to a transverse cervical foramen with color Doppler aliasing at the narrowed segment (*arrow*). Peak systolic velocity at the level of narrowing is 210 cm/s (*B*), compared with 62 cm/s in the proximal vertebral artery (*C*) on spectral Doppler interrogation. These findings indicate moderate-severe vertebral artery stenosis, possibly secondary to extrinsic compression from an osteophyte.

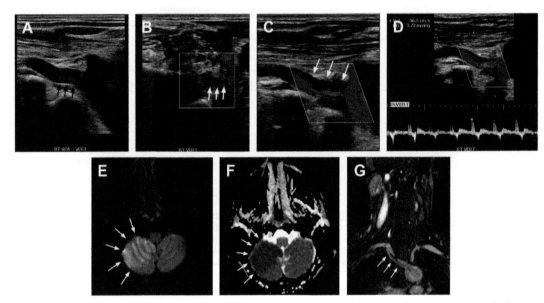

Fig. 10. A 43-year-old man with right facial droop, nystagmus, and double vision that is worse when looking to the right. (A) Sagittal grayscale image demonstrating echogenic intraluminal material (*arrows*) at the origin of the right vertebral artery. Axial (B) and sagittal (C) color Doppler images demonstrate absence of flow (color void) (*arrows*) within the corresponding region. (D) Spectral Doppler image showing an irregular waveform with mildly elevated peak systolic velocity (PSV) at the origin of the right vertebral artery. Peak systolic velocity is increased due to compression of the true lumen by the thrombosed false lumen or mural hematoma. Axial diffusion-weighted MR image (E) shows increased signal within the right inferior cerebellar hemisphere (*arrows*) with corresponding low signal (*arrows*) on the apparent diffusion coefficient map (F), consistent with an acute cerebellar infarct. (G) Coronal contrast-enhanced MR angiogram of the neck showed a dissection flap (*white arrows*) within the brachiocephalic artery, and a "flame shaped" smoothly tapering termination of the right vertebral artery lumen (*blue arrow*). The distal vertebral artery could not be visualized, likely related to occlusion or near complete occlusion. These findings are compatible with dissection of the right vertebral artery with a thrombosed false lumen or mural hematoma.

progression of neurologic symptoms, or an enlarging associated PSA despite adequate anticoagulation or antiplatelet treatment.[33,34]

Occlusion/Thrombosis

Absence of flow on color and spectral Doppler interrogation within the VA is suggestive, but not diagnostic of occlusion. False-positive examinations may occur due to poor technique, patient body habitus limiting evaluation, and hypoplastic or congenitally absent VAs. Flow within the V2 segment of the VA does not exclude occlusion at the origin, as the VA may be reconstituted by collaterals from the external carotid artery.[7] However, in such cases, one might expect to see low velocity flow or a tardus parvus waveform within the V2 segment of VA.

Aneurysm/Pseudoaneurysm

Vertebral artery aneurysms and PSAs (**Fig. 11**) are rare, and often occur because of penetrating or blunt trauma, including iatrogenic trauma from attempted internal jugular vein catheterization.

Other etiologies include chiropractic manipulation, dissections, and connective tissue disorders such as Ehlers-Danlos syndrome or fibromuscular dysplasia.[35] Varying combinations of VA dissection, PSA, and AVF may coexist in the same patient.[36] Vertebral artery PSAs have a similar appearance to PSAs elsewhere in the body, including a focal outpouching with a "yin-yang" appearance of slowly swirling blood flow on color Doppler within the PSA. If a thin neck is present, a "to-and-fro" spectral Doppler waveform pattern with flow heading toward the PSA sac during systole and away from the sac during diastole will be observed. However, the to-and-fro pattern may not be seen if the neck of the PSA is wide. Of note, when there is an associated AVF, a continuous swirling pattern of flow may be seen in the PSA sac,[37] and the to-and-fro pattern of flow may not be seen in the neck (**Fig. 12**). Dissection and PSA of the VA may also manifest as increased mean velocity and PSV in the intracranial VA because of vasospasm or narrowing of the true lumen by a thrombosed false lumen.[32,38] Because the course of the VA through the cervical

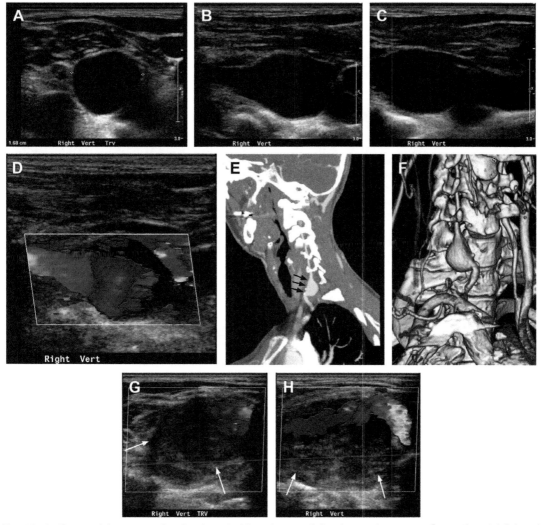

Fig. 11. A 42-year-old woman who developed vision changes following neck trauma. Grayscale axial (*A*) and sagittal (*B, C*) US images show marked dilatation of the right vertebral artery. (*D*) Sagittal color Doppler image shows flow within. Maximum intensity projection CT (*E*) and 3D reconstructions (*F*) demonstrate a pseudoaneurysm of the right vertebral artery (*arrows* in *E*). She was managed conservatively and followed using ultrasound. Axial (*G*) and sagittal (*H*) color Doppler ultrasound done 4 years after initial presentation shows partial thrombosis (*arrows*) of the vertebral artery pseudoaneurysm with a patent lumen.

transverse foramina greatly limits direct open surgical access, endovascular embolization treatments are a preferred alternative to open surgery.[39]

Arteriovenous Fistula

Trauma to the VA may result in creation of an AVF if the adjacent vertebral vein is also injured. Iatrogenic trauma during attempted central venous catheterization occurs more often during attempted internal jugular vein punctures than subclavian vein punctures.[36] Color and spectral Doppler waveforms may be used to delineate the AVF. Doppler US findings are similar to the findings of

AVFs occurring elsewhere and include increased PSV and EDV in the feeding VA with an arterialized pulsatile high-velocity waveform in the draining vertebral vein with reversal of flow (see **Fig. 12**). Coil embolization has been used to treat vertebral AVFs.[40]

SUMMARY

There has been a renewal of interest in ultrasound imaging of the VA, partly due to the increasing use of stent placement for treatment of VA stenosis. In addition, Doppler ultrasound of the VAs may provide valuable information about the proximal great vessels and posterior intracranial circulation.

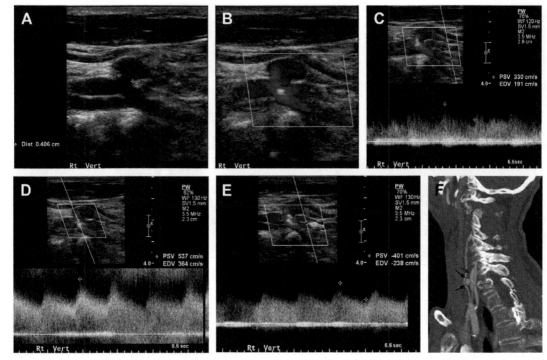

Fig. 12. A 71-year-old man who developed severe neck swelling immediately following attempted central line placement. An internal jugular vein laceration was noted, which was surgically repaired. A thrill was noted on physical examination 2 months later. Sagittal grayscale US image (*A*) demonstrated an anechoic 0.5 × 0.6-cm out-pouching arising from the proximal right cervical vertebral artery with an apparent neck (calipers) that filled on sagittal color Doppler image (*B*) with a "yin-yang" appearance, consistent with a pseudoaneurysm (PSA). However, spectral Doppler images showed a low-resistance waveform with increased peak systolic velocity (PSV) of 330 cm/s and spectral broadening in the proximal vertebral artery (*C*) and a similar-appearing waveform with a PSV of 537 cm/s close to the neck of the outpouching (*D*), rather than the normal waveform in the proximal vertebral artery and the "to-and-fro" waveform pattern in the neck that one would expect to see in the setting of a PSA. In addition, there was arterialization of the spectral Doppler waveform in the inferior (draining) right vertebral vein (*E*), which demonstrates high velocity pulsatile flow. (*F*) Coronal reconstructed maximum intensity projection of a CT angiogram demonstrates a PSA (*black arrows*) arising from the right vertebral artery (*red arrows*) as well as communication to the right vertebral vein (*blue arrow*) consistent with a co-existent arteriovenous fistula to the vertebral vein. The patient was managed conservatively, and a CTA of the neck 6 months later showed decreased size of the PSA and no residual arteriovenous fistula (not shown).

Knowledge of the normal and abnormal VA waveforms is important for the radiologist to identify specific pathologies affecting the VA as well as proximal and distal cerebrovascular circulation.

REFERENCES

1. AIUM practice parameter for the performance of an ultrasound examination of the extracranial cerebrovascular system. 2016. Available at: https://www.aium.org/resources/guidelines/extracranial.pdf. Accessed August 2, 2018.

2. Kalaria VG, Jacob S, Irwin W, et al. Duplex ultrasonography of vertebral and subclavian arteries. J Am Soc Echocardiogr 2005;18(10):1107–11.

3. Buckenham TM, Wright IA. Ultrasound of the extracranial vertebral artery. Br J Radiol 2004;77(913):15–20.

4. Yurdakul M, Tola M. Doppler criteria for identifying proximal vertebral artery stenosis of 50% or more. J Ultrasound Med 2011;30(2):163–8.

5. Cloud GC, Markus HS. Diagnosis and management of vertebral artery stenosis. QJM 2003;96(1):27–54.

6. Kim ES, Thompson M, Nacion KM, et al. Radiologic importance of a high-resistive vertebral artery Doppler waveform on carotid duplex ultrasonography. J Ultrasound Med 2010;29(8):1161–5.

7. Vicenzini E, Ricciardi MC, Sirimarco G, et al. Extracranial and intracranial sonographic findings in vertebral artery diseases. J Ultrasound Med 2010;29(12):1811–23.

8. Kliewer MA, Hertzberg BS, Kim DH, et al. Vertebral artery Doppler waveform changes indicating subclavian steal physiology. AJR Am J Roentgenol 2000;174(3):815–9.

9. Savitz SI, Caplan LR. Vertebrobasilar disease. N Engl J Med 2005;352:2618–26.

10. Bornstein NM, Norris JW. Subclavian steal: a harmless haemodynamic phenomenon? Lancet 1986;2:303–5.

11. Horrow MM, Stassi J. Sonography of the vertebral arteries: a window to disease of the proximal great vessels. AJR Am J Roentgenol 2001;177(1):53–9.

12. Sakima H, Wakugawa Y, Isa K, et al. Correlation between the degree of left subclavian artery stenosis and the left vertebral artery waveform by pulse Doppler ultrasonography. Cerebrovasc Dis 2011;31(1):64–7.

13. Tan TY, Schminke U, Lien LM, et al. Subclavian steal syndrome: can the blood pressure difference between arms predict the severity of steal? J Neuroimaging 2002;12(2):131–5

14. Chen SP, Hu YP, Fan LH, et al. Bidirectional flow in the vertebral artery is not always indicative of the subclavian steal phenomenon. J Ultrasound Med 2013;32:1945–50.

15. Kotval PS, Babu SC, Shah PM. Doppler diagnosis of partial vertebral/subclavian steals convertible to full steals with physiologic maneuvers. J Ultrasound Med 1990;9:207–13.

16. Ginat DT, Bhatt S, Sidhu R, et al. Carotid and vertebral artery Doppler ultrasound waveforms: a pictorial review. Ultrasound Q 2011;27(2):81–5.

17. Labropoulos N, Nandivada P, Bekelis K. Prevalence and impact of the subclavian steal syndrome. Ann Surg 2010;252(1):166 70.

18. Antoniou GA, Murray D, Georgiadis GS, et al. Percutaneous transluminal angioplasty and stenting in patients with proximal vertebral artery stenosis. J Vasc Surg 2012;55(4):1167–77.

19. Flossmann E, Rothwell PM. Prognosis of vertebrobasilar transient ischaemic attack and minor stroke. Brain 2003;126:1940–54.

20. Bamford J, Sandercock P, Dennis M, et al. Classification and natural history of clinically identifiable subtypes of cerebral infarction. Lancet 1991;337:1521–6.

21. Stayman AN, Nogueira RG, Gupta R. A systematic review of stenting and angioplasty of symptomatic extracranial vertebral artery stenosis. Stroke 2011;42:2212–6.

22. de Bray JM, Pasco A, Tranquart F, et al. Accuracy of color-Doppler in the quantification of proximal vertebral artery stenoses. Cerebrovasc Dis 2001;11(4):335–40.

23. Koch S, Romano JG, Park H, et al. Ultrasound velocity criteria for vertebral origin stenosis. J Neuroimaging 2009;19(3):242–5.

24. Skoda O, Kalvach P, Prochazka B, et al. Non-invasive evaluation of proximal vertebral artery stenosis using color Doppler sonography and CT angiography. J Neuroradiol 2014;41(5):336–41.

25. Hua Y, Meng XF, Jia LY, et al. Color Doppler imaging evaluation of proximal vertebral artery stenosis. AJR Am J Roentgenol 2009;193(5):1434–8.

26. Khan S, Rich P, Clifton A, et al. Noninvasive detection of vertebral artery stenosis. a comparison of contrast-enhanced MR angiography, CT angiography, and ultrasound. Stroke 2009;40:3499–503.

27. Jia L, Hua Y, Li J, et al. Optimal ultrasound criteria for defining the severity of vertebral artery in-stent restenosis. Ultrasound Med Biol 2015;41(3):775–80.

28. Lee VH, Brown RD, Mandrekar JN, et al. Incidence and outcome of cervical artery dissection: a population-based study. Neurology 2006;67:1809–12.

29. Chandra A, Suliman A, Angle N. Spontaneous dissection of the carotid and vertebral arteries: the 10-year UCSD experience. Ann Vasc Surg 2007;21(2):178–85.

30. Pugliese F, Crusco F, Cardaioli G, et al. CT angiography versus colour-Doppler US in acute dissection of the vertebral artery. Radiol Med 2007;112(3):435–43.

31. Flis CM, Jager HR, Sidhu PS. Carotid and vertebral artery dissections: clinical aspects, imaging features and endovascular treatment. Eur Radiol 2007;17:820–34.

32. Debette S, Leys D. Cervical-artery dissections: predisposing factors, diagnosis, and outcome. Lancet Neurol 2009;8(7):668–78.

33. Pham MH, Rahme RJ, Arnaout O, et al. Endovascular stenting of extracranial carotid and vertebral artery dissections: a systematic review of the literature. Neurosurgery 2011;68:856–66.

34. Alterman DM, Heidel RE, Daley BJ, et al. Contemporary outcomes of vertebral artery injury. J Vasc Surg 2013;57(3):741–6.

35. Cihangiroglu M, Rahman A, Yildirim H, et al. Iatrogenic vertebral artery pseudoaneurysm: US, CT and MRI findings. Eur J Radiol 2002;43(1):14–8.

36. Inamasu J, Guiot BH. Iatrogenic vertebral artery injury. Acta Neurol Scand 2005;112:349–57.

37. Wilkinson DL, Polak JF, Grassi CJ, et al. Pseudoaneurysm of the vertebral artery: appearance on color-flow Doppler sonography. AJR Am J Roentgenol 1988;151(5):1051–2.

38. Gottesman RF, Sharma P, Robinson KA, et al. Imaging characteristics of symptomatic vertebral artery dissection: a systematic review. Neurologist 2012;18(5):255–60.

39. Lee YJ, Ahn JY, Han IB, et al. Therapeutic endovascular treatments for traumatic vertebral artery injuries. J Trauma 2007;62(4):886–91.

40. Ricolfi F, Valiente E, Bodson F, et al. Arteriovenous fistulae complicating central venous catheterization: value of endovascular treatment based on a series of seven cases. Intensive Care Med 1995;21:1043–7.

Sonography of Acute Cholecystitis and Its Mimics

Daniel C. Oppenheimer, MD*, Deborah J. Rubens, MD

KEYWORDS

- Cholelithiasis • Acute cholecystitis • Gangrenous cholecystitis • GB perforation

KEY POINTS

- Gallstones appear as mobile, echogenic, intraluminal structures with posterior acoustic shadowing due to sound attenuation.
- The presence of cholelithiasis combined with a positive sonographic Murphy sign (maximal tenderness with transducer pressure over the GB) are the most specific sonographic findings of acute cholecystitis.
- Gangrenous cholecystitis is manifested sonographically by sloughed mucosal membranes, focal wall bulge, ulceration, and disruption. It is associated with increased risk of GB perforation.
- Intrahepatic ducts parallel the adjacent portal veins and should measure no greater than 40% of the diameter of the adjacent portal vein.
- When attempting to distinguish between portal vein thrombus and slow portal venous flow, technical parameters should be optimized for detecting slow flow. Increased Doppler frequency is more sensitive to slow flow; however, decreased frequency may be needed for improved penetration of deeper vessels.

ULTRASOUND IMAGING TECHNIQUE AND TECHNICAL CONSIDERATIONS

Optimal evaluation of the gallbladder (GB) is achieved with the patient fasting for at least 4 to 6 hours, although this may not always be possible in clinical practice.[1] Fasting ensures the GB is distended and reduces upper abdominal gas, which can impede acoustic windows.[2] The GB is typically scanned using a 3 to 5 MHz curvilinear transducer in both longitudinal and transverse planes, with the patient in both supine and decubitus positions, using a combination of subcostal and intercostal windows. When using the subcostal window, having the patient to take in and hold a deep breath will move the diaphragm caudally, which improves visualization of the inferior liver and GB.[3]

Gallstones appear as mobile, echogenic, intraluminal structures with posterior acoustic shadowing due to sound attenuation. Identifying posterior shadowing is an important distinguishing feature between stones and sludge; the latter does not demonstrate posterior shadowing. Optimizing technical parameters is essential to demonstrate shadowing, particularly with small stones.[4] Because sound absorption increases with higher frequency, using a higher frequency transducer will improve detection of shadowing. Correct positioning of the focal zone (the narrowest portion of the sound beam with the best lateral resolution) at the level of the stone ensures that the stone will absorb the greatest amount of the sound beam.[3] Real-time compounding can diminish the ability to detect shadowing and, therefore,

The authors have no conflicts of interest to disclose.
Department of Imaging Sciences, University of Rochester Medical Center, 601 Elmwood Avenue, Box 648, Rochester, NY 14642, USA
* Corresponding author.
E-mail address: Daniel_Oppenheimer@URMC.Rochester.edu

Radiol Clin N Am 57 (2019) 535–548
https://doi.org/10.1016/j.rcl.2019.01.002
0033-8389/19/© 2019 Elsevier Inc. All rights reserved.

removing compounding can improve the conspicuity of shadowing in small stones.[5] On the other hand, using tissue-harmonic imaging is helpful in demonstrating posterior shadowing of small gallstones, particularly in obese patients[6] (**Fig. 1**).

ACUTE CHOLECYSTITIS
Imaging Techniques and American College of Radiology Appropriateness

Acute cholecystitis (AC) is a potentially life-threatening condition, and prompt diagnosis and treatment are essential to reduce the rate of complications. Importantly, clinical history, physical examination, and laboratory analysis do not permit a definitive diagnosis of AC. Therefore, clinicians rely heavily on imaging to establish a diagnosis of AC, identify complications, or suggest an alternative diagnosis.[7] Numerous studies, including meta-analyses, have shown that GB scintigraphy has superior sensitivity and specificity for AC compared with ultrasound (US).[8] However, US remains the initial test of choice for imaging patients with suspected AC because it is widely available, fast, portable, permits real-time imaging, does not emit ionizing radiation, readily identifies gallstones and biliary ductal dilatation, and is capable of identifying complications of AC or alternative diagnoses.[1]

Scintigraphy may be helpful in triaging patients with suspected AC in whom findings on US are equivocal. It has also been suggested that scintigraphy can predict the severity of cholecystitis and the likelihood of complications with laparoscopic cholecystectomy.[9] However, scintigraphy is limited by examination time and logistical issues, particularly after-hours and weekends, when nuclear medicine staff and availability of radiotracer may be limited.

Computed tomography (CT) is not the preferred initial imaging test in patients with acute right upper quadrant (RUQ) pain; however, CT can be helpful if US findings are inconclusive, or if US is not available in after hours or underserved locations. A recent study comparing diagnostic accuracy for AC showed that CT is more sensitive for the diagnosis of AC than US, although the investigators acknowledge the nonblinded retrospective nature of the study, predominately obese male US Department of Veterans Affairs patient population, and small sample size are potential sources of bias and confounding.[10] CT is particularly useful in assessing for complications such as gas formation and perforation, and can also stratify patients, which may require open cholecystectomy.[11] CT may also identify alternative diagnoses that may not be seen on US, such as pancreatitis, peptic ulcer, bowel obstruction, or gastroenteritis.

Although MR imaging, like CT, is not a first-line imaging modality in the evaluation of RUQ pain, the reported sensitivity and specificity for AC on MR imaging is similar to that of US.[8] MR imaging enables detailed evaluation of the extrahepatic bile ducts, which may not be optimally visualized sonographically in nonmobile or obese patients.[12] MR imaging is also preferred to scintigraphy or CT in pregnant patients who have an inconclusive US.[1,13]

Uncomplicated Calculous Acute Cholecystitis

Up to 95% of cases of AC are caused by obstruction of the GB neck or cystic duct by cholelithiasis, resulting in increased intraluminal pressure and progressive GB distension.[14] Inflammation ensues due to bile stasis, chemical injury to the GB mucosa by bile salts, and superimposed infection.[15] The principal treatment of AC is laparoscopic cholecystectomy; however, patients who are too ill to undergo surgery may be temporarily managed with percutaneous cholecystostomy.[16]

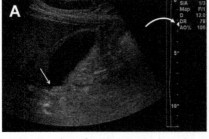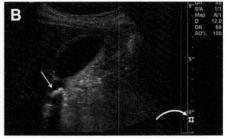

Fig. 1. Cholelithiasis, value of optimizing technical parameters. (*A*) Sagittal greyscale image with focal zone inappropriately placed too shallow (*curved arrow*). The stone in the GB neck is not easily appreciated and does not show posterior shadowing (*arrow*). (*B*) Sagittal greyscale image with improved focal zone positioning and using harmonic imaging (*curved arrow*) shows improved conspicuity of the stone and strong posterior shadowing (*arrow*).

The sonographic findings of AC are presented in **Box 1**. The presence of cholelithiasis combined with a positive sonographic Murphy sign (maximal tenderness with transducer pressure over the GB) is the most specific sonographic findings of AC[17] (**Fig. 2**). GB distension (>4 cm transverse and 10 cm in length) and an impacted stone or stones in the GB neck or cystic duct are additional findings suggestive of AC.[14] For this reason, we instruct our sonographers to specifically identify the GB neck or cystic duct in all patients who are scanned for RUQ pain, using both intercostal and subcostal acoustic windows. Unless the patient is sedated or otherwise uncooperative, the patient should be imaged in left lateral decubitus, sitting up, or standing position, in addition to supine imaging, to assess for gallstone mobility or impaction. GB wall thickening measuring greater than 3 mm and pericholecystic fluid are additional findings that can be seen with AC; however, they are less specific than the signs previously described.[17]

Acalculous Cholecystitis

Acalculous cholecystitis accounts for a minority of all cases of AC but is associated with higher morbidity and mortality than calculus AC. It typically occurs in patients in the intensive care unit who are victims of trauma or burns, status after major surgery, suffer prolonged fasting, are being treated with total parenteral nutrition, or who have diabetes mellitus or severe vascular disease. GB ischemia is believed to be the underlying pathophysiology.[18] The sonographic findings are nonspecific and include GB wall thickening, pericholecystic fluid, and GB distension (in the absence of gallstones)[3] (**Fig. 3**). Sonographic Murphy sign is often difficult to assess in these patients who frequently have altered mental status or are medicated or sedated due to their underlying condition. Treatment of acalculous cholecystitis is with percutaneous cholecystostomy to decompress the GB.[14]

Gangrenous Cholecystitis

Gangrenous cholecystitis (GC) results from ischemia and necrosis of the GB wall due to increased intraluminal pressure. GC is manifested sonographically by sloughed mucosal membranes, focal wall bulge, ulceration, and disruption. It is associated with increased risk of GB perforation[19] (**Fig. 4**). A high index of suspicion is necessary because the sonographic Murphy sign is negative in most patients with GC, which is believed to be related to denervation of the GB from gangrenous changes.[20] Findings on CT and MR imaging include intraluminal membranes, irregular mural enhancement or hypoenhancement, wall ulceration, bulge, or frank defect.[21] Urgent cholecystectomy is advocated because of the increased risk of GB perforation, which can result in generalized peritonitis and is associated with a worse prognosis. The GB fundus is the most common area to perforate because it is the least vascularized portion of the GB wall.[3]

Emphysematous Cholecystitis

Emphysematous cholecystitis (EC) occurs from gas-forming bacteria in the GB wall and lumen. EC is commonly seen in diabetic male patients and ischemia is the primary etiologic factor.[22] Sonographically, gas in the GB lumen or wall appears as curvilinear echogenic reflectors, which may have dirty shadowing and ring-down artifact[23] (**Fig. 5**). Occasionally, it can be difficult to distinguish gas in the GB in the setting of EC from a GB full of stones (wall-echo-shadow sign) or porcelain GB with a diffusely calcified GB wall. This distinction is important because EC carries an increased risk of perforation.[24] In cases that are unclear, CT will distinguish between gas and calcification in the GB wall. Due to risk of perforation, the treatment is cholecystectomy, although percutaneous cholecystostomy can be used temporarily in patients who are too ill to undergo surgery.

CLINICAL MIMICS OF ACUTE CHOLECYSTITIS: OTHER CAUSES OF RIGHT UPPER QUADRANT PAIN

In addition to acute GB disease, a variety of other pathologic processes can cause RUQ pain and simulate AC clinically. US can often suggest an alternative diagnosis and may be diagnostic, obviating further imaging and allowing prompt treatment.

Box 1
Sonographic findings of acute cholecystitis

Gallstones, particularly if impacted in neck

Sonographic Murphy sign

GB distension

Pericholecystic fluid

GB wall thickening greater than 3 mm

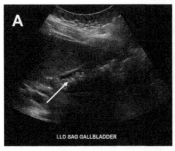 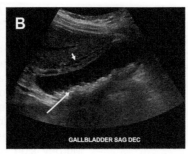 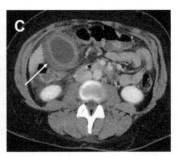

Fig. 2. AC. (*A*) Sagittal greyscale image of the GB demonstrates cholelithiasis (*arrows*) with posterior acoustic shadowing without GB wall thickening or GB distension. Sonographic Murphy sign was negative. (*B*) Sagittal greyscale image of the GB obtained 6 weeks later when the patient developed acute onset RUQ abdominal pain demonstrates cholelithiasis (*arrows*) with posterior acoustic shadowing (*asterisk*), now with GB wall thickening (*short arrow*) and GB distension. Sonographic Murphy sign was positive. (*C*) Axial contrast-enhanced (CE) CT (CECT) image demonstrates GB distension with marked wall thickening (*arrow*) and adjacent inflammatory changes. Note that the gallstones are not visible on CT.

Acute Hepatitis

Acute hepatitis is an inflammatory response in the liver that has many potential causes, including viral infection, drugs or toxins, autoimmune disease, and fat deposition. Patients may present with abdominal pain, fever, and elevated serum aspartate aminotransferase and alanine aminotransferase.[25] Imaging findings are nonspecific and must be correlated with patient history, physical examination, and laboratory tests to arrive at the correct diagnosis. Sonographic features of acute hepatitis include hepatomegaly, GB wall thickening, periportal edema, increased attenuation of the portal vein walls, and diffusely decreased hepatic echogenicity, producing the starry sky appearance (**Fig. 6**).[26] CT and MR imaging may show hepatomegaly, GB wall thickening, periportal edema, and periportal lymphadenopathy.[27]

Nonalcoholic fatty liver disease deserves specific mention because it is now the most common cause of chronic liver disease worldwide, and nonalcoholic steatohepatitis is among the most common indications for liver transplantation.[28] Several emerging techniques permit accurate noninvasive hepatic fat quantitation (proton density fat fraction) and measurement of hepatic fibrosis (magnetic resonance elastography and US elastography),[29,30] which may decrease the need for tissue diagnosis with liver biopsy.

Gallbladder Cancer

GB cancer is believed to be related to chronic irritation of the GB wall by stones and is most

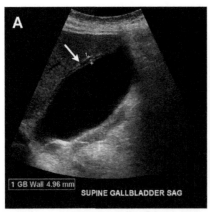 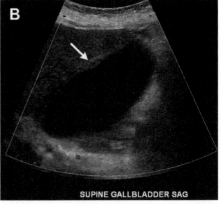

Fig. 3. Acalculous cholecystitis in an intensive care unit patient with sepsis. Sagittal greyscale (*A*) and color Doppler (*B*) images of the GB show a distended GB with wall thickening measuring 5 mm (*arrows*). No gallstones were visualized. Subsequent hydroxyiminodiacetic acid scan (not shown) demonstrated nonvisualization of the GB, consistent with acalculous cholecystitis.

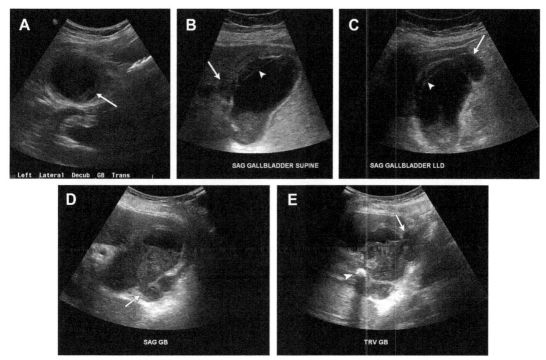

Fig. 4. GC in 3 patients. (*A*) Transverse greyscale image in the first patient shows sloughed mucosal membranes (*arrow*). (*B, C*) Sagittal greyscale images of the GB in another patient demonstrate GB distension with layering echogenic debris and sloughed membranes (*arrowheads*). There are areas of mural irregularity and focal bulges (*arrows*), consistent with perforation or impending perforation. Sagittal (*D*) and transverse (*E*) greyscale images of the GB in the third patient demonstrate echogenic intraluminal material with GB wall thickening, focal areas of discontinuity in the GB wall (*arrows*), and a gallstone located outside of the GB lumen (*arrowhead*), consistent with perforated AC. Decub, decubitus; LLD, left lateral decubitus; Sag, sagittal; Trans, transverse; TRV, transverse.

frequently seen in elderly women. The prognosis for patients is generally poor, with the 5-year survival rate less than 20% because most patients have direct tumor invasion of the adjacent liver, bile ducts, hepatic vasculature, or spread to regional lymph nodes at the time of diagnosis.[31] The sonographic findings of GB cancer include a soft tissue mass that partially or completely obliterates the GB lumen, or, less commonly, focal or diffuse GB wall thickening (usually irregular and asymmetric) (**Fig. 7**). A polypoid intramural mass is rarely GB cancer (it is much more likely to be a cholesterol polyp); however, cancer should be considered if the polyp measures larger than 1 cm and is sessile rather than pedunculated.[32]

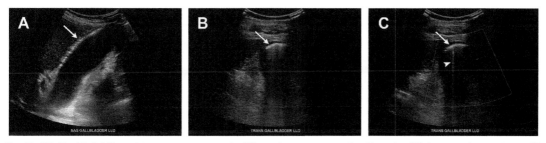

Fig. 5. EC. Sagittal (*A*) and transverse greyscale (*B*), and transverse color Doppler (*C*) images demonstrate GB distension with bright echogenic reflectors in the nondependent GB wall (*arrows*). There is associated ringdown artifact on the transverse images (*arrowhead*). Note the lack of color Doppler flow in the GB wall in this patient.

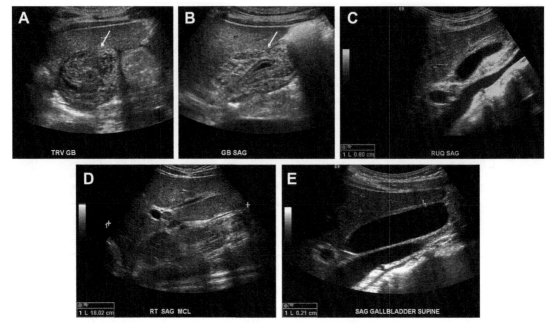

Fig. 6. GB wall thickening secondary to hepatitis. Transverse (*A*) and sagittal (*B*) greyscale sonographic images of a 17 year male who recently began a course of trimethoprim-sulfamethoxazole antibiotics demonstrates marked GB wall thickening > 1 cm (*arrow*) and near complete obliteration of the GB lumen. LFTs were severely elevated and he was subsequently diagnosed with drug-induced hepatitis. Sagittal greyscale images (*C, D*) in a 14 year old female demonstrates GB wall thickening up to 0.8 cm (between calipers) without cholelithiasis, as well as hepatomegaly. She was subsequently diagnosed with acute mononucleosis, and the GB wall thickening resolved on follow-up exam performed 2 weeks later (*E*). LFTs, liver function tests; MCL, mid clavicular line; RT, right.

Biliary Obstruction

Biliary ductal obstruction is usually characterized by biliary ductal dilatation. Intrahepatic ducts parallel the adjacent portal veins and should measure no greater than 40% of the diameter of the adjacent portal vein. Dilated intrahepatic ducts lack Doppler signal, are usually tortuous, and may demonstrate wall irregularity.[33] The common bile duct (CBD) is generally considered dilated when it measures more than 7 mm (measured from inner-inner wall), although the

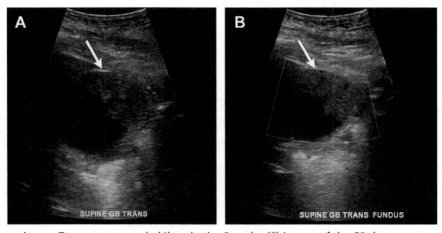

Fig. 7. GB carcinoma. Transverse greyscale (*A*) and color Doppler (*B*) images of the GB demonstrate an eccentric lobulated area of echogenic material involving the GB wall extending into the lumen at the fundus, with associated vascularity (*arrows*). The patient was subsequently diagnosed with GB carcinoma.

duct progressively dilates with patient age and following cholecystectomy.[34]

Choledocholithiasis

Choledocholithiasis is a common cause of biliary obstruction and acute pancreatitis, and usually results in RUQ pain. Most choledocholiths are located in the distal common duct (CD) near the ampulla of Vater.[35] Identifying the extrahepatic duct and choledocholithiasis sonographically requires an understanding of anatomy at the porta hepatis and pancreatic head. The portal vein is a useful landmark for identifying the CD. At the porta, the CD runs anterior to the main portal vein (MPV) and the right hepatic artery. The hepatic artery arises from the celiac axis and courses anterior to the portal vein and medial to the CD. This produces the classic Mickey Mouse appearance: Mickey's head is the MPV, his right ear is the CD, and his left ear is the hepatic artery.

The proximal CD is best seen with the patient left posterior oblique (LPO) or left lateral decubitus and scanning from a right subcostal approach.[36] The distal CD is located at the posterior and lateral aspect of the head of the pancreas and can be visualized with an anterior epigastric approach angling right from the superior mesenteric vein when viewed longitudinally. Alternatively, placing the patient in LPO or right posterior oblique to eliminate duodenal gas and using a semicoronal right lateral or anterolateral approach, or using the GB as a window, can be useful to identify the CD.[35] Asking the patient to drink water can also be useful to displace bowel gas and improve visualization of the distal duct (Fig. 8). Similarly, a transverse scan through the pancreatic head can be useful to compress bowel gas and visualize the distal duct.

CD stones are identified sonographically as round or oval echogenic intraductal structures with posterior shadowing[37] (Fig. 9). However, a substantial minority of intraductal stones do not shadow even when technical parameters are optimized.[33] Scanning both longitudinal and transverse to the duct can increase the confidence that a suspected choledocholith is truly within the lumen of the duct. False-negative results are usually secondary to failure to visualize the distalmost CD. However, most patients with dilated ducts and no sonographically apparent cause of biliary obstruction will subsequently be referred for magnetic resonance cholangiopancreatography, which has excellent sensitivity for detecting distal CD stones.[38] If the sonogram clearly shows choledocholithiasis, the patient can be immediately referred for endoscopic retrograde cholangiopancreatography, sphincterotomy, and stone extraction.

Ascending Cholangitis

Ascending cholangitis results from infection of an obstructed biliary system. Patients are usually febrile, jaundiced, and complain of RUQ pain. Choledocholithiasis is the most common cause of cholangitis, with benign strictures (sclerosing cholangitis, trauma, liver transplant) and malignant strictures (cholangiocarcinoma) representing less common causes.[39] The sonographic findings of ascending cholangitis include bile duct wall thickening and intraductal debris, often with associated biliary ductal dilatation[14] (Fig. 10). Treatment of ascending cholangitis includes IV fluids, antibiotics, and endoscopic or percutaneous decompression of the biliary tract.

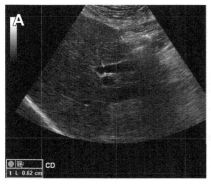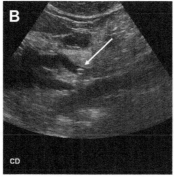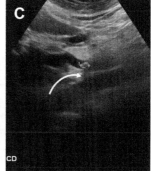

Fig. 8. Choledocholithiasis: importance of patient positioning and technique. (A) Sagittal greyscale image demonstrates visualization of the proximal common hepatic duct at the hilum measuring 0.6 cm (calipers) but the distal extrahepatic duct is obscured by bowel gas. (B) Sagittal greyscale image obtained in right posterior oblique positioning after asking the patient to drink a glass of water demonstrates visualization of the distal CBD with a small choledocholith (arrow). (C) Sagittal greyscale image obtained with the addition of harmonics demonstrates improved conspicuity of the intraductal stone (calipers) and a strong posterior shadow (curved arrow).

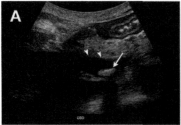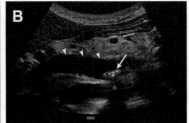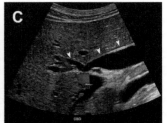

Fig. 9. Choledocholithiasis. Sagittal greyscale (*A*) and color Doppler (*B, C*) images of the CBD demonstrate marked dilatation of the extrahepatic and central intrahepatic ducts (*arrowheads*). There is an oval shaped echogenic intraductal structure in the distal duct with posterior acoustic shadowing and twinkle artifact (*arrows*), compatible with choledocholithiasis.

Cholecystoenteric Fistula

Inflammation of the GB may lead to chronic perforation and fistulous communication with the adjacent duodenum or hepatic flexure of the colon.[40] The fistula permits gas to reflux from the gastrointestinal tract into the GB and bile ducts, and stones to pass from the GB into the bowel. When stones enter the lumen of the bowel, they can result in mechanical obstruction, usually in the ileum (gallstone ileus) or in the duodenum (Bouveret syndrome). Gas within the GB lumen in the setting of cholecystoenteric fistula can be misinterpreted on US as normal bowel loops or EC, and CT may be required to make a definitive diagnosis[14] (**Fig. 11**).

Portal Vein Thrombosis

Acute portal vein thrombosis can be highly variable in clinical severity, ranging from incidental and asymptomatic to life-threatening ischemia and infarction. Portal vein thrombosis most frequently results from slow portal flow secondary to portal hypertension but can also occur in patients with intestinal infection or inflammation (ie, appendicitis, diverticulitis, or inflammatory bowel disease), hypercoagulable states, or from direct invasion by tumor[41] (**Fig. 12**). Portal vein thrombus ranges in echogenicity from anechoic or hypoechoic to hyperechoic.[42] Identifying an area of absent intraluminal flow in the portal vein on color Doppler is particularly useful when the thrombus is isoechoic to the adjacent normal portal vein.[43] When attempting to distinguish between portal vein thrombus and slow portal venous flow, technical parameters should be optimized for detecting slow flow. Increased Doppler frequency is more sensitive to slow flow; however, decreased frequency may be needed for improved penetration of deeper vessels. Additionally, manually compressing the lower abdomen can augment mesenteric or portal venous flow and may improve detection of slow flow. The patient can also be rescanned after a meal because portal venous flow normally increases in the postprandial state.[3] A contrast-enhanced study (CT, MR imaging, or US) can be used to confirm portal vein patency in challenging cases.

Hepatic Abscess

Hepatic abscesses represent walled off collections of purulent material in the liver parenchyma in response to infection by bacterial, fungal, or

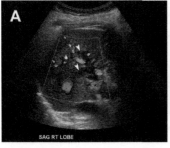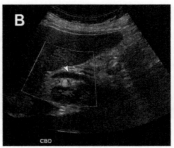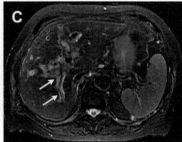

Fig. 10. Cholangitis. Sagittal color Doppler images of the right hepatic lobe (*A*) and CBD (*B*) demonstrate mild intrahepatic ductal dilatation with wall thickening and debris in the intrahepatic and extrahepatic ducts (*arrowheads*). T2-weighted fat suppressed MR image (*C*) in the same patient demonstrates intrahepatic duct wall thickening and periductal edema (*arrows*).

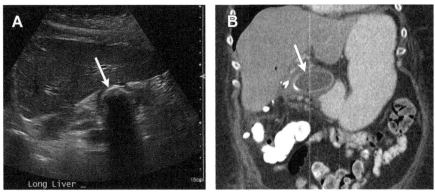

Fig. 11. Gastric outlet obstruction secondary to obstructing gallstone, Bouveret syndrome. Sagittal greyscale image of the RUQ (A) demonstrate an echogenic shadowing structure adjacent to the liver compatible with a gallstone (arrows). However, this patient had a history of recent cholecystectomy and the location of the gallstone is not typical. Coronal CECT image (B) demonstrates a large ectopic gallstone in the distal stomach (arrow), resulting in gastric outlet obstruction. The patient returned to the OR for removal of the obstructing stone.

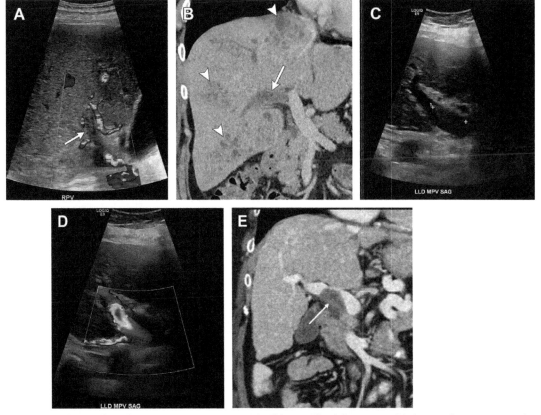

Fig. 12. Portal vein thrombosis in 2 patients. Sagittal color Doppler (A) sonographic image demonstrates echogenic material filling the central right portal vein with lack of color Doppler flow (arrow). Coronal CECT (B) demonstrates right portal vein thrombosis (arrow), and several ill-defined multiloculated fluid collections in the liver (arrowheads). The patient was diagnosed with septic thrombophlebitis with hepatic abscesses secondary to sigmoid diverticulitis. Sagittal greyscale (C) and color Doppler images (D) in another patient with cirrhosis and portal hypertension demonstrates mildly hyperechoic partially occlusive thrombus in the MPV (calipers) with lack of color Doppler flow in this segment of the vessel. Corresponding coronal CECT (E) demonstrates partially occlusive MPV thrombus (arrow). Also note the nodular liver contour and large portosystemic collaterals in the gastrohepatic ligament.

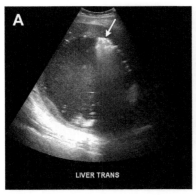
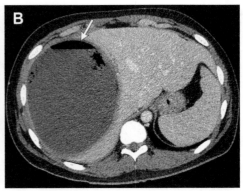

Fig. 13. Hepatic abscess. Transverse greyscale image of the liver (*A*) demonstrates a large hypoechoic mass in the right hepatic lobe with numerous bright echogenic reflectors (*arrow*) and ring-down artifact. Corresponding CECT (*B*) demonstrates a large fluid attenuation mass in the right hepatic lobe containing gas (*arrow*), consistent with hepatic abscess. The patient was subsequently treated with percutaneous drainage.

parasitic organisms.[44] Common causes of pyogenic hepatic abscess include gastrointestinal infection or inflammation (eg, appendicitis, diverticulitis, or inflammatory bowel disease), cholangitis, endocarditis, and osteomyelitis. Fungal abscesses are more common in immunocompromised patients, whereas parasitic abscesses are usually seen in patients from endemic regions.[45]

Pyogenic hepatic abscesses have a variable sonographic appearance, including complex fluid collections of heterogeneous echogenicity, thick-walled cystic lesions with or without septations, or cystic lesions with fluid-fluid levels. Occasionally, hepatic abscess can mimic a solid hepatic mass; however, the presence of increased through transmission can be a clue to liquefied rather than solid composition.[46] Gas can form within abscesses and appears as bright echogenic reflectors with dirty shadowing or ring-down artifact (**Fig. 13**). Although the clinical presentation combined with US findings is often suggestive of the

diagnosis, CT or MR imaging are more capable of evaluating the full extent of infection within the liver and adjacent structures.

Benign and Malignant Hepatic Masses

Any large hepatic mass may cause RUQ pain due to stretching of the liver capsule. Acute onset of pain usually occurs when the mass undergoes rupture or hemorrhage.[47] Hepatocellular adenoma and hepatocellular carcinoma are the 2 most common primary hepatic lesions to undergo spontaneous hemorrhage[48] (**Fig. 14**). However, hepatic metastatic disease is more common than primary liver neoplasms and RUQ pain is occasionally the first presenting symptom, even in the absence of hemorrhage (**Fig. 15**). Detailed discussion of the spectrum of benign and malignant hepatic lesions is beyond the scope of this article, and definitive characterization of solid liver lesions is often not possible without a contrast-enhanced study.

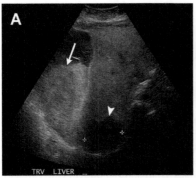
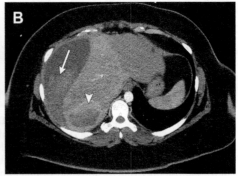

Fig. 14. Ruptured hepatic adenoma. Transverse greyscale image (*A*) demonstrates a hypoechoic mass in the right hepatic lobe (*arrowhead*, between calipers) and a large mixed echogenicity subcapsular hematoma (*arrow*). Corresponding axial CECT (*B*) demonstrates a centrally low attenuation peripherally enhancing mass in the right hepatic lobe (*arrowhead*) with rupture resulting in subcapsular hematoma (*arrow*).

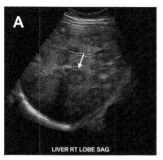
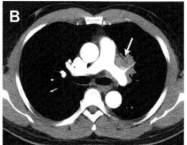
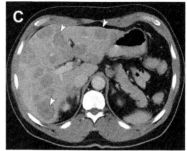

Fig. 15. Hepatic metastases. Sagittal greyscale images of the right hepatic lobe (*A*) demonstrate numerous targetoid lesions in the liver (*arrow*). Corresponding CECT of the chest (*B*) demonstrates a soft tissue mass in the left hilum (*arrow*). CECT of the abdomen (*C*) demonstrates numerous hypoattenuating hepatic metastases (*arrowheads*).

However, the patient age and clinical history can be suggestive of the correct diagnosis. For example, a heterogeneous hepatic mass in a young female patient on oral contraception with associated subcapsular hematoma or hemoperitoneum is suggestive of hepatic adenoma, whereas a heterogeneous mass in a patient with morphologic features of cirrhosis (nodular liver contour, atrophy of the right hemiliver, and hypertrophy of the left hemiliver and caudate lobe) is suggestive of hepatocellular carcinoma.

Free Air or Duodenal Ulcer

CT is the preferred imaging test for detecting and evaluating the cause of pneumoperitoneum; however, sonography may be the first imaging test obtained if the ordering provider does not suspect perforated hollow viscus in a patient presenting with RUQ pain. On US, pneumoperitoneum appears as nondependent echogenic reflectors with dirty shadowing or ring-down artifact (Fig. 16). The echoes deep to the abdominal wall often obscure a portion of the liver when the transducer is applied to the anterior abdomen with the patient

positioned supine. The echogenic reflectors will move to nondependent portions of the abdomen with changes in patient positioning, and are particularly well seen between the abdominal wall and liver with the patient in left lateral decubitus position.[49]

Pyelonephritis

Pyelonephritis represents infection of the renal parenchyma and collecting system, usually secondary to ascending infection from the lower urinary tract. Patients usually present with flank pain, fever, and leukocytosis but symptoms may overlap with those of AC or other causes of RUQ pain. The sonographic findings of pyelonephritis are most often normal; however, the diagnosis may be suggested in the appropriate clinical setting when identifying urothelial thickening, unilateral or bilateral renal enlargement, patchy areas of increased or decreased echogenicity, or focal areas of decreased color or power Doppler flow secondary to vasoconstriction[50] (Fig. 17). Identifying obstructing stones or complications such as pyonephrosis, renal parenchymal, or

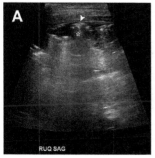
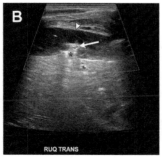
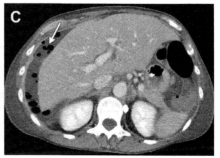

Fig. 16. Free intraperitoneal air. Sagittal greyscale (*A*) and transverse color Doppler images (*B*) of the RUQ demonstrate complex hyperechoic and hypoechoic material surrounding the liver (*arrowheads*) with dirty shadowing (*asterisk*) and twinkle artifacts (*arrow*). Axial CECT (*C*) demonstrates numerous foci of free intraperitoneal air (*arrow*) and perihepatic ascites. Perforated duodenal ulcer was subsequently confirmed at surgery.

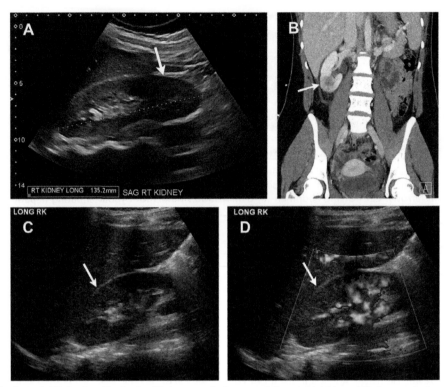

Fig. 17. Pyelonephritis in 2 patients. Sagittal greyscale image of the right kidney (*A*) demonstrates mild renal enlargement (13.5-cm length) with a region of decreased echogenicity in the lower pole (*arrow*). Coronal CECT image (*B*) demonstrates patchy hypoenhancement in the right kidney lower pole (*arrow*), compatible with pyelonephritis. Sagittal greyscale (*C*) and power Doppler (*D*) images of the right kidney in a different patient demonstrate a focal region of increased echogenicity in the upper pole with corresponding decreased power Doppler flow (*arrows*). RK, right kidney.

perinephric abscess have important treatment implications because patients may require a procedure to relieve the obstructing stone, percutaneous drainage, or surgical debridement.[51] Renal abscesses appear as complex fluid collections or cystic masses but occasionally can appear solid and mimic renal cell carcinoma (**Fig. 18**). Perinephric abscesses appear as complex echogenicity

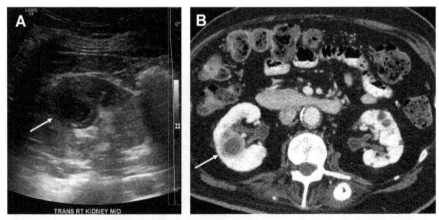

Fig. 18. Renal abscess in a patient with spinal cord injury and chronic indwelling Foley catheter. Transverse greyscale image of the right kidney (*A*) demonstrates a complex mass in the right mid kidney with thick echogenic rim and low-level internal echoes centrally (*arrow*). (*B*) Corresponding CECT demonstrates a rim-enhancing mass in the right kidney (*arrow*). Also note bilateral urothelial thickening and enhancement, and several tiny cysts in the left kidney.

perinephric collections and the diagnosis is usually suspected based on clinical history.

SUMMARY

Sonography is the first-line imaging test for evaluating patients with RUQ pain. Sonography has high sensitivity and specificity for diagnosing AC and can also suggest alternative causes of RUQ pain. The radiologist must be able to optimize technical parameters when performing RUQ sonography and be familiar with the sonographic appearance of AC and its mimics.

REFERENCES

1. Yarmish GM, Smith MP, Rosen MP, et al. ACR appropriateness criteria right upper quadrant pain. J Am Coll Radiol 2014;11(3):316–22.
2. Laing FC, Federle MP, Jeffrey RB, et al. Ultrasonic evaluation of patients with acute right upper quadrant pain. Radiology 1981;140:449–55.
3. Middleton WD, Hertzberg BS. "Gallbladder." Ultrasound: the requisites. Elsevier; 2016.
4. Bortoff GA, Chen MYM, Ott DJ, et al. Gallbladder stones: imaging and intervention. Radiographics 2000;20:751–66.
5. Oktar SO, Yücel C, Ozdemir H, et al. Comparison of conventional sonography, real-time compound sonography, tissue harmonic sonography, and tissue harmonic compound sonography of abdominal and pelvic lesions. AJR Am J Roentgenol 2003; 181(5):1341–7.
6. Choudhry S, Gorman B, Charboneau JW, et al. Comparison of tissue harmonic imaging with conventional US in abdominal disease. Radiographics 2000;20(4):1127–35.
7. Trowbridge RL, Rutkowski NK, Shojania KG. Does this patient have acute cholecystitis? JAMA 2003; 289:80–6.
8. Kiewiet JJ, Leeuwenburgh MM, Bipat S, et al. A systematic review and meta-analysis of diagnostic performance of imaging in acute cholecystitis. Radiology 2012;264(3):708–20.
9. Cho JY, Han HS, Yoon YS, et al. Hepatobiliary scan for assessing disease severity in patients with cholelithiasis. Arch Surg 2011;146:169–74.
10. Wertz JR, Lopez JM, Olson D, et al. Comparing the diagnostic accuracy of ultrasound and CT in evaluating acute cholecystitis. AJR Am J Roentgenol 2018;211:W1–6.
11. Fuks D, Mouly C, Robert B, et al. Acute cholecystitis: preoperative CT can help the surgeon consider conversion from laparoscopic to open cholecystectomy. Radiology 2012;263:128–38.
12. Hakansson K, Leander P, Ekberg O, et al. MR imaging in clinically suspected acute cholecystitis. A comparison with ultrasonography. Acta Radiol 2000;41:322–8.
13. Oto A, Ernst RD, Ghulmiyyah LM, et al. MR imaging in the triage of pregnant patients with acute abdominal and pelvic pain. Abdom Imaging 2009;34: 243–50.
14. Hanbidge AE, Buckler PM, O'Malley ME, et al. From the RSNA refresher courses: imaging evaluation for acute pain in the right upper quadrant. Radiographics 2004;24(4):1117–35.
15. Jivegord I, Thornell E, Svanvik J. Pathophysiology of acute obstructive cholecystitis: implications for nonoperative management. Br J Surg 1987;74: 1084–6.
16. Strasberg SM. Clinical practice. Acute calculous cholecystitis. N Engl J Med 2008;358:2804.
17. Ralls PW, Colletti PM, Lapin SA, et al. Real time sonography in suspected acute cholecystitis: prospective evaluation of primary and secondary signs. Radiology 1985;155:767–71.
18. Mirvis SE, Vainright JR, Nelson AW, et al. The diagnosis of acute acalculous cholecystitis: a comparison of sonography, scintigraphy, and CT. AJR Am J Roentgenol 1986;147:1171–5.
19. Jeffrey RB, Laing FC, Wong W, et al. Gangrenous cholecystitis: diagnosis by ultrasound. Radiology 1983;148:219–21.
20. Simeone JF, Brink JA, Mueller PR, et al. The sonographic diagnosis of acute gangrenous cholecystitis: importance of the Murphy sign. AJR Am J Roentgenol 1989;152:289–90.
21. Watanabe Y, Nagayama M, Okumura A, et al. MR imaging of acute biliary disorders. Radiographics 2007;27(2):477–95.
22. Grayson DE, Abbott RM, Levy AD, et al. Emphysematous infections of the abdomen and pelvis: a pictorial review. Radiographics 2002;22:543–61.
23. Parulekar SG. Sonographic findings in acute emphysematous cholecystitis. Radiology 1982;145: 117–9.
24. Mentzer RM, Golden GT, Chandler JG, et al. A comparative appraisal of emphysematous cholecystitis. Am J Surg 1975;124:10–5.
25. Han SH, Saab S, Martin P. Acute viral hepatitis. Curr Treat Options Gastroenterol 2000;3(6):481–6.
26. Heller MT, Tublin ME. The role of ultrasonography in the evaluation of diffuse liver disease. Radiol Clin North Am 2014;52(6):1163–75.
27. Mortele KJ, Ros PR. Imaging of diffuse liver disease. Semin Liver Dis 2001;21:195–212.
28. Caussy C, Reeder SB, Sirlin CB, et al. Non-invasive, quantitative assessment of liver fat by MRI-PDFF as an endpoint in NASH trials. Hepatology 2018;68(2): 763–72.
29. Reeder SB, Sirlin C. Quantification of liver fat with magnetic resonance imaging. Magn Reson Imaging Clin N Am 2010;18(3):337–57.

30. Srinivasa Babu A, Wells ML, Teytelboym OM, et al. Elastography in chronic liver disease: modalities, techniques, limitations, and future directions. Radiographics 2016;36(7):1987–2006.

31. Stinson LM, Shaffer EA. Epidemiology of gallbladder disease: cholelithiasis and cancer. Gut Liver 2012;6: 172–87.

32. Bach AM, Loring LA, Hann LE, et al. Gallbladder cancer: can ultrasonography evaluate extent of disease? J Ultrasound Med 1998;17:303–9.

33. Rosenthal SJ, Cox GG, Wetzel LH, et al. Pitfalls and differential diagnosis in biliary sonography. Radiographics 1990;10:285–311.

34. Matcuk GR, Grant EG, Ralls PW. Ultrasound measurements of the bile ducts and gallbladder: normal ranges and effects of age, sex, cholecystectomy, and pathologic status. Ultrasound Q 2014;30:41–8.

35. Laing FC, Jeffrey RB, Wing VW. Improved visualization of choledocholithiasis by sonography. AJR Am J Roentgenol 1984;143:949–52.

36. Behan M, Kazam E. Sonography of the common bile duct: value of the right anterior oblique view. AJR Am J Roentgenol 1978;130:701–9.

37. Parulekar SG. Transabdominal sonography of bile ducts. Ultrasound Q 2002;18:187–202.

38. Griffin N, Charles-Edwards G, Grant LA. Magnetic resonance cholangiopancreatography: the ABC of MRCP. Insights Imaging 2012;3(1):11–21.

39. Catalano OA, Sahani DV, Forcione DG, et al. Biliary infections: spectrum of imaging findings and management. Radiographics 2009;29(7): 2059–80.

40. Oikarinen H, Paivansalo M, Tikkakoski T, et al. Radiological findings in biliary fistula and gallstone ileus. Acta Radiol 1996;37:917–22.

41. Parikh S, Shah R, Kapoor P. Portal vein thrombosis. Am J Med 2010;123(2):111–9.

42. Robinson KA, Middleton WD, Al-Sukaiti R, et al. Doppler sonography of portal hypertension. Ultrasound Q 2009;25:3–13.

43. Tessler FN, Gehring BJ, Gomes AS, et al. Diagnosis of portal vein thrombosis: value of color Doppler imaging. AJR Am J Roentgenol 1991;157:293–6.

44. Huang CJ, Pitt HA, Lipsett PA, et al. Pyogenic hepatic abscess. Ann Surg 1996;223:600–9.

45. Mortelé KJ, Segatto E, Ros PR. The infected liver: radiologic-pathologic correlation. Radiographics 2004;24(4):937–55.

46. Benedetti NJ, Desser TS, Jeffrey RB. Imaging of hepatic infections. Ultrasound Q 2004;24:267–78.

47. Casillas VJ, Amendola MA, Gascue A, et al. Imaging of nontraumatic hemorrhagic hepatic lesions. Radiographics 2000;20(2):367–78.

48. Irshad A, Anis M, Ackerman SJ. Current role of ultrasound in chronic liver disease: surveillance, diagnosis and management of hepatic neoplasms. Curr Probl Diagn Radiol 2012;41:43–51.

49. Goudie A. Detection of intraperitoneal free gas by ultrasound. Australas J Ultrasound Med 2013;16(2): 56–61.

50. Cavorsi K, Prabhakar P, Kirby C. Acute pyelonephritis. Ultrasound Q 2010;26:103–5.

51. Haddad MC, Hawary MM, Khoury NJ, et al. Radiology of perinephric fluid collections. Clin Radiol 2002;57(5):339–46.

Ultrasound of Diffuse Liver Disease Including Elastography

Richard G. Barr, MD, PhD, FACR, FSRU, FAIUM

KEYWORDS

- Diffuse liver disease • Liver stiffness • Elastography • Cirrhosis • Liver fibrosis • Ultrasound
- Portal hypertension • Chronic liver disease

KEY POINTS

- Elastography can accurately stage the degree of liver fibrosis allowing for appropriate treatment and surveillance.
- For accurate assessment of liver stiffness, adherence to a strict protocol is required.
- The combination of the conventional ultrasound examination and elastography is a powerful tool in the assessment of chronic liver disease.
- At liver stiffness values of 2.6 to 2.9 m/s (20–25 kPa), there is a high probability of clinically significant portal hypertension.

INTRODUCTION

Chronic diffuse liver disease is a world-wide problem. Any disease that incites liver inflammation can lead to fibrosis, which can progress to cirrhosis. Major causes are hepatitis B, hepatitis C, nonalcoholic steatohepatitis, alcoholic liver disease, autoimmune, and primary biliary cirrhosis. **Box 1** lists major causes of liver inflammation. The major cause varies depending on the region of the world, with the viral causes more prevalent in Asia and Africa,[1] whereas nonalcoholic liver disease more prevalent in North America.[2]

Chronic liver damage from any cause results in hepatic fibrosis characterized by an increase in extracellular matrix produced by fibroblast-like cells. The major consequence is increasing deposition of fibrous tissue leading to the development of portal hypertension, hepatic insufficiency, and hepatocellular carcinoma (HCC). Liver fibrosis can progress to cirrhosis with distortion of the normal liver architecture and resultant portal hypertension. The time needed to progress to cirrhosis varies with the inciting cause.[3]

The stage of liver fibrosis is important to determine prognosis and surveillance and to prioritize for treatment. The process of fibrosis is dynamic, and regression of fibrosis is possible with treatment of the underlying conditions.[4]

With increasing fibrosis, the liver becomes stiffer, eventually resulting in portal hypertension. Previously, the only method of quantifying the degree of fibrosis was a random liver biopsy. This is an imperfect reference standard.[4] Conventional ultrasound is limited in the detection of degrees of fibrosis less than cirrhosis. Recently, shear wave elastography (SWE) has become widely clinically available and can assess and monitor liver stiffness.[4] For accurate stiffness measurements a strict protocol is required and is discussed at length in this article.

Disclosures: Research Grants: Siemens Ultrasound, Philips Ultrasound, Supersonic Imagine, B and K Ultrasound, GE Ultrasound. Speakers Bureau: Siemens Ultrasound, Philips Ultrasound, Mindray, Canon Medical Systems. Royalties: Thieme Publishers.
Northeastern Ohio Medical University, Southwoods Imaging, 7623 Market Street, Youngstown, OH 44512, USA
E-mail address: rgbarr@zoominternet.net

Radiol Clin N Am 57 (2019) 549–562
https://doi.org/10.1016/j.rcl.2019.01.003
0033-8389/19/© 2019 Elsevier Inc. All rights reserved.

Box 1
Common causes of hepatic inflammation that progress to fibrosis

Hepatitis B (chronic)

Hepatitis C

Nonalcoholic fatty liver disease/nonalcoholic steatohepatitis

Alcohol abuse

Drugs (eg, methotrexate and some chemotherapy agents)

Primary biliary cirrhosis

Hemochromatosis

Autoimmune hepatitis

Wilson disease

Alpha-1 antitrypsin deficiency

Sclerosing cholangitis

Postgastric bypass

Schistosomiasis

IMAGING PROTOCOLS

When evaluating patients with chronic liver disease, a full ultrasound evaluation of the liver should be performed. The examination should be performed with a curved linear transducer optimized for abdominal imaging. The frequency of the transducer should be adjusted as needed for the patient's body habitus. Generally, the left lobe of the liver is best imaged in a supine position using a subcostal approach, whereas the right lobe is best imaged using a left lateral decubitus position through an intercostal window. In order to visualize the dome of the liver, the patient is asked to take in a breath. A small sector probe can also be helpful in anatomically difficult locations. Vascular landmarks should be included so position of the images can be identified according to the Couinaud classification.[5] The biliary system should also be evaluated. The examination should include evaluation of the liver echotexture, a high-resolution image of the liver capsule, assessment of the size of the right lobe of the liver and caudate lobe, and portal vein diameter. Doppler evaluation with spectral analysis of the portal vein and hepatic veins should performed. Detection and characterization of focal liver lesions should be included but is not discussed in this paper. The splenic size and evaluation for varcies should also be evaluated particularly in patients with cirrhosis. **Table 1** lists the conventional ultrasound protocol for chronic liver disease.

Elastography should be performed to determine the liver stiffness. The stiffness value can be used to estimate the degree of liver fibrosis; however, other factors that affect the stiffness value are discussed later. Some systems also allow for evaluation of the attenuation of the liver, which can provide some information on the degree of steatosis. The combination of elastography and a standard ultrasound of the abdomen is a powerful tool in the assessment of diffuse liver disease.

Shear Wave Imaging

There are several types of elastography that can assess liver fibrosis. These include transient elastography (TE), magnetic resonance elastography (MRE), and acoustic radiation force impulse (ARFI) ultrasound techniques.[4,6,7] TE is a nonimaging technique that uses a mechanical push to

Table 1
Typical scanning protocol for patients with chronic liver disease

Mode		Anatomic Location	Key Findings
B-mode	Curved linear probe	Entire liver Bile ducts/gallbladder	Echo pattern Capsule nodularity Liver size (right lobe and caudate lobe) Focal liver lesions
	Linear probe		Liver capsule—smooth or nodular
Color Doppler with spectral analysis		Portal vein Hepatic vein Splenic vein Inferior vena cava Aorta	Portal vein size and flow pattern Hepatic vein patency Varices present or not
Elastography		Liver stiffness Splenic stiffness	Liver stiffness Spleen stiffness in cirrhotic patients

generate shear waves and single-line ultrasound is used to estimate the shear wave speed. MRE uses a mechanical device to create standing waves in the liver and special sequences are used to calculate the liver stiffness. These 2 techniques are discussed in detail elsewhere and will not be discussed further.[4]

There are 2 ARFI techniques clinically available to estimate liver stiffness: point SWE (p-SWE) and 2D SWE (2D-SWE). **Fig. 1** shows representative images from p-SWE and 2D-SWE. p-SWE determines the liver stiffness in an approximately 1 cc volume where 2D-SWE evaluates a larger area (around 20 cc). A detailed description of the basic science of these 2 techniques can be found elsewhere.[4,7] There are differences between systems, with reports of approximately 12% variability between systems in the same patient.[8] These differences are greater at higher degrees of fibrosis.[9]

The technique for both p-SWE and 2D-SWE are similar. Adherence to a strict protocol is required for accurate measurements.[4] Patients should fast for 4 hours before the examination because food ingestion increases blood flow to the liver that elevates the liver stiffness. The examination should be performed in the supine or slight left lateral position with the patient's right arm raised above the head to increase the intercostal spaces. Measurements should be taken through an intercostal approach at the location of the best acoustical window (**Fig. 2**). Measurements taken in the left lobe of the liver or by a substernal approach are usually inaccurate. Measurements should be taken in a neutral breath hold. Measurements should be taken 1.5 to 2.0 cm below the liver capsule to avoid reverberation artifact (**Fig. 3**).

The transducer should be placed perpendicular to the liver capsule in both planes. Placement of the region of interest (ROI) should avoid large blood vessels and bile ducts.

Number of Measurements Required

The number of measurements that should be taken varies with which technique is used. For p-SWE, 10 measurements are recommended with the median value used. For 2D-SWE, if a quality measure is used, 5 high-quality measurements are recommended, using the median value for the result. For both systems the interquartile range/median (IQR/M) should be used as a quality assessment. An IQR/M of less than 0.3 (30%) suggests a good set of measurements. If the IRQ/M is greater than 0.3, mention should be made that the data set may be inaccurate. An IQR/M greater than 0.3 can occur in patients with cirrhosis due to attenuation of the ARFI pulse. In this case, if all the measurements suggest cirrhosis, the measurement should be considered accurate. The IQR/M can also be used as a quality control within the department or of the sonographers. The results can be reported either as the shear wave speed (which is what is measured on all systems) in meters/second (m/s) or converted to pressure measurements (Young modulus) in kiloPascals (kPa) making some assumptions.[4,7]

Confounding Factors

There are multiple confounding factors that need to be considered when performing liver elastography. These are listed in **Box 2**. During breathing, the hepatic venous pressure changes leading to

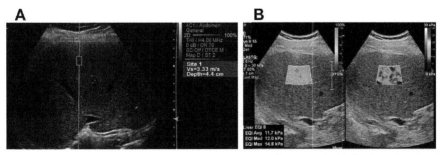

Fig. 1. (*A*) Representative image of p-SWE. The fixed-size region of interest (ROI) (box) is placed at least 1.5 to 2.0 cm from the liver capsule. The transducer is placed perpendicular to the liver capsule. The patient holds their breath in a neutral position during the measurement. In this case, the liver stiffness is 3.33 m/s (32 kPa) consistent with cirrhosis. With p-SWE, 10 similar measurements are taken and the median value is used as the result. (*B*) A representative image of 2D-SWE. A large field of view (FOV), which on most systems can be varied, is placed similar to p-SWE. 2D-SWE can be a single shot or real-time imaging depending on vendor. An ROI can then be placed within the FOV to obtain the liver stiffness value. The map on the right is the velocity map and the map on the left is the quality map. The quality map can be used to locate the areas of highest quality shear waves (green) for placement of the ROI. With 2D-SWE with a quality measure, 5 measurements should be taken with the median used as the liver stiffness. In this case, the liver stiffness is 12.0 kPa (2.0 m/s), which suggests severe fibrosis.

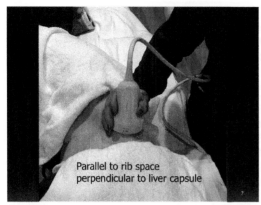

Parallel to rib space
perpendicular to liver capsule

Fig. 2. The technique to be used in obtaining accurate elastography of the liver. The patient should be positioned in the supine or left lateral decubitus position and measurements should be taken intercostal with the transducer perpendicular to the liver capsule. The location should be at the site of the best B-mode image without shadowing artifacts. The B-mode is used to track the shear waves, so a good B-mode is required for accurate shear wave speed estimation.

Box 2
Confounding factors for accurate liver stiffness values with elastography
Method of performing examination (MRE, TE, SWE)
Type of equipment (hardware and software)
Patient factors
Obesity
Ascites
Medications
Fasting
Laboratory values (aspartate aminotransferase, alanine aminotransferase)
Comorbidities
Acute on chronic disease
Vascular congestion (congestive heart failure, fluid overload)
Pretest and posttest probability
Technologist experience

changes in liver stiffness. This is especially true during a Valsalva maneuver (**Fig. 4**). Therefore, it is recommended that the patient hold their breath in a neutral position (not inhaling or exhaling) when measurements are being taken. Taking measurements at the same breathing position are necessary for consistent results.

After eating there is increased blood flow through the portal vein, which also increases the liver stiffness. It is recommended that the patient

be fasting for 4 hours before measurements are taken. Note that eating will only increase the liver stiffness. So, if the patient ate before the examination and the liver stiffness value is normal, a repeat examination is not required. Small amounts of water will not affect the measurements.

Acute inflammation of the liver, which can be identified as elevated liver enzymes, will also elevate the stiffness of the liver, so the amount of fibrosis will be overestimated.[10] Usually this is not critical until the transaminase levels are 5 times normal. Other causes of overestimating the degree of liver fibrosis include increased right heart pressure from congestive heart failure or fluid overload and extrahepatic cholestasis.[4]

The scanning protocol for liver elastography is summarized in **Box 3**. There are several consensus and guidelines available regarding the use of SWE in the staging of liver fibrosis.[4,7,11,12]

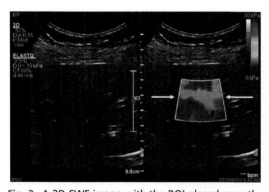

Fig. 3. A 2D-SWE image with the ROI placed near the liver capsule. Note the red and green area (*arrows*). This is the reverberation artifact from the liver capsule. Measurements should not be taken in this area because they are artificially elevated. With p-SWE this is not visualized, so it is critical that the ROI be placed 1.5 to 2.0 cm below the liver capsule. However, the ROI should be placed as close to 4.5 cm from the transducer AND avoiding this artifact.

IMAGING FINDINGS/PATHOLOGY

In addition to the chronic diffuse liver disease already discussed, there are several acute diffuse liver diseases. These include viral hepatitis and acute Budd–Chiari syndrome. In acute hepatitis of any cause, there is hepatomegaly, hypoechoic parenchyma, and increased periportal echoes. Color Doppler and spectral Doppler findings remain normal. The liver stiffness will be increased due to the inflammation (not due to fibrosis). It

A   **B**

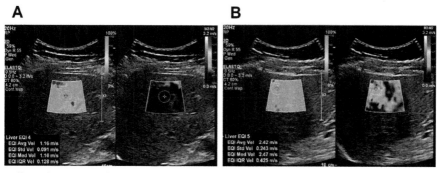

Fig. 4. Controlling the patient's breathing is critical for an accurate shear wave speed estimate. Measurements should be taken in a neutral breathing position (not during inhale or exhale). In (*A*) the measurement was taken in the neutral position with a liver stiffness of 1.16 m/s (normal). In (*B*) the measurement was taken during a deep breath with a liver stiffness of 2.42 m/s (cirrhosis). Therefore, controlling breathing to the same neutral position is essential to obtain an accurate shear wave estimate.

should be noted that for the viral causes, only chronic infections progress to fibrosis. Although 5% to 15% of hepatitis B acute infections become chronic, 75% to 85% of acute hepatitis C infections become chronic.

In acute Budd–Chiari syndrome there will be hepatomegaly and heterogeneity of the liver due to congestion. The venous occlusion will be identified on Color Doppler. There may be development of small intrahepatic venous collaterals. In chronic Budd–Chiari syndrome there is usually peripheral liver atrophy with central hypertrophy and regenerating nodules.

Liver biopsy has been regarded as the gold standard for assessment of fibrosis stage, grading steatosis, necrosis, and inflammation activity. However, it is an imperfect histologic reference standard with considerable interobserver variability.[4] Liver stiffness assessed by SWE has replaced the need for random liver biopsies except in confounding cases.

Fatty Liver Disease

Hepatic steatosis (fatty infiltration) can be caused by several pathologic processes. The differential diagnosis for diffuse fatty infiltration of the liver are listed in Box 4. Diffuse fatty infiltration results in increased echogenicity of the liver. This leads to poor or nonvisualization of the diaphragm, intrahepatic vessels, and posterior part of the right hepatic lobe. Grading can be made using a qualitative grading system of mild, moderate, or severe.[13] Mild (Grade 1) has a diffuse slight increase in fine echoes with normal visualization of the diaphragm and intrahepatic vessels borders. Moderate (Grade 2) has moderate diffuse increase in fine echoes with slightly impaired visualization of the intrahepatic vessels and diaphragm. Marked (Grade 3) is represented by a marked increase in

fine echoes with poor or no visualization of the intrahepatic vessel borders, diaphragm, and posterior portion of the right lobe of the liver (Fig. 5).

A more qualitative method of staging liver steatosis is the sonographic hepatorenal index[13,14] (Fig. 6). This is based on comparison of the echogenicity of the liver to the normal kidney. If this is not available on the ultrasound system, a suitable image can be exported and analyzed with proprietary software or public domain programs such as ImageJ (National Institutes of Health, Bethesda, MD, USA). Several studies have found this technique has significant correlation to histologic steatosis. A recent study using 3T MR imaging as the gold standard found that cut-off values of 1.21, 1.28, and 2.15 had a 100% sensitivity for diagnosis of greater than 5%, 25%, and 50% respectively with a specificity of greater than 70%.[14]

Fibrosis

Fibrosis is a common pathway for numerous causes of hepatic inflammation leading to cirrhosis. The cause of the hepatic inflammation can be from infections, metabolic, toxins, autoimmune, or other causes. Common causes leading to fibrosis are listed in Table 1. Fibrosis is an abnormal increase in collagen fibers and other components of the extracellular matrix in response to chronic injury. Cirrhosis is a diffuse process, characterized by fibrosis and the conversion of normal liver architecture into structurally abnormal nodules.[15]

The speckle pattern changes with both steatosis and fibrosis. Quantifying the acoustic structure using acoustic structure quantification (ASQ) can be used to assess the speckle pattern. ASQ does not perform as well as SWE techniques in grading fibrosis but can be used for quantification of steatosis.[16]

Box 3
Strict protocol for acquiring accurate liver stiffness values

Patient should fast for at least 4 hours.

Examination should be performed in the supine or slight left lateral position with the arm raised above the head to increase the intercostal space.

Measurements should be taken through an intercostal approach at the location of the best acoustical window.

Measurements should be taken 1.5 to 2.0 cm below the liver capsule to avoid reverberation artifact. The optimal location for maximum shear wave generation is 4.0 to 4.5 cm from the transducer.

The transducer should be perpendicular to the liver capsule in both planes.

Placement of the ROI should avoid large blood vessels, bile ducts, and masses.

Ten measurements should be obtained from 10 independent images, in the same location, with the median value used for TE and pSWE techniques.

Three or five measurements may be appropriate for 2-D SWE when a quality assessment parameter is used.

The IQR/M should be used as a measure of quality. For kPa measurements the IQR/M should be <0.3 and for m/s it should be <.15 for an accurate data set.

For TE the appropriate transducer should be selected based on patient's body habitus.

Box 4
Causes of diffuse hepatic steatosis

Obesity

Hyperlipidemia

Nonalcoholic fatty liver disease/nonalcoholic steatohepatitis

Chronic alcohol ingestion

Steroid use

Amiodarone

Hepatitis B

Hepatitis C

Some chemotherapy agents

Valproic acid

Glycogen storage diseases

Hemochromatosis

Wilson disease

Total parenteral nutrition

Cystic fibrosis

Conventional ultrasound features that have been used to grade liver fibrosis include liver parenchymal echotexture, liver surface, liver edge, liver size, portal vein diameter, spleen size, and portal vein Doppler. The liver parenchymal echotexture becomes course with the development of fibrosis. However, this finding is subjective, operator dependent, a function of the equipment, and is complicated when fatty infiltration of the liver is present. Therefore, this sign is neither sensitive nor specific.[17]

As fibrosis progresses to cirrhosis the liver becomes nodular. The nodularity can be described as micronodular or macronodular.[18] Nodules less than 3 mm are classified as micronodular, whereas larger ones are classified as macronodular. The nodularity of the liver can be best detected by evaluating the liver surface (**Fig. 7**). The surface should be a smooth echogenic line measuring less than 1 mm.[17,19] The best way to evaluate the liver surface is to use a high-frequency linear probe. The presence of ascites may make the surface nodularity more apparent. Interruption of the normal liver capsule line is termed the "dotted-line sign" and has been described as characteristic for micronodular cirrhosis.[17]

The right lobe of the liver tends to be more involved than the left lobe and caudate lobe. The caudate lobe often becomes hypertrophic to compensate for the cirrhotic right lobe (**Fig. 8**).[20–22] The use of the ratio greater than 0.65 of the transverse diameter of the caudate to the right lobe has been reported to yield a sensitivity of 84% and specificity of 100%.[21]

Splenomegaly is usually considered present if the spleen is greater than 12 cm in longitudinal diameter or greater than 45 cm^2 in maximum cross-sectional area. Cirrhosis and portal hypertension are associated with splenomegaly.[23]

Portal Hypertension

As the degree of fibrosis increases, the portal pressures also increase to overcome the increased resistance to flow. Cirrhosis causes intrahepatic portal hypertension. Portal hypertension leads to complications of varices, ascites, hepatic encephalopathy, splenomegaly, thrombocytopenia, and anemia.[24]

The most reproducible method is measurement of the hepatic venous pressure gradient (HVPG).

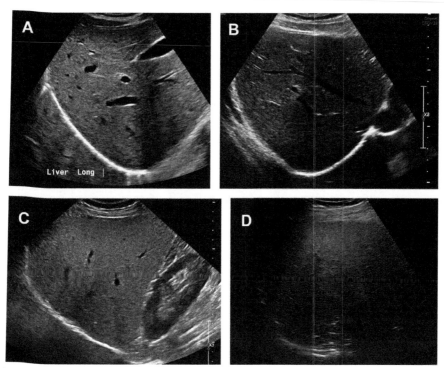

Fig. 5. With increasing steatosis (fatty deposition), the echogenicity of the liver increases and visualization of the vascular structures changes. (*A*) Normal, (*B*) Grade 1, (*C*) Grade 2, (*D*) Grade 3. Note the difference in visualization of the vessels at the various grades of liver steatosis.

This is an invasive test where a catheter is inserted into the superior vena cava and manipulated into a hepatic vein. The pressure is measured by the following equation:

$$HVPG = WHVP - FHVP$$

where WHVP is the wedged (occluded) hepatic venous pressure (WHVP) and is a measure of hepatic sinusoidal pressure. FHVP is the free hepatic venous pressure and is a measure of systemic blood pressure (internal zero). Normal HVPG is 3 to 5 mm Hg. The WHVP correlates well with liver biopsy in chronic hepatitis.[25]

For cirrhotic patients an HVPG greater than or equal to 6 mm Hg is more accurate than fibrosis score at predicting short-term decompensation.[26] HVPG greater than or equal to 10 mm Hg is an independent predictor of decompensation in

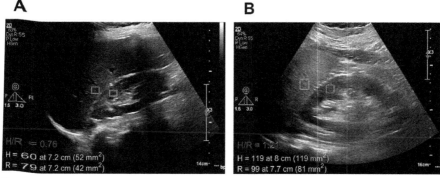

Fig. 6. Another way of grading the degree of steatosis is to calculate the hepatorenal index. An ROI is placed in the liver parenchyma and another in the renal cortex. The system then calculated the ratio of the echogenicities correcting for gain compensation. Note that each vendor may use a different algorithm and cut-off values may vary depending on system. Two representative images are presented in (*A*) and (*B*).

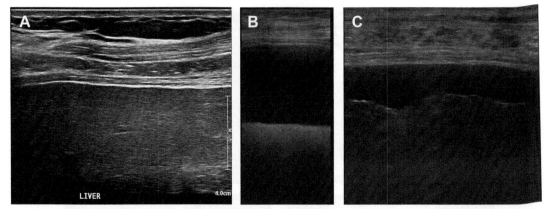

Fig. 7. As fibrosis increases to the point of cirrhosis, nodularity of the liver is noted. This is best visualized by using a high-frequency linear transducer to evaluate the liver surface. When ascites is present it aids in the visualization. In (*A*) a normal well-defined liver capsule is noted without nodularity. In (*B*) the liver capsule is less well defined and has mild nodularity. In (*C*) a markedly nodular liver surface is present.

patients with compensated cirrhosis.[27] Clinically significant portal hypertension (CSPH) is defined as an HVPG greater than 10 mm Hg.[28] This pressure predicts the development of varcies and clinical decompensation. In patients with compensated cirrhosis, a reduction in HVPG

Fig. 8. In cirrhosis the right lobe of the liver is usually involved more than the caudate lobe. The caudate lobe also hypertrophies leading to an increased caudate to right lobe ratio. An axial slice immediately below the bifurcation of the main portal vein is used to perform the measurement. A parasagittal line is drawn through the right lateral border of the portal vein. A second parasagittal line is drawn through the left lateral border of the caudate lobe. A line orthogonal to the 2 parasagittal lines between the portal vein and the inferior vena cava is drawn to the right liver edge. The measurements of the right lobe and caudate are taken on this orthogonal line. In this example, the ratio is 0.47, which suggests a noncirrhotic liver. Based on other features, this patient had cirrhosis pointing out that the specificity of this sign is high, but the sensitivity is less.

greater than 10% at 1 year protects against the development of varices.[29] In patients with large varices that have not bled, a decrease in HVPG greater than 10% improves outcomes.[30]

The normal portal vein diameter is less than 13 mm. The normal portal venous flow is hepatopedal with a velocity of 20 to 33 cm per second. With portal hypertension, the diameter of the portal vein increases while the velocity decreases (**Fig. 9**). The hepatic artery flow usually increases as a compensatory response to the decreased portal flow. As the portal hypertension increases, the portal flow can become to and fro. Eventually the portal flow becomes hepatofugal (reversed), a sign of severe portal hypertension. The slow flow state in portal hypertension can cause portal vein thrombosis (**Fig. 10**).

Varices occur at sites of portosystemic communication; common varices are a recanalized umbilical vein, coronary or left gastric, and splenorenal shunt.[31] Variceal bleeding is one of the major causes of death in cirrhotic patients.[32] Upper gastrointestinal endoscopy is the gold standard for diagnosis of esophageal varices. Ultrasound finding include lower esophageal Doppler signals, left gastric vein hepatofugal flow, and paraumbilical vein recanalization (**Fig. 11**).

Evaluation of the intraabdominal portion of the esophagus in patients with cirrhosis and portal hypertension has been reported to have an accuracy of 95% in detecting esophageal varices. The mean thickness of the esophageal was reported as 3.7 mm in normal and 7.3 mm in those with esophageal varices and 8.86 mm in those with varices at risk for bleeding.[33]

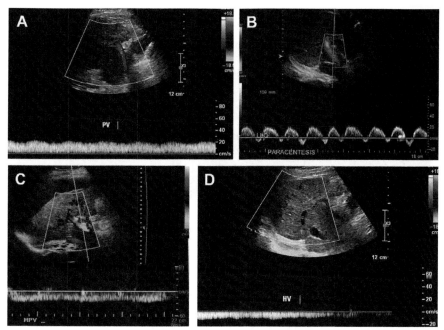

Fig. 9. With increasing liver fibrosis portal venous flow is affected due to the increased resistance to flow. The normal portal vein flow (A) should be hepatopedal with a velocity of 20 to 33 cm/s. As fibrosis increases the portal venous flow can become (B) "to and fro" (antegrade and retrograde) or can completely reverse (C). With increased liver fibrosis the hepatic vein flow can become monophasic (D).

Preliminary studies have found that splenic stiffness may be better than liver stiffness in diagnosing CSPH.[34–36] At the time of this article, there is no consensus on the cut-off values of splenic stiffness for diagnosis of CSPH.

DIAGNOSTIC CRITERIA

There is significant overlap of stiffness values for the varying degrees of liver fibrosis.[4] The population being evaluated also needs to be taken into consideration. In populations with a high prevalence it is important to not miss the diagnosis so false negatives are bad. In a population with a low prevalence of disease false positives are bad. Therefore, it is important to use cut-off values obtained from the appropriate population. All techniques have high accuracy for normal patients and most patients with cirrhosis. However, degrees of liver stiffness between these 2 extremes overlap substantially.[4]

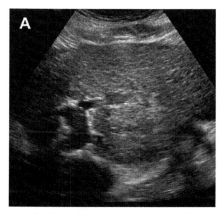
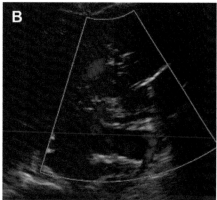

Fig. 10. Portal vein thrombosis. B-mode image (A) shows nonmobile echoes in the portal vein. Color Doppler image (B) shows only partial filling of the portal vein lumen with Doppler signal.

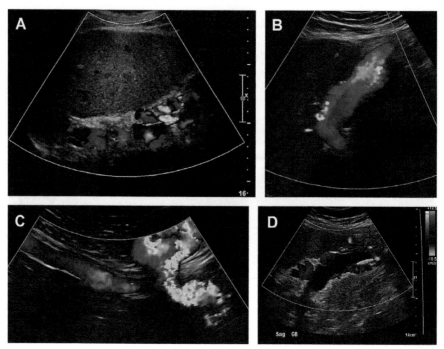

Fig. 11. Varices develop with increasing portal hypertension. Some representative samples of varies that can be seen with color Doppler are splenic varices (*A*), recannulated umbilical vein at the liver (*B*) extending to the umbilicus (*C*), and gallbladder varices (*D*).

One approach is to use a cut-off value system as recommended by the Society of Radiologists in Ultrasound, with a low cut-off below which there is a high probability of being normal or minimal fibrosis and a high cut-off value where there is a high probability of significant fibrosis or cirrhosis.[4] Some patients with biopsy-proven cirrhosis have had relatively low stiffness values in many studies so correlation with other imaging findings and laboratory findings should be performed. Therefore, the use of METAVIR cut-off values has been discouraged.[4,12]

Another clinical approach to interpreting liver stiffness values would be in keeping with that recommended for TE by the Baveno VI Conference.[37] The so-called "rule of 5" (Young modulus 5, 10, 15, and 20 kPa) could be recommended (Table 2): liver stiffness value less than 5 kPa has high probability of being normal; liver stiffness value less than 10 kPa, in the absence of other known clinical signs, rules out compensated advanced chronic liver disease (cACLD). Values between 10 and 15 kPa suggest cACLD but need further testing for confirmation. Values greater than 15 kPa highly suggest cACLD. Values greater than or equal to 20 to 25 kPa can rule in CSPH.

At this time the interpretation of liver stiffness is the same regardless of inciting cause due to

the lack of adequate studies on the various causes.[12]

DIFFERENTIAL DIAGNOSIS

Although multiple diseases lead to liver inflammation, they all lead to the same process of fibrosis with progression to cirrhosis. Each cause has a

Table 2
Suggested liver stiffness interpretation based on Baveno VI

Liver Stiffness	Interpretation
<5 kPa (1.2 m/s)	High probability of being normal
5 kPa-10 kPa (1.2–1.8 m/s)	In the absence of other known clinical signs, rules out cACLD
10 kPa-15 kPa (1.8–2.2 m/s)	Suggests cACLD but need further test for confirmation
>15 kPa (2.2 m/s)	Highly suggests cACLD
>20–25 kPa (2.6–2.9 m/s)	Can rule in CSPH

Abbreviations: cACLD, compensated advanced chronic liver disease, CSPH, Clinically significant portal hypertension.

different time of progression to cirrhosis with its resultant complications.[3] In general, the disease that incited chronic liver disease cannot be determined from the imaging findings.

PEARLS, PITFALLS, VARIANTS

It is important to remember that elastography measures liver stiffness NOT liver fibrosis. When confounding factors are present using cut-off values can over- or underestimate the degree of liver fibrosis.

B-mode imaging is used to measure the shear wave speed. Therefore, it is important to have the best B-mode image possible without artifacts to get an accurate shear wave measurement. A strong B-mode image implies that the optimal acoustical energy is getting to the liver. In this case, the ARFI push will also have optimal energy for creating strong shear waves leading to more accurate assessment of their speed.

For accurate liver stiffness measurements with elastography decreasing motion from both the patient and the technologists are important. Resting your arm on the patient while performing the examination is helpful in holding the transducer still. Controlling patient breathing is critical for accurate measurements. Practicing breathing with the patient before collecting results is helpful for the patient to understand how to hold their breath for the examination. Also, watching the monitor (B-mode) image helps to confirm the patient is holding their breath before starting the acquisition. In real-time 2D-SWE systems, watching the liver motion is also helpful in confirming that the stiffness value is collected at the same point in respiration.

For most systems the ARFI pulse is maximized at 4.0 to 4.5 cm from the transducer. Therefore, the ROI for liver stiffness measurements ideally should be placed at least 1.5 to 2.0 cm from the liver capsule and at 4.0 to 4.5 cm from the transducer. For patients with increased body mass index this is not possible. Although most systems allow measurements to be taken to 8 cm from the transducer, the strength of the ARFI pulse is usually attenuated significantly less than 6 cm, especially in steatosis and cirrhotic livers, leading to less accurate measurements.[4] Most systems have a broad band transducer for ARFI imaging. As the ARFI pulse traverses the liver, it is attenuated with the higher frequencies affected greater than the lower frequencies. Thus, the mean frequency of the ARFI pulse varies as it traverses the liver particularly in steatotic and cirrhotic livers. The shear wave speed varies with the ARFI frequency so it is important to obtain the

measurements at the same location for repeat examinations.

If the patient eats before the examination it leads to an increase in portal flow and liver stiffness. This increase the liver stiffness may lead to overestimating the degree of liver fibrosis. If the patient's liver stiffness values are not elevated (normal), there is no need to repeat the examination. If the values are increased commenting that the stiffness value may be increased due to eating should be mentioned in the report.

Because there is variability between systems, when a patient returns for a repeat examination the same system should be used. In general the variability is on the order of 10% and is increases with liver stiffness.[9]

The IQR/M has been shown to be a good-quality measure for the liver stiffness assessment.[4,7] An IQR/M of less than 0.3 (30%) suggests that the data set is accurate. In patients with cirrhosis the IQR/M may be greater than 0.3 but if all measurements suggest cirrhosis it can be assumed the data set is satisfactory. If the IQR/M is greater than 0.3 (in a noncirrhotic patient) a statement should be included in the report that the result may not be accurate. For example, *"The variance in the measurements is large (i.e. IQR/M>0.3) and therefore the accuracy of the measurement may be in question."*

WHAT THE REFERRING PHYSICIAN NEEDS TO KNOW

Fibrosis stage METAVIR 4 (cirrhosis) is the only fibrosis stage independently associated with liver-related mortality.[38] Cirrhosis consists of at least 2 distinct clinical stages: compensated and decompensated cirrhosis.[39] Decompensated cirrhosis is an easy diagnosis because the patients present with ascites, jaundice, encephalopathy, and/or variceal hemorrhage. However, compensated cirrhosis is not easily diagnosed clinically. The mean survival time of compensated cirrhosis patients is more than 12 years, whereas for decompensated cirrhosis it is less than 2 years.[39] In compensated cirrhosis 2 subpopulations can be identified based on the presence or absence of varices. Those with no varices have 1% 1-year mortality, whereas those with varices have a 3% 1-year mortality.[39] In patients with hepatitis C virus cirrhosis, probability of death and decompensation is greater in those with varices than in those without varices.[40]

Therefore, the noninvasive assessment of patients with chronic liver disease should try to answer the following questions:

- Does the patient have cirrhosis?
- If compensated cirrhosis is present, does the patient have clinically significant portal hypertension?
- If compensated cirrhosis is present, are gastroesophageal varices present or absent?
- In patients on therapy is there improvement with therapy?

Most clinicians take a stepwise approach to diagnosing cirrhosis. If on a physical examination the complications of cirrhosis are present (stigmata, enlarged left lobe of liver, splenomegaly and/or platelets <100,000, and AST > ALT) the patient is clinically diagnosed with cirrhosis.

If the stigmata of cirrhosis are not present, usually a complete blood count, liver profile, and imaging are performed. A fibrosis assessment with elastography or fibrosis serum panel is done. If there is agreement with the clinical, laboratory, and imaging regarding presence of cirrhosis, the patient is diagnosed with cirrhosis. If there is disagreement or diagnostic uncertainty, a liver biopsy may be ordered. Using this approach, the number of random liver biopsies is substantially decreased, and the diagnosis made with noninvasive methods.

For patients without cirrhosis but diagnosed with one of the causes known to progress to cirrhosis noninvasive monitoring of liver stiffness provides information on when treatment should be instituted. For example, many insurance companies will not cover antiviral treatment for hepatitis C until a certain level of fibrosis is present. The time of progression to cirrhosis varies with the inciting cause.[41]

For patients receiving treatment for liver fibrosis, noninvasive liver stiffness assessment can monitor if fibrosis is progressing or regressing on treatment. With the advent of treatments for hepatitis C, it is clear that regression of the fibrosis or cirrhosis is possible over the time course of years.[42] However, even with sustained viral response and decrease in fibrosis, the risk of HCC is still present and the patient needs continued monitoring for HCC.[43,44]

SUMMARY

Chronic liver disease is a substantial world-wide problem. Any process that incites liver inflammation can lead to liver fibrosis and progress to cirrhosis. It is now known that treating the inciting cause can stop the progress of fibrosis or even reverse it. Therefore, a noninvasive method that can accurately stage the degree of fibrosis is needed to assess the degree of fibrosis, determine when treatment should be initiated, monitor treatment, and evaluate for complication.

With a combination of B-mode, color Doppler and SWE patients can be classified into the degree of fibrosis for appropriate treatment and identify complications. It is important for the radiologist to know what information the referring doctor needs to know to properly treat the patient and limit complications. SWE using ARFI technology has been shown to be an accurate method of assessing liver stiffness. The technique requires a strict protocol. Most systems are now using a quality measure assessing the displacement curves used to estimate the shear wave speed, allowing greater confidence in the stiffness measurement.

REFERENCES

1. World Health Organization. Viral hepatitis. Report from the secretariat. World health assembly, 63. Geneva (Switzerland): World Health Organization; 2010.
2. Angulo P. Nonalcoholic fatty liver disease. N Engl J Med 2002;346(16):1221–31.
3. Poynard T, Munteanu M, Deckmyn O, et al. Validation of liver fibrosis biomarker (FibroTest) for assessing liver fibrosis progression: proof of concept and first application in a large population. J Hepatol 2012;57(3):541–8.
4. Barr RG, Ferraioli G, Palmeri ML, et al. Elastography assessment of liver fibrosis: society of radiologists in ultrasound consensus conference statement. Ultrasound Q 2016;32(2):94–107.
5. Fasel JH, Schenk A. Concepts for liver segment classification: neither old ones nor new ones, but a comprehensive one. J Clin Imaging Sci 2013;3:48.
6. Shiina T, Nightingale KR, Palmeri ML, et al. WFUMB guidelines and recommendations for clinical use of ultrasound elastography: Part 1: basic principles and terminology. Ultrasound Med Biol 2015;41(5): 1126–47.
7. Ferraioli G, Filice C, Castera L, et al. WFUMB guidelines and recommendations for clinical use of ultrasound elastography: Part 3: liver. Ultrasound Med Biol 2015;41(5):1161–79.
8. Palmeri M, Nightingale K, Fielding S, et al. RSNA QIBA ultrasound shear wave speed Phase II phantom study in viscoeastic media. Paper presented at: 2015 IEEE Ultrasonics Symosium International. Taipei (Taiwan), October 21–24, 2015.
9. Ferraioli G, De Silvestri A, Lissandrin R, et al. Evaluation of inter-system variability in liver stiffness measurements. Ultraschall Med 2018. [Epub ahead of print].
10. Zeng J, Zheng J, Jin JY, et al. Shear wave elastography for liver fibrosis in chronic hepatitis B:

adapting the cut-offs to alanine aminotransferase levels improves accuracy. Eur Radiol 2019;29(2): 857–65.

11. Cosgrove D, Piscaglia F, Bamber J, et al. EFSUMB guidelines and recommendations on the clinical use of ultrasound elastography. Part 2: clinical applications. Ultraschall Med 2013;34(3):238–53.

12. Ferraioli G, Wong VW, Castera L, et al. Liver ultrasound elastography: an update to the WFUMB guidelines and recommendations. Ultrasound Med Biol 2018;44(12):2419–40.

13. Gerstenmaier JF, Gibson RN. Ultrasound in chronic liver disease. Insights Imaging 2014;5(4):441–55.

14. Marshall RH, Eissa M, Bluth EI, et al. Hepatorenal index as an accurate, simple, and effective tool in screening for steatosis. AJR Am J Roentgenol 2012;199(5):997–1002.

15. Anthony PP, Ishak KG, Nayak NC, et al. The morphology of cirrhosis: definition, nomenclature, and classification. Bull World Health Organ 1977; 55(4):521–40.

16. Ricci P, Marigliano C, Cantisani V, et al. Ultrasound evaluation of liver fibrosis: preliminary experience with acoustic structure quantification (ASQ) software. Radiol Med 2013;118(6):995–1010.

17. Di Lelio A, Cestari C, Lomazzi A, et al. Cirrhosis: diagnosis with sonographic study of the liver surface. Radiology 1989;172(2):389–92.

18. Freeman MP, Vick CW, Taylor KJ, et al. Regenerating nodules in cirrhosis: sonographic appearance with anatomic correlation. AJR Am J Roentgenol 1986; 146(3):533–6.

19. Simonovsky V. The diagnosis of cirrhosis by high resolution ultrasound of the liver surface. Br J Radiol 1999;72(853):29–34.

20. Giorgio A, Amoroso P, Lettieri G, et al. Cirrhosis: value of caudate to right lobe ratio in diagnosis with US. Radiology 1986;161(2):443–5.

21. Harbin WP, Robert NJ, Ferrucci JT Jr. Diagnosis of cirrhosis based on regional changes in hepatic morphology: a radiological and pathological analysis. Radiology 1980;135(2):273–83.

22. Tchelepi H, Ralls PW, Radin R, et al. Sonography of diffuse liver disease. J Ultrasound Med 2002;21(9): 1023–32 [quiz: 1033–4].

23. Bolognesi M, Merkel C, Sacerdoti D, et al. Role of spleen enlargement in cirrhosis with portal hypertension. Dig Liver Dis 2002;34(2):144–50.

24. Berzigotti A. Advances and challenges in cirrhosis and portal hypertension. BMC Med 2017;15(1): 200.

25. van Leeuwen DJ, Howe SC, Scheuer PJ, et al. Portal hypertension in chronic hepatitis: relationship to morphological changes. Gut 1990;31(3):339–43.

26. Blasco A, Forns X, Carrion JA, et al. Hepatic venous pressure gradient identifies patients at risk of severe

hepatitis C recurrence after liver transplantation. Hepatology 2006;43(3):492–9.

27. Ripoll C, Groszmann R, Garcia-Tsao G, et al. Hepatic venous pressure gradient predicts clinical decompensation in patients with compensated cirrhosis. Gastroenterology 2007;133(2):481–8.

28. Nagula S, Jain D, Groszmann RJ, et al. Histological-hemodynamic correlation in cirrhosis-a histological classification of the severity of cirrhosis. J Hepatol 2006;44(1):111–7.

29. Groszmann RJ, Garcia-Tsao G, Bosch J, et al. Beta-blockers to prevent gastroesophageal varices in patients with cirrhosis. N Engl J Med 2005;353(21): 2254–61.

30. Villanueva C, Aracil C, Colomo A, et al. Acute hemodynamic response to beta-blockers and prediction of long-term outcome in primary prophylaxis of variceal bleeding. Gastroenterology 2009;137(1): 119 28.

31. Sharma M, Rameshbabu CS. Collateral pathways in portal hypertension. J Clin Exp Hepatol 2012;2(4): 338–52.

32. Mallet M, Rudler M, Thabut D. Variceal bleeding in cirrhotic patients. Gastroenterol Rep (Oxf) 2017; 5(3):185–92.

33. Abd Elrazek MA, Mahfouz H, Afifi M, et al. Detection of risky esophageal varices by two-dimensional ultrasound: when to perform endoscopy. Am J Med Sci 2014;347(1):28–33.

34. Colecchia A, Montrone L, Scaioli E, et al. Measurement of spleen stiffness to evaluate portal hypertension and the presence of esophageal varices in patients with HCV-related cirrhosis. Gastroenterology 2012;143(3):646–54.

35. Takuma Y, Nouso K, Morimoto Y, et al. Measurement of spleen stiffness by acoustic radiation force impulse imaging identifies cirrhotic patients with esophageal varices. Gastroenterology 2013;144(1): 92–101 e102.

36. Takuma Y, Nouso K, Morimoto Y, et al. Portal hypertension in patients with liver cirrhosis: diagnostic accuracy of spleen stiffness. Radiology 2016;279(2):609–19.

37. de Franchis R, Baveno VIF. Expanding consensus in portal hypertension: Report of the Baveno VI Consensus Workshop: Stratifying risk and individualizing care for portal hypertension. J Hepatol 2015;63(3):743–52.

38. Younossi ZM, Stepanova M, Rafiq N, et al. Pathologic criteria for nonalcoholic steatohepatitis: interprotocol agreement and ability to predict liver-related mortality. Hepatology 2011;53(6):1874–82.

39. D'Amico G, Garcia-Tsao G, Pagliaro L. Natural history and prognostic indicators of survival in cirrhosis: a systematic review of 118 studies. J Hepatol 2006;44(1):217–31.

40. Bruno S, Zuin M, Crosignani A, et al. Predicting mortality risk in patients with compensated HCV-

induced cirrhosis: a long-term prospective study. Am J Gastroenterol 2009;104(5):1147–58.

41. Poynard T, de Ledinghen V, Zarski JP, et al. Relative performances of FibroTest, Fibroscan, and biopsy for the assessment of the stage of liver fibrosis in patients with chronic hepatitis C: a step toward the truth in the absence of a gold standard. J Hepatol 2012;56(3):541–8.

42. Marcellin P, Gane E, Buti M, et al. Regression of cirrhosis during treatment with tenofovir disoproxil fumarate for chronic hepatitis B: a 5-year open-label follow-up study. Lancet 2013;381(9865): 468–75.

43. Fattovich G, Stroffolini T, Zagni I, et al. Hepatocellular carcinoma in cirrhosis: incidence and risk factors. Gastroenterology 2004;127(5 Suppl 1):S35–50.

44. Maan R, Feld JJ. Risk for hepatocellular carcinoma after hepatitis C virus antiviral therapy with direct-acting antivirals: case closed? Gastroenterology 2017;153(4):890–2.

Ultrasound Evaluation in Patients at Risk for Hepatocellular Carcinoma

David T. Fetzer, MD[a],*, Shuchi K. Rodgers, MD[b],
James H. Seow, MBBS, FRANZCR[c], Adrian A. Dawkins, MD[d],
Gayatri Joshi, MD[e], Helena Gabriel, MD[f], Aya Kamaya, MD[g]

KEYWORDS

- Ultrasound • Cirrhosis • HCC • Screening • Surveillance • Contrast-enhanced ultrasound
- LI-RADS

KEY POINTS

- Ultrasound (US) is useful in chronic liver disease for identifying features of cirrhosis and stigmata of portal hypertension, both of which influence management.
- US is considered the primary screening/surveillance test for hepatocellular carcinoma (HCC) in at-risk patients, which includes those with cirrhosis, and subsets of patients with hepatitis B without cirrhosis.
- The US Liver Imaging Reporting and Data System (LI-RADS) algorithm for screening and surveillance uses both a US category (determines follow-up) and US visualization score (conveys expected examination sensitivity).
- Contrast-enhanced US LI-RADS defines an algorithm for definitive diagnosis of HCC in at-risk patients by contrast-enhanced ultrasound, which offers distinct advantages over CT/MR imaging.

INTRODUCTION

Ultrasound (US) is the first-line imaging modality when evaluating patients with known or suspected chronic liver disease (CLD); can demonstrate hepatic steatosis, features of fibrosis, and frank cirrhosis; and can simultaneously assess for biliary pathology and stigmata of portal hypertension. In patients with cirrhosis and subsets of those with noncirrhotic hepatitis B virus (HBV), the risk of hepatocellular carcinoma (HCC) development warrants screening and surveillance US to detect

Disclosure Statement: No author reports conflicts of interest directly related to this work. The following disclosures are included: D.T. Fetzer—Research agreements, Philips Ultrasound, Inc, and Siemens Medical Solutions, USA; Speaker's bureau, Philips Healthcare North America, LLC, and Siemens Medical Solutions, USA. None (S.K. Rodgers, J.H. Seow, A.A. Dawkins, G. Joshi, H. Gabriel); and A. Kamaya—Book royalties, Amirsys.
[a] Department of Radiology, UT Southwestern Medical Center, 5323 Harry Hines Boulevard, Dallas, TX 75390-9316, USA; [b] Abdominal Radiology, Department of Radiology, Sidney Kimmel Medical College, Thomas Jefferson University, Einstein Medical Center, 5501 Old York Road, Philadelphia, PA 19141, USA; [c] Department of Radiology, Royal Perth Hospital, Wellington Street, Perth, Western Australia 6000, Australia; [d] Department of Radiology, University of Kentucky, 800 Rose Street, Room HX-318A, Lexington, KY 40536-0293, USA; [e] Department of Radiology and Imaging Sciences, Emory University Hospital Midtown, Emory University School of Medicine, 550 Peachtree Street Northeast, Atlanta, GA 30308, USA; [f] Department of Radiology, Feinberg School of Medicine, Northwestern University, 676 North St. Clair Avenue, Suite 800, Chicago, IL 60611, USA; [g] Department of Radiology, Stanford University Medical Center, 300 Pasteur Drive H1307, Stanford, CA 94305, USA
* Corresponding author. 5323 Harry Hines Boulevard, Dallas, TX 75390-9316.
E-mail address: David.Fetzer@utsouthwestern.edu

HCC at an early, potentially curable stage. When a focal liver lesion is identified, contrast-enhanced US (CEUS), which has several distinct advantages in comparison to CT and MR imaging, may then be used for definitive characterization. This article provides an overview of the use of US in CLD, focusing on cirrhosis and portal hypertension and the associated risks of HCC, and introduces recently published additions to the American College of Radiology (ACR) Liver Imaging Reporting and Data System (LI-RADS) for HCC detection and definitive diagnosis by US.

CHRONIC LIVER DISEASE AND HEPATOCELLULAR CARCINOMA

CLD is a worldwide health issue estimated to affect more than 45 million individuals worldwide and more than 4.4 million in North America alone, as reported by the Global Burden of Disease Study of 2016.[1] CLD is defined as any process that causes progressive destruction of hepatic parenchyma over a period of greater than 6 months,[2] with repeated liver injury leading to necroinflammation and fibrogenesis, which, if not halted, may progress to cirrhosis.[3,4] Death may result from decompensation related to associated portal hypertension or hepatocyte failure or may be secondary to the development of primary liver cancer (HCC and cholangiocarcinoma). Each year, more than 1.2 million deaths in the world are attributed to cirrhosis and other complications of CLD, more than 800,000 of which are attributable to liver cancer. These cancers may also arise in patients with noncirrhotic CLD, in particular, HCC in select populations with HBV.[5] The annual risk of HCC in patients with cirrhosis is estimated to be 1% to 6% per year, which confers a cumulative 10-year risk ranging from 9% to 45%.[6,7]

In North America, alcohol is the leading cause of liver-related mortality (35.2%), followed by hepatitis C virus (HCV) (32.5%), with HBV constituting a minority of cases (8.7%).[1] More recently, nonalcoholic fatty liver disease (NAFLD) has become a major health issue. Although NAFLD is not fully reflected in the Global Burden of Disease 2016 data, it is now estimated that 25.2% of the world population is affected by hepatic steatosis, and NAFLD has become the leading cause of CLD in Western countries.[5] NAFLD is defined as the presence of greater than or equal to 5% hepatic steatosis, without secondary causes, such as alcohol consumption, medications (eg, steroids and tamoxifen), and monogenic hereditary disorders. Patients with NAFLD have increased mortality, particularly from cardiovascular disease, compared with the general population.[8]

An important subcategory of NAFLD is nonalcoholic steatohepatitis (NASH), where there is superimposed inflammation and hepatocyte damage, with or without fibrosis, and an associated increased risk of HCC.[8] The true prevalence of NASH is difficult to determine due to the need for histologic diagnosis by liver core biopsy,[9] although it is considered to comprise a significant proportion of what has been previously considered cryptogenic cirrhosis[10] and is likely to overtake HCV as the leading cause of liver transplantation in the United States.[11,12]

ULTRASOUND AND HEPATIC STEATOSIS

A US practitioner should be comfortable with the features of fatty liver because the presence of significant steatosis may have an impact on the quality of a liver US examination, affecting both the detection and diagnosis of HCC. The presence of intracellular lipid vacuoles within hepatocytes results in greater sonoreflectivity as well as attenuation of the US beam, perceived as increased relative echogenicity (brightness) of the hepatic parenchyma and reduced through-transmission (increased attenuation).

The right kidney is a convenient internal reference for the liver, with the liver normally equally to or slightly more echogenic than the normal kidney (Fig. 1). Steatosis is inferred if the liver is significantly brighter than the kidney; however, difficulties may arise if the echogenicity of the kidney is abnormally increased due to intrinsic renal disease (Fig. 2A), and, in this situation, comparison with the spleen is an alternative, which in normal patients is brighter than the liver. This usually requires use of split-screen imaging while maintaining identical imaging parameters between the 2 images. Secondary features include focal fatty sparing at typical sites, such as the gallbladder fossa (Fig. 2B) or adjacent to the falciform ligament; loss of the normal echogenicity of the portal walls or gallbladder wall; and poor visualization of the diaphragm.

Qualitative grading of hepatic steatosis has been well documented,[13] with mild steatosis (grade 1) (Fig. 3) resulting in increased parenchymal echogenicity alone, moderate steatosis (grade 2) (Fig. 4) obscuring hepatic and portal vein walls, and severe steatosis (Grade 3) (Fig. 5) resulting in reduced through-transmission, thereby impairing visualization of a significant proportion of the deep aspects of the liver and/or diaphragm. These categories seem to correlate well with MR spectroscopy,[14] although performance relative to histology has been shown to be stronger for moderate to severe steatosis compared with mild or no steatosis.[15–18]

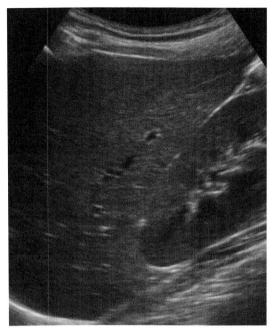

Fig. 1. Nonsteatotic liver—normal liver to kidney echogenicity. A 21-year-old man evaluated for abnormal liver function tests (LFTs). B-mode image of the right lobe liver shows similar echogenicity of the hepatic parenchyma relative to the right renal cortex.

DIAGNOSIS OF CIRRHOSIS

A diagnosis of cirrhosis has significant implications in patient management, given the need to enroll cirrhotic patients in HCC screening and surveillance programs. Pathologically, cirrhosis refers to the end stage of chronic hepatocyte injury, characterized by bridging fibrosis and nodular regeneration. Although biopsy is considered the gold standard in grading liver fibrosis and confirming hepatic cirrhosis, US can be used as a cost-effective, readily available tool to identify patients with chronic morphologic changes of cirrhosis without biopsy.[19] The noninvasive measurement of tissue stiffness, a surrogate marker of hepatic fibrosis, whether by transient elastography, shear wave elastography, or MR elastography, is discussed elsewhere in this issue.

Morphologic Changes by Ultrasound

Classic B-mode US findings of cirrhosis include a small liver with nodular contour and heterogeneous or coarsened parenchymal echotexture, although this constellation of findings may be present to varying degrees. When hepatic volume redistribution is observed, the classic appearance involves right hepatic lobe atrophy (particularly posterior segments 6 and 7), with a relatively hypertrophy of the caudate lobe (Fig. 6) and left hepatic lobe (in particular, segments 2 and 3).[19–21] Ratios of caudate lobe size or volume relative to the right hepatic lobe have been used to diagnose cirrhosis; however, sensitivity and accuracy of this method have been reported as 43% and 79%, respectively.[20,22–24] Exaggerated indentation along the posterior aspect of the liver may be observed at the junction of the atrophied right hepatic lobe and hypertrophied caudate lobe, typically near the hepatorenal interface, an appearance coined the notch sign (Fig. 7) and, in the cirrhotic liver, is more commonly seen with underlying chronic viral infection compared with chronic alcohol use.[21,25,26] Lobar atrophy can result in a widened appearance of the periportal region or expanded appearance of the gallbladder fossa or interlobar fissures (Fig. 8).[27]

In some cases, surface nodularity may be the only gray-scale US finding to indicate cirrhosis. Use of a high-frequency linear array transducer

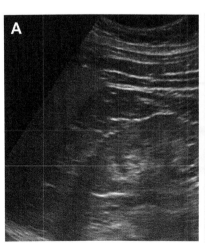
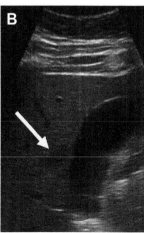

Fig. 2. Steatotic liver and abnormally echogenic kidney. A 45-year-old man with new renal impairment. B-mode image with both liver and right kidney (A) shows similar echogenicity of liver and renal cortex; however, both are abnormally echogenic—the liver due to steatosis and the kidney due to intrinsic/medical renal disease. Note both are echogenic relatively to the intervening intra-abdominal fat. In the same patient, image of the liver and gallbladder (B) demonstrates focal fatty sparing along the gallbladder fossa (arrow), confirming the presence of hepatic steatosis.

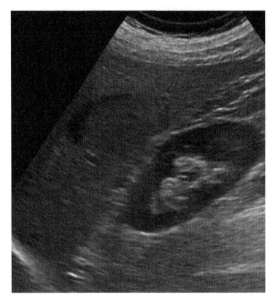

Fig. 3. Qualitative grading of hepatic steatosis—mild. A 57-year-old man with HBV. Longitudinal B-mode view of the right lobe of the liver shows that the liver is of greater echogenicity than expected compared with the right kidney.

can improve sensitivity in detecting subtle surface nodularity (**Fig. 9**).[20,28–30] Nodularity can be asymmetrically distributed, and assessment of the anterior and posterior margins of the liver should be

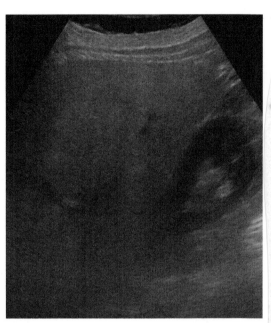

Fig. 5. Qualitative grading of hepatic steatosis—severe. A 66-year-old woman with NAFLD. Longitudinal B-mode view of the liver shows marked US attenuation resulting in poor visualization of the diaphragm. In addition, there is obscuration of the portal walls and increased echogenicity relative to the kidney.

performed (**Fig. 10**). Presence of ascites can improve detection of surface nodularity as well. Careful evaluation of the hepatic parenchyma with the higher-resolution high-frequency linear

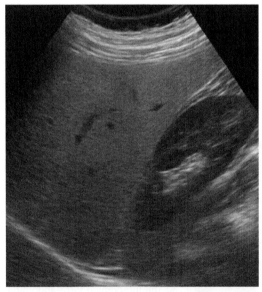

Fig. 4. Qualitative grading of hepatic steatosis—moderate. A 40-year-old man with HBV. Longitudinal B-mode view of the right lobe of the liver shows increased echogenicity of the liver, resulting in obscuration of the normally echogenic walls of the portal veins.

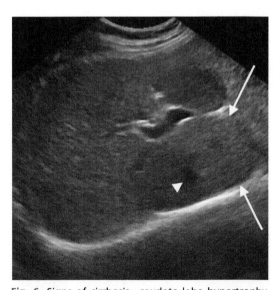

Fig. 6. Signs of cirrhosis—caudate lobe hypertrophy. A 56-year-old man with alcoholic cirrhosis. Transverse B-mode sonographic image shows enlargement of the caudate lobe with rounded, convex margins (*arrows*), surrounding the intrahepatic IVC (*arrowhead*).

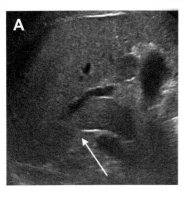
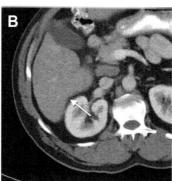

Fig. 7. Signs of cirrhosis posterior notch sign. A 55-year-old man with NASH-related cirrhosis. Transverse B-mode sonographic image of the right lobe of liver (*A*) shows the posterior hepatic notch sign (*arrow*). Corresponding axial contrast-enhanced CT image (*B*) shows exaggerated indentation at the junction of the atrophied posterior right hepatic lobe and hypertrophied caudate lobe (*arrow*).

transducer may reveal cirrhosis-associated nodules that are less conspicuous with the lower-frequency curved transducers (**Fig. 11**).

Portal Hypertension

Identifying signs of portal hypertension may assist in diagnosis of end-stage CLD/cirrhosis and should be included in a US examination performed for the evaluation of CLD.

Portal vein parameters
Enlargement of the portal vein has long been believed an indicator of portal hypertension, with diameters of 13 mm and 15 mm commonly used as thresholds; however, these values have more recently been shown to be unreliable predictors.[31,32] Decreased portal venous velocity (<16 cm/s), when combined with an increasing diameter, is a stronger indicator of portal hypertension, commonly expressed as the congestion index.[33] Reversed (hepatofugal) portal venous flow may be seen in severe portal hypertension,[34] often associated with diminutive portal venous caliber and increased hepatic arterial caliber (**Fig. 12**).[35,36]

Venous collaterals
Portal hypertension often leads to the development of collateral vascular pathways in an attempt to circumvent the high-pressure intrahepatic circulation. These collateral pathways typically involve the distention of normal tributaries of the splenoportal venous system, various systemic veins, and paraumbilical veins, resulting in the formation of varices (**Fig. 13**).

Splenic parameters
Splenomegaly and hypersplenism result from splenic congestion, hyperplasia, and fibrosis.[37] Splenic length has been shown to correlate well with overall volume and, therefore, is frequently used as a surrogate.[38] Noting that splenic size varies with gender, height, and weight, Chow and colleagues[39] showed that when a craniocaudal length of 12 cm is used as the upper limit of normal, 25% of normal men and 6% of normal women within their study population were erroneously labeled as having splenomegaly; therefore, most institutions use a threshold of 13 cm. Gamna-Gandy bodies, iron-laden (siderotic) splenic nodules, may occasionally be seen sonographically as nonshadowing echogenic foci.[40] In addition, more recently, US elastography assessment of splenic stiffness has been shown superior in predicting portal hypertension than liver stiffness.[41]

Ascites
Portal hypertension often results in the development of ascites,[42] due to vasodilation of the splanchnic circulation coupled with sodium and

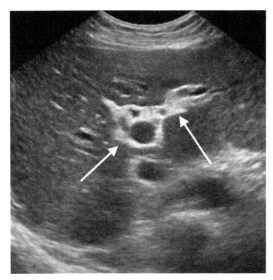

Fig. 8. Signs of cirrhosis—fissural widening. A 55-year-old woman with HCV-related cirrhosis. Transverse B-mode image shows increased quantity of echogenic fat within the porta hepatis (*arrows*) due to interlobar atrophy.

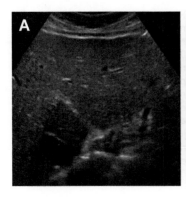 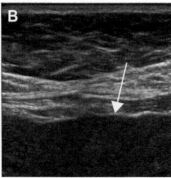

Fig. 9. Signs of cirrhosis—capsular nodularity. A 65-year-old woman with HCV-related cirrhosis. Transverse B-mode image of the left hepatic lobe using a curved transducer (A) shows only subtle contour lobulation. B-mode image in the same patient using a higher-frequency linear array transducer (B) shows improved near-field resolution, revealing surface nodularity of the liver (arrow).

water retention and hypoalbuminemia. In the supine position, ascites is typically noted within the hepatorenal recess (Morison pouch) (Fig. 14), within the paracolic gutters, and in the dependent pelvis. The presence of ascites is an indicator of decompensation and is a prognostic finding, with 15% of patients succumbing within the first year and 44% within 5 years.[43] Ascites may be further complicated by spontaneous bacterial peritonitis, associated with a 20% to 40% rate of mortality if untreated.[44] Hepatic hydrothorax is a less common complication of portal hypertension, characterized by a chronic, recurrent pleural effusion, most frequently right-sided.[45]

HEPATOCELLULAR CARCINOMA SCREENING AND SURVEILLANCE

HCC is now the second leading cause of cancer death worldwide and the fastest growing cause of cancer death in the United States.[6] Cirrhosis from CLD is the greatest risk factor for HCC, present in 80% to 90% of HCC cases. HCC if left untreated is uniformly deadly; however, if detected at an early stage, HCC potentially can be cured with liver transplantation, resection, or targeted liver-directed therapies.

One large-scale randomized controlled trial evaluated the use of US and serum α-fetoprotein in the early detection of HCC.[46] In this study, US surveillance showed a significant reduction in mortality of 37% in patients with chronic HBV, despite poor study compliance. Because of these and other smaller-scale studies, a majority of hepatology societies and HCC practice guidelines endorse the use of US every 6 months in screening and surveillance for HCC.[47–50] Screening is defined as the initial application of a test, whereas surveillance is defined as the repeated application of the same test in a population that is at risk for the disease. α-Fetoprotein has recently been reintroduced by the American Association for the Study of Liver Diseases (AASLD) as an optional supplement to US.[47]

Most societies agree that the target at-risk population includes those with cirrhosis from any cause and subsets of patients with chronic HBV (Table 1).[51–53] For this reason, a diagnosis of cirrhosis by US, whether by primary gray-scale features or findings of portal hypertension, remains paramount. The most recent AASLD guidelines further delineate that patients with Child-Pugh class C cirrhosis who are not transplant candidates should not be included in screening and surveillance given the limited life expectancy and lower anticipated survival benefits even with screening.[47] Furthermore, AASLD does not provide a specific screening or surveillance

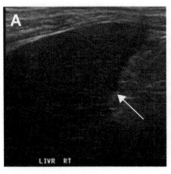 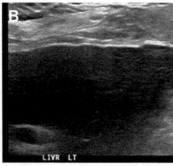

Fig. 10. Signs of cirrhosis—capsular nodularity. B-mode image through the right hepatic lobe (A) shows nodularity along the posterior margin (arrow) with relatively smooth superficial margin. B-mode image through the left hepatic lobe in the same patient (B) shows surface nodularity along the superficial margin.

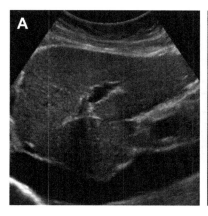
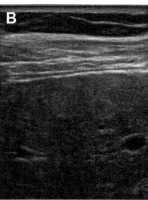

Fig. 11. Signs of cirrhosis—parenchymal heterogeneity. A 65-year-old woman with HCV-related cirrhosis. B-mode image of the right hepatic lobe using a curved transducer (A) shows no obvious morphologic changes of CLD. B-mode image of the liver parenchyma in the same patient using a higher-frequency linear array transducer (B) reveals diffusely heterogeneous echogenicity and coarsened echotexture with presence of regenerating nodules.

strategy for liver transplant candidates, given the lack of evidence to indicate the best strategy in this population.[47] Debate remains as to whether screening/surveillance is effective in other liver disease populations, such as NAFLD/NASH, hemochromatosis, and chronic cardiogenic passive congestion without cirrhosis.

A meta-analysis reported a pooled sensitivity of US to be 94% for detection of HCC at any stage, although a 63% detection rate in early HCC (improved to 70.1% when less than or equal to 6-months' interval surveillance was performed).[54] In comparison, a retrospective study looking at explanted cirrhotic livers showed CT and MR imaging sensitivity for early-stage HCC to be 65% and 72%, respectively.[55] Given the user dependence of US and the limitations and mitigating techniques unique to this modality, a renewed focus on US examination technique and image quality is needed to optimize US as a screening and surveillance test.

Ultrasound Liver Imaging Reporting and Data System

US remains the recommended screening and surveillance modality by all major international hepatology societies. Until recently, however, there has been a paucity of guidance regarding protocol and technical requirements/recommendations, study interpretation, and reporting of these screening/surveillance examinations. The latest version of the ACR LI-RADS includes a new component that specifically addresses US-based HCC screening/surveillance (US LI-RADS). This system provides a lexicon, guidelines for interpretation, and recommendations for reporting and follow-up. Published online,[56] and discussed in several recent publications,[57,58] US LI-RADS also includes technical standards and recommendations, an example reporting template, and image examples.

The following sections provide a short description of the critical components of US LI-RADS. Briefly, US LI-RADS involves the assignment of 2 assessments: study category and visualization score. The study category describes the findings of the US study, is applied to the entire study based on the most suspicious observation identified, and determines the management recommendations. Fig. 15 provides a decision tree for assigning the US LI-RADS category, the details of which are discussed later. The second component is the visualization score, a qualitative evaluation of the US study quality.

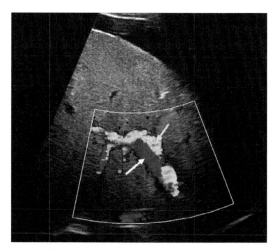

Fig. 12. Signs of portal hypertension—reversal of portal vein flow. A 36-year-old man with alcohol induced cirrhosis. B-mode image of the liver at the level of the portal vein with color Doppler overlay shows retrograde portal venous flow (white arrow) with associated hypertrophy of the hepatic artery (yellow arrow), both features of portal hypertension.

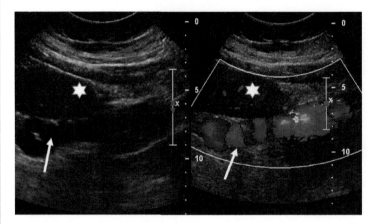

Fig. 13. Signs of portal hypertension—portosystemic collaterals. A 53-year-old man with chronic HCV. Sagittal B-mode image, with (right) and without (left) color Doppler overlay, obtained within the left upper quadrant shows the inferior edge of the spleen (star). Large, tortuous vascular collaterals are noted at the inferior aspect, consistent with a splenorenal shunt (arrow).

This new system is designed to facilitate data collection on performance and outcomes. As these data and experience accrue, future LI-RADS versions will include further refinements of the US LI-RADS system.

US LI-RADS Exam Categories

The study category classifies the observations, is applied to the entire study (as opposed to individual observations) and is determined by the most suspicious observation. An observation generally describes a distinctive area relative to the background liver and is the term preferred by LI-RADS because it does not convey a judgment of whether a finding is benign or malignant. Three categories are possible.

The US LI-RADS category US-1, Negative, indicates that there is no evidence of HCC. No focal observations or only definitely benign observations are identified. Definitely benign observations include nodules previously characterized as benign (for example, hemangiomas) and classic benign observations, including simple cysts and focal sparing or deposition of fat (Fig. 16).

The US LI-RADS category US-2, Subthreshold, is applied when an observation is identified that measures less than 10 mm in maximum diameter (and is it not definitely benign) (Fig. 17). If an observation remains stable for 2 years or greater, it may be considered benign and the study categorized

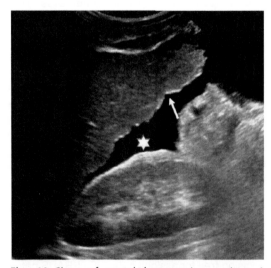

Fig. 14. Signs of portal hypertension—ascites. A 50-year-old woman with HCV cirrhosis. Transverse B-mode image of the abdomen demonstrates anechoic free fluid within Morison pouch (star). Nodular liver contour is also noted (arrow).

Table 1
Target population for hepatocellular carcinoma screening and surveillance

AASLD Target Population	Adults with compensated cirrhosis of any cause
	Subsets of adult patients with chronic HBV infection even in the absence of cirrhosis:
	• Asian male HBV carriers over age 40
	• Asian female HBV carriers over age 50
	• HBV carrier with family history of HCC
	• African or North American blacks with HBV

Depending on geographic region, local recommendations may differ. LI-RADS defers to regional practice guidelines for the operational definition of the target population for HCC surveillance based on local practice guidelines.[53,57,58]

Adapted from Fetzer DT, Rodgers SK, Harris AC, et al. Screening and surveillance of hepatocellular carcinoma: an introduction to ultrasound liver imaging reporting and data system. Radiol Clin North Am 2017;55(6):1209; with permission.

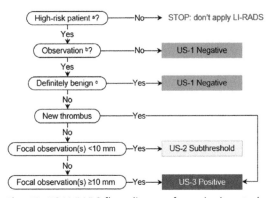

Fig. 15. US LI-RADS flow diagram for assigning study category. A US category is only assigned in high-risk patients and applies to the whole study based on the most suspicious observation. An observation may be a distinct nodule or an area of parenchymal distortion, defined as an area greater than or equal to 10 mm with 1 of the following features: ill-defined area of heterogeneity, refractive edge shadows, and/ or loss of normal hepatic architecture. [a] High risk patient: In general, this includes patients with cirrhosis of any cause or with chronic HBV infection even in absence of cirrhosis. [b] Observation: Distinctive area compared to background liver. [c] Examples of definitely benign observations: Simple cyst, focal fat sparing around gallbladder, previously confirmed hemangioma. (Adapted from https://www.acr.org/ Clinical-Resources/Reporting-and-Data-Systems/LI-RADS. Accessed July 31, 2018; with permission.)

as US-1, Negative, if no other suspicious observations are present.

For the US LI-RADS category US-3, Positive, an observation greater than or equal to 10 mm in maximum diameter is identified (not definitely benign), a new thrombus-in-vein is identified (regardless of whether bland thrombus or tumor-in-vein is suspected), or an ill-defined area of parenchymal distortion distinct from background liver, with refractive edge shadows or loss of normal hepatic architecture, is identified (an appearance often attributed to infiltrative/diffuse subtype of HCC) (Figs. 18–20).

Visualization Score

The visualization score is also applied to the entire study and helps convey the expected level of sensitivity of the examination, based on factors that may influence complete visualization of the liver parenchyma. These factors may include marked hepatic parenchymal nodularity that may have an impact on detection of a distinct observation; poor acoustic penetration due to abdominal wall and/or hepatic beam attenuation; or parenchymal obscuration by lung, rib, or bowel gas. Table 2 summarizes the visualization scores. Three scores are possible.

For US LI-RADS Visualization A, no or few/mild limitations are present that may affect the sensitivity for detecting HCC. This score may be applied

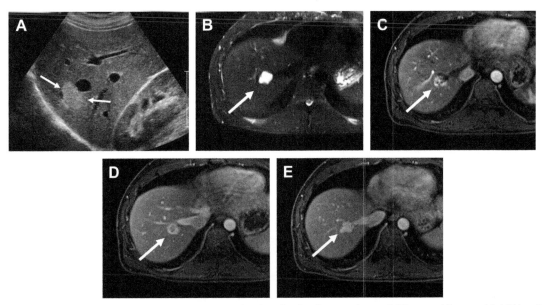

Fig. 16. US LI-RADS category US-1, negative examination; benign hemangioma. A 39-year-old man with HBV and HIV. Longitudinal B-mode image through the right lobe of liver (A) shows a homogeneous, hyperechoic nodule with subtle posterior acoustic enhancement (arrows). An abdominal MR imaging performed for pain several months prior shows features classic for a hemangioma with T2 hyperintense signal (B), peripheral nodular enhancement during the arterial phase (C), and progressive centripetal fill-in by the portal-venous (D) and delayed (E) phases of enhancement.

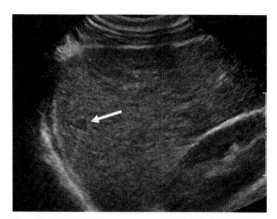

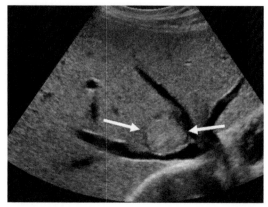

Fig. 17. US LI-RADS category US-2, Subthreshold. A 31-year-old man with alcoholic cirrhosis. Longitudinal B-mode image of right lobe of liver shows a small, 7-mm hypoechoic nodule near the dome (*arrow*).

Fig. 18. US LI-RADS category US-3, Positive. A 63-year-old man with HCV-related cirrhosis and α-fetoprotein level of 1796. Transverse B-mode image of the liver shows a slightly heterogeneous, isoechoic solid observation measuring 2.5 cm, interposed between the right and middle hepatic veins (*arrows*).

if there is up to mild or moderate parenchymal heterogeneity or acoustic attenuation, but the liver is visualized in its near entirety (**Fig. 21**).

For US LI-RADS Visualization B, limitations are encountered that may result in decreased sensitivity for small observations. These limitations may include a moderately heterogeneous or nodular liver in which a small observation may be difficult to discern or moderate acoustic attenuation in which small portions of the liver are not visualized or may occur in patients in whom small portions of the liver are obscured by lung, rib, or bowel gas (**Figs. 22** and 23).

For US LI-RADS Visualization C, limitations are present that have a significant impact on visualization of the liver and severely limit detection of even large observations. Examples include severe parenchymal heterogeneity/nodularity, severe loss of acoustic penetration that precludes visualization of the deepest portions of the liver obscuring greater than 50% of the diaphragm, and obscuration of large portions of the liver (>50% of the volume) (**Figs. 24** and 25).

Management

Recommendations, such as follow-up interval or further work-up, are based on the US category.

For US-1, Negative, the patient returns to 6-month US surveillance, based on practice guidelines and multiple societal endorsements.[48,49,53]

For US-2, Subthreshold, patients should undergo short-interval US follow-up (3–6 months), based on current AASLD guidelines, with flexibility inherent in the recommendation to accommodate situations such as patient or provider preference, risk factors, and availability of local resources. It is not recommended that subthreshold observations undergo further work-up by a contrast-enhanced study, because these small observations are commonly encountered in cirrhosis, are often benign, and frequently are too small to definitively characterize. Therefore, a short-interval follow-up US is recommended to assess for observation stability, resolution, or growth.

For US-3, Positive, these patients are recommended to undergo a diagnostic, contrast-enhanced test (CEUS, CT, or MR imaging) for characterization of the observation.

Although the visualization score is intended to convey the expected level of sensitivity of the

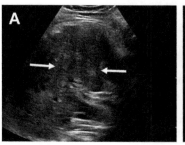
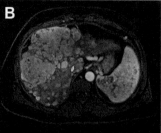

Fig. 19. US LI-RADS category US-3, Positive. A 56-year-old man with cirrhosis. Transverse B-mode image of the liver (*A*) shows marked parenchymal distortion and refractive shadowing (*arrows*). Image from a subsequent contrast-enhanced MR imaging (*B*) shows a large area of confluent arterial phase hyperenhancement that showed subsequent washout (not shown), consistent with diffuse, multifocal HCC.

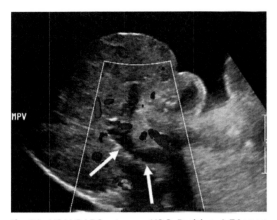

Fig. 20. US LI-RADS category US-3, Positive. A 74-year-old man presenting with decompensated cirrhosis. Longitudinal B-mode image shows a frankly cirrhotic liver, ascites and a right pleural effusion, and lack of color Doppler signal from the main portal vein (*arrows*), a new finding. Spectral Doppler evaluation confirmed these findings (not shown).

screening/surveillance examination, it currently does not influence management recommendations. As performance and outcomes data accumulate, future versions may incorporate the visualization score into these recommendations. Until then, for patients with visualization score B or C, local practice preferences may be applied, and difficult cases may warrant a multidisciplinary discussion to determine the optimal follow-up for a specific patient.

HEPATOCELLULAR CARCINOMA DIAGNOSIS BY CONTRAST-ENHANCED ULTRASOUND

CEUS is an imaging technique combining intravenously administered a microbubble-based contrast agent with a contrast-specific, low mechanical index imaging mode (contrast mode). CEUS has been extensively performed and studied in Canada, Europe, and Asia. In 2016, the Food and Drug Administration approved the use of sulfur hexafluoride lipid-type A microspheres (Bracco Diagnostics Inc, Monroe Township,

Table 2
US LI-RADS visualization score

Score	Concept	Examples
A, no or minimal limitations	Limitations, if any, are unlikely to meaningfully affect sensitivity.	Liver homogeneous or minimally heterogeneous Minimal beam attenuation or shadowing Liver visualized in near entirety
B, moderate limitations	Limitations may obscure small masses.	Liver moderately heterogeneous Moderate beam attenuation or shadowing Some portions of liver or diaphragm not visualized
C, severe limitations	Limitations significantly lower sensitivity for focal liver lesions.	Liver severely heterogeneous Severe beam attenuation or shadowing Majority (>50%) of liver not visualized Majority (>50%) of diaphragm not visualized

Applied to the entire study, the visualization score is a qualitative assessment of factors that may influence the sensitivity of the examination for HCC.[57,58]

Abbreviations: LI-RADS, Liver Imaging Reporting and Data System; US, ultrasound.

Adapted from Fetzer DT, Rodgers SK, Harris AC, et al. Screening and surveillance of hepatocellular carcinoma: an introduction to ultrasound liver imaging reporting and data system. Radiol Clin North Am 2017;55(6):1209; with permission.

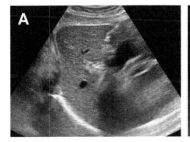
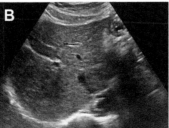

Fig. 21. US LI-RADS visualization score A. A 58-year-old woman with HBV. B-mode images of the left (*A*) and right (*B*) lobes of liver show near-complete visualization of the hepatic parenchyma with good penetration and mild parenchymal coarsening.

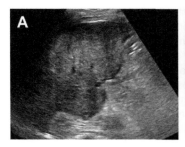 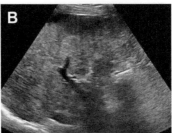

Fig. 22. US LI-RADS visualization score B. A 42-year-old man with alcoholic cirrhosis. B-mode images of the right lobe of liver in longitudinal (*A*) and transverse (*B*) orientations show near-complete visualization with, however, moderate hepatic parenchymal heterogeneity and incomplete visualization of the hepatic dome.

New Jersey), a purely intravascular US contrast agent, for characterization of focal liver lesions. Another similar contrast agent perflutren lipid microspheres (Lantheus Medical Imaging, North Billerica, Massachusetts) is also used extensively for CEUS. The following sections review the advantages and disadvantages, indications, and technique as well as examination interpretation in the context of patients with CLD or cirrhosis.

Advantages and Disadvantages

Advantages of CEUS include its low cost, high temporal and spatial resolution, the safety profile of CEUS contrast agents (eg, no nephrotoxicity), high patient tolerance, allowance for continuous imaging during the arterial phase, the ability to perform multiple contrast injections over a short interval, and the ability to perform at bedside. Disadvantages and limitations of CEUS include its operator dependency, limited evaluation of subdiaphragmatic or deep observations, limited use in large patients, and poor penetration in patients with severe steatosis. In patients with known malignancy, such as HCC, CEUS is not suitable for complete disease staging.

Indications

Specific indications of CEUS in liver imaging include the following[59,60]:

1. To characterize a greater than or equal to 10-mm observation detected at screening or surveillance US, prior to multiphase contrast-enhanced CT or MR imaging, or after CT/MR imaging fails to visualize or characterize the observation
2. To determine the presence of arterial-phase hyperenhancement (APHE) in an observation suspected of having a mistimed arterial phase or misregistration artifact on prior multiphase contrast-enhanced CT/MR imaging
3. To characterize an indeterminate liver observation identified by another modality (example: CT/MR LI-RADS LR-3, LR-4, and LR-M observations)
4. To characterize a liver observation in a patient with renal insufficiency that precludes administration of iodinated or gadolinium contrast
5. To guide biopsy of observation occult on B-mode imaging or those containing necrotic areas
6. To differentiate tumor-in-vein from bland thrombus

Contrast-enhanced Ultrasound Technique

Details describing the specific CEUS imaging technique for liver imaging are available on the ACR LI-RADS Web site online[56] and discussed in several recent publications.[59,61] Briefly, intravenous access is needed. A 22 gauge or larger intravenous needle is preferred, and the

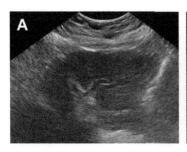 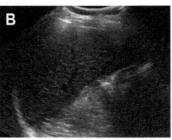

Fig. 23. US LI-RADS visualization score B. A 79-year-old man with cirrhosis. B-mode images of the left (*A*) and right (*B*) lobes of liver show mildly decreased penetration, moderate to severe hepatic parenchymal heterogeneity, and incomplete visualization of the hepatic dome.

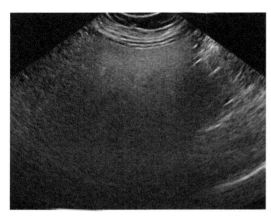

Fig. 24. US LI-RADS visualization score C. A 60-year-old man with CLD. Longitudinal B-mode image of the right lobe of liver shows marked beam attenuation resulting in poor penetration and nonvisualization of the diaphragm and the deepest 50% of the lobe.

left antecubital fossa should be used when available (because the scanning is performed from the patient's right side). A 3-way stopcock is connected (with minimal intervening tubing), with a saline flush oriented perpendicular and the contrast agent parallel to the direction of flow—this minimizes turbulent flow and inadvertent bubble destruction.

The liver observation or area of interest is then localized using gray-scale and color Doppler ultrasound. The use of sagittal imaging maximizes continual visualization of the observation with the patient breathing. With contrast mode active, a dual-screen, side-by-side B-mode and contrast image layout allows anatomic localization, because the contrast image is virtually devoid of signal prior to contrast injection. The US contrast is hand injected using a bolus technique followed immediately by a 5-mL to 10-mL saline flush. A contrast timer is initiated at the start of the saline flush.

The dynamic contrast-enhanced portion of the examination consists of arterial (10–45 seconds),

portal venous (30–120 seconds), and late phases (>120 seconds) of enhancement, with the total scan lasting approximately 5 minutes to 6 minutes. The examination may be repeated if another series of images in a different imaging plane is desired, if accurate recording of the arterial phase was not achieved with the initial injection, or if another observation requires characterization.

CEUS LI-RADS

Introduction
LI-RADS was originally intended to standardize the performance and interpretation of multiphase contrast-enhanced CT/MR imaging studies of the liver in patients at risk for HCC. In 2016, the ACR CEUS LI-RADS working group published an algorithm for the performance and interpretation of CEUS of the liver, adding US as a third diagnostic test for HCC. The algorithm is available on the ACR LI-RADS Web site online and reviewed in recently published articles.[59,61]

Although the diagnostic performance of CEUS is comparable to multiphase contrast-enhanced CT/MR imaging in characterizing focal liver observations,[62–64] the AASLD removed CEUS from the diagnostic algorithm in 2010 due to concern that intrahepatic cholangiocarcinoma (ICC) could be mistaken for HCC. Subsequent studies have shown, however, that ICC has distinguishable patterns of arterial enhancement and washout.[65,66] As a result, the 2017 AASLD guidelines have acknowledged that CEUS may be used to diagnose HCC noninvasively in expert centers but that additional studies are needed.[47,63]

Contrast-enhanced ultrasound examination interpretation
Recent CEUS LI-RADS articles[59,61] and the ACR CEUS LI-RADS Web site[56] describe the CEUS examination in detail. Major features in the ACR CEUS LI-RADS imaging algorithm include the size of an observation; the presence, type, and

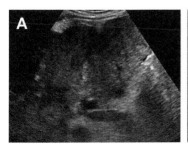
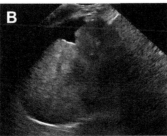

Fig. 25. US LI-RADS visualization score C. A 45-year-old woman with cirrhosis. B-mode images of the right lobe of liver in longitudinal (A) and transverse (B) orientations show marked parenchymal heterogeneity, obscuration of portions of the liver by rib shadow and poor penetration, the combination of which could obscure visualization of a large mass.

Table 3
CEUS LI-RADS exam categories

Exam Category	Concept	Example
CEUS LR-NC	Not categorizable	Inadequate study due to image degradation or omission of the observation from the acquisition
CEUS LR-1	Definitely benign	Hemangioma Simple cyst Focal fat sparing or deposition
CEUS LR-2	Probably benign	Distinct isoenhancing solid nodule <10 mm Non–mass-like isoenhancing observation of any size, not typical for hepatic fat deposition/sparing CEUS LR-3 nodules with size stability ≥2 y
CEUS LR-3	Intermediate probability of malignancy	Observations with no APHE or washout Observations that are <20 mm with late and mild washout without APHE Observations <10 mm with nonrim and nonperipheral globular discontinuous APHE with no washout
CEUS LR-4	Probably HCC	Observations that are ≥20 mm that have no APHE but have late and mild washout Observations that are <10 mm that have nonrim and nonperipheral globular discontinuous APHE and late to mild washout Observations that are ≥10 mm with nonrim and nonperipheral globular discontinuous APHE with no washout
CEUS LR-5	Definitely HCC	Observation that is ≥10 mm with nonrim and nonperipheral globular discontinuous APHE with late and mild washout
CEUS LR-M	Probably or definitely malignant, not specific for HCC	Observation with rim-APHE Early washout (<60 s) Marked washout before 2 min Differential includes HCC, ICC, and metastasis
CEUS LR-TIV	Tumor in vein	Echogenicity within a vessel on gray-scale imaging that enhances on the arterial phase

The concept behind each of 8 categories with description and examples of each provided.
Abbreviations: CEUS, contrast-enhanced ultrasound; LI-RADS, Liver Imaging Reporting and Data System.

degree of APHE; and the presence, timing, and degree of washout.[59] To accurately assess arterial enhancement, the observation should be continuously imaged during the entire arterial phase for up to a minute. Several benign patterns of APHE are known, such as the peripheral globular discontinuous enhancement seen in hemangiomas. Rim-APHE should specifically be noted because this pattern can be attributed to ICC.

To minimize bubble destruction after visualization of the arterial phase, the observation is reimaged every 30 seconds to 60 seconds, up to a total of 5 minutes to 6 minutes or until all bubbles are cleared from the image plane. Washout is defined as a decrease in echogenicity on the contrast image relative to the background liver. Images are evaluated for presence, timing (less than or greater than 60 seconds), and degree of washout (mild or marked; partial or complete). Classically, HCC shows late (>60 seconds) and mild washout, whereas early (<60 seconds) or marked washout prior to 2 minutes suggests the possibility of a non-HCC malignancy.

The observation can be measured on the images that best shows its margins (B-mode or contrast image). Key differences between CEUS LI-RADS and CT/MR imaging LI-RADS are the timing and degree of washout, the inability of CEUS to accurately evaluate more than 3 observations, and the inability of CEUS to completely stage a patient with known malignancy.[61]

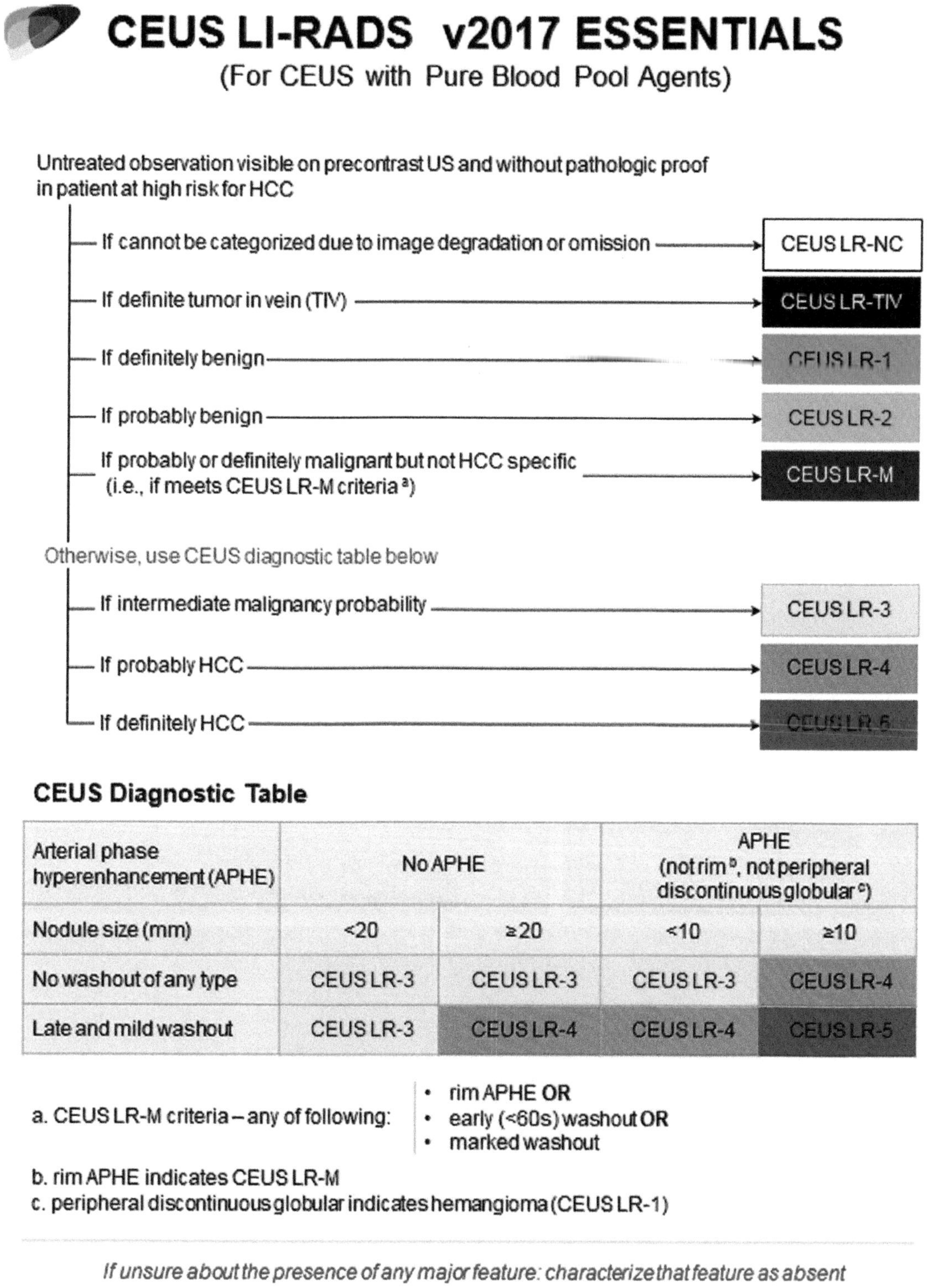

CEUS LI-RADS v2017 ESSENTIALS
(For CEUS with Pure Blood Pool Agents)

Untreated observation visible on precontrast US and without pathologic proof in patient at high risk for HCC

- If cannot be categorized due to image degradation or omission ⟶ **CEUS LR-NC**
- If definite tumor in vein (TIV) ⟶ **CEUS LR-TIV**
- If definitely benign ⟶ **CEUS LR-1**
- If probably benign ⟶ **CEUS LR-2**
- If probably or definitely malignant but not HCC specific (i.e., if meets CEUS LR-M criteria[a]) ⟶ **CEUS LR-M**

Otherwise, use CEUS diagnostic table below

- If intermediate malignancy probability ⟶ **CEUS LR-3**
- If probably HCC ⟶ **CEUS LR-4**
- If definitely HCC ⟶ **CEUS LR-5**

CEUS Diagnostic Table

Arterial phase hyperenhancement (APHE)	No APHE		APHE (not rim[b], not peripheral discontinuous globular[c])	
Nodule size (mm)	<20	≥20	<10	≥10
No washout of any type	CEUS LR-3	CEUS LR-3	CEUS LR-3	CEUS LR-4
Late and mild washout	CEUS LR-3	CEUS LR-4	CEUS LR-4	CEUS LR-5

a. CEUS LR-M criteria – any of following:
- rim APHE **OR**
- early (<60s) washout **OR**
- marked washout

b. rim APHE indicates CEUS LR-M

c. peripheral discontinuous globular indicates hemangioma (CEUS LR-1)

If unsure about the presence of any major feature: characterize that feature as absent

Fig. 26. CEUS LI-RADS imaging algorithm essentials summary slide. (*From* https://www.acr.org/Clinical-Resources/Reporting-and-Data-Systems/LI-RADS. Accessed July 31, 2018; with permission.)

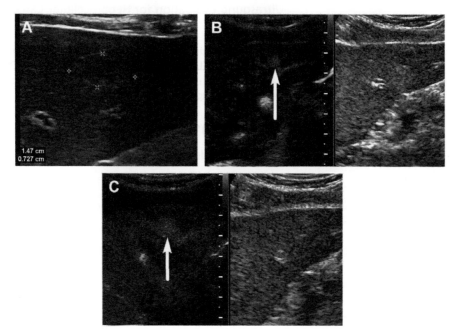

Fig. 27. CEUS LR-1 observation; hemangioma. A 60-year-old man with HCV cirrhosis. B-mode high-frequency image (*A*) shows a mixed echogenicity nodule in the left lobe of the liver, a US LI-RADS category US-3, positive observation (calipers). Arterial-phase CEUS side-by-side image with contrast-only (*left*) and B-mode (*right*) panels, at 21 seconds (*B*) shows discontinuous peripheral nodular enhancement (*arrow*). Portal venous-phase CEUS image at 1 minute (*C*) shows complete homogeneous hyperenhancement of the nodule compared with the background liver. There was no washout on delayed phases (not shown). The patient can resume surveillance imaging in 6 months.

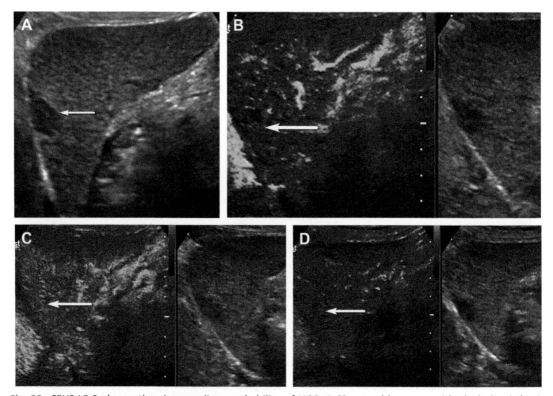

Fig. 28. CEUS LR-3 observation, intermediate probability of HCC. A 62-year-old woman with alcoholic cirrhosis. Sagittal B-mode US image of the left lobe (*A*) shows a 14-mm hypoechoic observation (*arrow*) initially detected on surveillance US imaging (US-3, positive). Side-by-side contrast (*left*) and B-mode (*right*) US images (*B–D*) show a small component that is isoenhancing to the liver in arterial phase (*arrow [B]*), isoenhancement of entire observation in venous phase (*arrow [C]*), and no washout in delayed phase (*arrow [D]*). Management options include a repeat diagnostic test in 3 months and/or possible biopsy.

CEUS LI-RADS Categories

There are 8 CEUS LI-RADS categories, descriptions of and examples for which are provided in **Table 3**.

The diagnostic algorithm is shown in **Fig. 26**. After ensuring a diagnostic-quality study and excluding tumor-in-vein, a CEUS LI-RADS (LR) category LR-1 to LR-5 or LR-M is assigned based on observation size, presence, and pattern of APHE and presence, timing, and degree of washout.[59,61] Briefly, the various CEUS examination categories are:

- CEUS LR-NC, not categorizable—this category is applied most commonly when there is a study failure.
- CEUS LR-1 to LR-5—these categories rate an observation's probability of HCC, from LR-1 (definitely benign) to LR-5 (definitely HCC) (**Figs. 27–29**).
- CEUS LR-M, probably or definitely malignant, not specific for HCC—this category should be used when findings of malignancy, such as washout, are identified; however, features may suggest or overlap with a non-HCC malignancy (**Fig 30**).

- CEUS LR-TIV, tumor in vein—this category is applied when tumor invasion of a hepatic vein or portal vein is identified (**Fig 31**).

Pitfalls

Similar to every imaging modality, CEUS study quality depends on appropriate technique, and image artifacts may confound accurate diagnoses.[67] Pitfalls of CEUS include lack of adequate enhancement, which may be due to unintentional bubble loss (eg, injection under a closed stop-cock or resistance during intravenous injection, which may lead to bubble destruction) or from poor visualization (eg, markedly steatotic liver, target observation very deep in the liver, or obscuration of the observation by rib or lung shadow). Nonlinear signal from background tissues or an inappropriately high gain setting may result in an artifact known as pseudoenhancement (signal not from bubbles), potentially resulting in inappropriate diagnosis of enhancement in nonenhancing structures. Pseudo-washout is a result of rapid bubble loss in the plane of imaging due to continuous scanning over a single

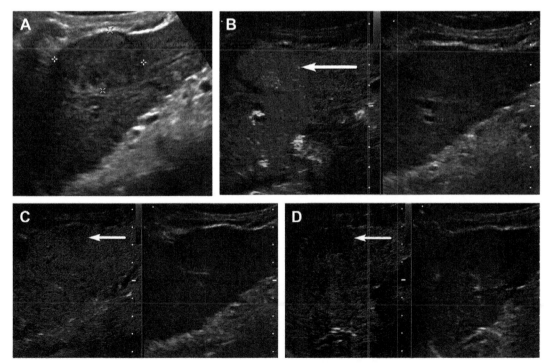

Fig. 29. CEUS LR-5 observation, definitely HCC. An 80-year-old man with HCV cirrhosis. Sagittal B-mode image (*A*) shows a solid isoechoic to hypoechoic observation (calipers) in the subcapsular left lobe, bulging the liver contour. Sagittal side-by-side contrast (*left*) and B-mode (*right*) images at 26 seconds (*B*) shows diffuse APHE (*arrow*), a small area of mild washout in the portal venous phase at 1 minute 58 seconds (*arrow* [*C*]), and larger area of progressive washout at 4 minutes 3 seconds (*arrow* [*D*]).

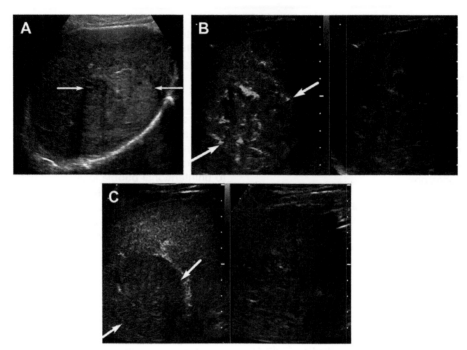

Fig. 30. CEUS LR-M, probably or definitely malignant, not specific for HCC. A 68-year-old man with chronic HCV cirrhosis. Transverse B-mode image (*A*) shows an echogenic solid liver mass (*arrows*) with areas of refractive shadowing. Transverse side-by-side contrast (*left*) and B-mode (*right*) image in the arterial phase at 21 seconds (*B*) and late arterial/portal venous phase at 44 seconds (*C*) shows dysmorphic APHE of the observation (*arrows* [*B*]) and early washout (*arrows* [*C*]), a feature not specific for HCC. Management includes performing a different diagnostic test or possible biopsy.

area, or inappropriately high-output power. Finally, centrally necrotic HCC may mimic rim-enhancement APHE pattern attributable to ICC.

SUMMARY

In summary, US is an important, cost-effective tool to evaluate patients with CLD. US may diagnose underlying liver disease, such as steatosis and cirrhosis, and identify complications of CLD, such as portal hypertension and decompensation. US is considered the primary screening and surveillance tool in the detection of HCC in high-risk patients. CEUS allows for characterization of observed focal liver lesions. Through standardization of technique and reporting provided by the US LI-RADS and CEUS LI-RADS algorithms, US practitioners can improve study quality and confidently influence the management of these at-risk patients.

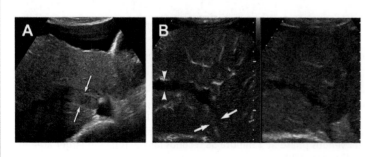

Fig. 31. CEUS LR-TIV, tumor in vein. A 68-year-old man with HCV cirrhosis. Transverse B-mode image of the right lobe (*A*) shows echoes within the right hepatic vein (*arrows*). Transverse side-by-side contrast (*left*) and B-mode (*right*) image in the arterial phase at 7 seconds (*B*) shows enhancing thrombus in the right hepatic vein (*arrows*) as well as nonenhancing, bland thrombus (*arrowheads*).

REFERENCES

1. Institute for Health Metrics and Evaluation. Global health data exchange 2018. Available at: http://ghdx.healthdata.org/gbd-results-tool. Accessed June 12, 2018.

2. Oxford Medical Education. Chronic liver disease (CLD) - compensated. 2015. Available at: http://www.oxfordmedicaleducation.com/gastroenterology/chronic-liver-disease-cld-compensated/. Accessed June 9, 2018.

3. Tsochatzis EA, Bosch J, Burroughs AK. Liver cirrhosis. Lancet 2014;383(9930):1749–61.

4. Marcellin P, Kutala BK. Liver diseases: a major, neglected global public health problem requiring urgent actions and large-scale screening. Liver Int 2018;38(Suppl 1):2 6.

5. Tang A, Hallouch O, Chernyak V, et al. Epidemiology of hepatocellular carcinoma: target population for surveillance and diagnosis. Abdom Radiol (NY) 2018;43(1):13–25.

6. Ferlay J, Soerjomataram I, Dikshit R, et al. Cancer incidence and mortality worldwide: sources, methods and major patterns in GLOBOCAN 2012. Int J Cancer 2015;136(5):E359–86.

7. El-Serag HB. Epidemiology of viral hepatitis and hepatocellular carcinoma. Gastroenterology 2012; 142(6):1264–73.e1.

8. Chalasani N, Younossi Z, Lavine JE, et al. The diagnosis and management of nonalcoholic fatty liver disease: Practice guidance from the American Association for the Study of Liver Diseases. Hepatology 2018;67(1):328–57.

9. Younossi ZM, Koenig AB, Abdelatif D, et al. Global epidemiology of nonalcoholic fatty liver disease-Meta-analytic assessment of prevalence, incidence, and outcomes. Hepatology 2016;64(1):73–84.

10. Mohamad B, Shah V, Onyshchenko M, et al. Characterization of hepatocellular carcinoma (HCC) in non-alcoholic fatty liver disease (NAFLD) patients without cirrhosis. Hepatol Int 2016;10(4):632–9.

11. Estes C, Razavi H, Loomba R, et al. Modeling the epidemic of nonalcoholic fatty liver disease demonstrates an exponential increase in burden of disease. Hepatology 2018;67(1):123–33.

12. Wong RJ, Aguilar M, Cheung R, et al. Nonalcoholic steatohepatitis is the second leading etiology of liver disease among adults awaiting liver transplantation in the United States. Gastroenterology 2015;148(3): 547–55.

13. Ma X, Holalkere NS, Kambadakone RA, et al. Imaging-based quantification of hepatic fat: methods and clinical applications. Radiographics 2009;29(5): 1253–77.

14. Kramer H, Pickhardt PJ, Kliewer MA, et al. Accuracy of liver fat quantification with advanced CT, MRI, and ultrasound techniques: prospective comparison with MR spectroscopy. AJR Am J Roentgenol 2017; 208(1):92–100.

15. Esterson YB, Grimaldi GM. Radiologic imaging in nonalcoholic fatty liver disease and nonalcoholic steatohepatitis. Clin Liver Dis 2018;22(1):93–108.

16. Zhang YN, Fowler KJ, Hamilton G, et al. Liver fat imaging-a clinical overview of ultrasound, CT, and MR imaging. Br J Radiol 2018;91:20170959.

17. Kelly EM, Feldstein VA, Etheridge D, et al. Sonography predicts liver steatosis in patients with chronic hepatitis B. J Ultrasound Med 2017;36(5):925–32.

18. Hernaez R, Lazo M, Bonekamp S, et al. Diagnostic accuracy and reliability of ultrasonography for the detection of fatty liver: a meta-analysis. Hepatology 2011;54(3):1082–90.

19. Schuppan D, Afdhal NH. Liver cirrhosis. Lancet 2008;371(9615):838 51.

20. Tchelepi H, Ralls PW, Radin R, et al. Sonography of diffuse liver disease. J Ultrasound Med 2002;21(9): 1023–32 [quiz: 1033–4].

21. Tan KC. The right posterior hepatic notch sign. Radiology 2008;248(1):317–8.

22. Giorgio A, Amoroso P, Lettieri G, et al. Cirrhosis: value of caudate to right lobe ratio in diagnosis with US. Radiology 1986;161(2):443–5.

23. Middleton WD, Kurtz AB, Hertzberg BS. Ultrasound the requisites. 2nd edition. St Louis (MO): Mosby; 2004.

24. Awaya H, Mitchell DG, Kamishima T, et al. Cirrhosis: modified caudate-right lobe ratio. Radiology 2002; 224(3):769 74.

25. Indiran V, Jagannathan K. Right posterior hepatic notch sign. Abdom Radiol (NY) 2017;42(11): 2780.

26. Okazaki H, Ito K, Fujita T, et al. Discrimination of alcoholic from virus-induced cirrhosis on MR imaging. AJR Am J Roentgenol 2000;175(6):1677–81.

27. Ito K, Mitchell DG, Gabata T, et al. Expanded gallbladder fossa: simple MR imaging sign of cirrhosis. Radiology 1999;211(3):723–6.

28. Di Lelio A, Cestari C, Lomazzi A, et al. Cirrhosis: diagnosis with sonographic study of the liver surface. Radiology 1989;172(2):389–92.

29. Ladenheim JA, Luba DG, Yao F, et al. Limitations of liver surface US in the diagnosis of cirrhosis. Radiology 1992;185(1):21–3 [discussion: 23–4].

30. Simonovsky V. The diagnosis of cirrhosis by high resolution ultrasound of the liver surface. Br J Radiol 1999;72(853):29–34.

31. Bolondi L, Gandolfi L, Arienti V, et al. Ultrasonography in the diagnosis of portal hypertension: diminished response of portal vessels to respiration. Radiology 1982;142(1):167–72.

32. Vilgrain V, Lebrec D, Menu Y, et al. Comparison between ultrasonographic signs and the degree of portal hypertension in patients with cirrhosis. Gastrointest Radiol 1990;15(3):218–22.

33. Haag K, Rossle M, Ochs A, et al. Correlation of duplex sonography findings and portal pressure in 375 patients with portal hypertension. AJR Am J Roentgenol 1999;172(3):631–5.

34. Wachsberg RH, Bahramipour P, Sofocleous CT, et al. Hepatofugal flow in the portal venous system: pathophysiology, imaging findings, and diagnostic pitfalls. Radiographics 2002;22(1):123–40.

35. Bookstein JJ, Cho KJ, Davis GB, et al. Arterioportal communications: observations and hypotheses concerning transsinusoidal and transvasal types. Radiology 1982;142(3):581–90.

36. Ralls PW. Color Doppler sonography of the hepatic artery and portal venous system. AJR Am J Roentgenol 1990;155(3):517–25.

37. Bolognesi M, Merkel C, Sacerdoti D, et al. Role of spleen enlargement in cirrhosis with portal hypertension. Dig Liver Dis 2002;34(2):144–50.

38. Lamb PM, Lund A, Kanagasabay RR, et al. Spleen size: how well do linear ultrasound measurements correlate with three-dimensional CT volume assessments? Br J Radiol 2002;75(895):573–7.

39. Chow KU, Luxembourg B, Seifried E, et al. Spleen size is significantly influenced by body height and sex: establishment of normal values for spleen size at US with a cohort of 1200 healthy individuals. Radiology 2016;279(1):306–13.

40. Bhatt S, Simon R, Dogra VS. Gamna-Gandy bodies: sonographic features with histopathologic correlation. J Ultrasound Med 2006;25(12):1625–9.

41. Takuma Y, Nouso K, Morimoto Y, et al. Portal hypertension in patients with liver cirrhosis: diagnostic accuracy of spleen stiffness. Radiology 2016;279(2):609–19.

42. Gines P, Quintero E, Arroyo V, et al. Compensated cirrhosis: natural history and prognostic factors. Hepatology 1987;7(1):122–8.

43. Planas R, Montoliu S, Balleste B, et al. Natural history of patients hospitalized for management of cirrhotic ascites. Clin Gastroenterol Hepatol 2006;4(11):1385–94.

44. Tandon P, Garcia-Tsao G. Bacterial infections, sepsis, and multiorgan failure in cirrhosis. Semin Liver Dis 2008;28(1):26–42.

45. Kim YK, Kim Y, Shim SS. Thoracic complications of liver cirrhosis: radiologic findings. Radiographics 2009;29(3):825–37.

46. Zhang BH, Yang BH, Tang ZY. Randomized controlled trial of screening for hepatocellular carcinoma. J Cancer Res Clin Oncol 2004;130(7):417–22.

47. Marrero JA, Kulik LM, Sirlin C, et al. Diagnosis, staging and management of hepatocellular carcinoma: 2018 practice guidance by the American Association for the Study of Liver Diseases. Hepatology 2018;68(2):723–50.

48. European Association for the Study of the Liver, European Organisation for Research and Treatment of Cancer. EASL-EORTC clinical practice guidelines: management of hepatocellular carcinoma. J Hepatol 2012;56(4):908–43.

49. Omata M, Lesmana LA, Tateishi R, et al. Asian Pacific Association for the Study of the Liver consensus recommendations on hepatocellular carcinoma. Hepatol Int 2010;4(2):439–74.

50. Kudo M, Izumi N, Kokudo N, et al. Management of hepatocellular carcinoma in Japan: Consensus-Based Clinical Practice Guidelines proposed by the Japan Society of Hepatology (JSH) 2010 updated version. Dig Dis 2011;29(3):339–64.

51. Marrero JA. Screening tests for hepatocellular carcinoma. Clin Liver Dis 2005;9(2):235–51, vi.

52. El-Serag HB, Davila JA. Surveillance for hepatocellular carcinoma: in whom and how? Therap Adv Gastroenterol 2011;4(1):5–10.

53. Bruix J, Sherman M, American Association for the Study of Liver Diseases. Management of hepatocellular carcinoma: an update. Hepatology 2011;53(3):1020–2.

54. Singal A, Volk ML, Waljee A, et al. Meta-analysis: surveillance with ultrasound for early-stage hepatocellular carcinoma in patients with cirrhosis. Aliment Pharmacol Ther 2009;30(1):37–47.

55. Yu NC, Chaudhari V, Raman SS, et al. CT and MRI improve detection of hepatocellular carcinoma, compared with ultrasound alone, in patients with cirrhosis. Clin Gastroenterol Hepatol 2011;9(2):161–7.

56. American College of Radiology. Liver imaging reporting & data system 2017. Available at: https://www.acr.org/Clinical-Resources/Reporting-and-Data-Systems/LI-RADS. Accessed July 27, 2018.

57. Morgan TA, Maturen KE, Dahiya N, et al. US LI-RADS: ultrasound liver imaging reporting and data system for screening and surveillance of hepatocellular carcinoma. Abdom Radiol (NY) 2018;43(1):41–55.

58. Fetzer DT, Rodgers SK, Harris AC, et al. Screening and surveillance of hepatocellular carcinoma: an introduction to ultrasound liver imaging reporting and data system. Radiol Clin North Am 2017;55(6):1197–209.

59. Lyshchik A, Kono Y, Dietrich CF, et al. Contrast-enhanced ultrasound of the liver: technical and lexicon recommendations from the ACR CEUS LI-RADS working group. Abdom Radiol (NY) 2018;43(4):861–79.

60. Jo PC, Jang HJ, Burns PN, et al. Integration of contrast-enhanced us into a multimodality approach to imaging of nodules in a cirrhotic liver: how I do it. Radiology 2017;282(2):317–31.

61. Wilson SR, Lyshchik A, Piscaglia F, et al. CEUS LI-RADS: algorithm, implementation, and key differences from CT/MRI. Abdom Radiol (NY) 2018;43(1):127–42.

62. Hanna RF, Miloushev VZ, Tang A, et al. Comparative 13-year meta-analysis of the sensitivity and positive predictive value of ultrasound, CT, and MRI for detecting hepatocellular carcinoma. Abdom Radiol (NY) 2016;41(1):71–90.

63. Heimbach JK, Kulik LM, Finn RS, et al. AASLD guidelines for the treatment of hepatocellular carcinoma. Hepatology 2018;67(1):358–80.

64. Zhang J, Yu Y, Li Y, et al. Diagnostic value of contrast-enhanced ultrasound in hepatocellular carcinoma: a meta-analysis with evidence from 1998 to 2016. Oncotarget 2017;8(43): 75418–26.

65. Li R, Yuan MX, Ma KS, et al. Detailed analysis of temporal features on contrast enhanced ultrasound may help differentiate intrahepatic cholangiocarcinoma from hepatocellular carcinoma in cirrhosis. PLoS One 2014;9(5):e98612.

66. Wildner D, Bernatik T, Greis C, et al. CEUS in hepatocellular carcinoma and intrahepatic cholangiocellular carcinoma in 320 patients - early or late washout matters: a subanalysis of the DEGUM multicenter trial. Ultraschall Med 2015;36(2):132–9.

67. Fetzer DT, Rafailidis V, Peterson C, et al. Artifacts in contrast-enhanced ultrasound: a pictorial essay. Abdom Radiol (NY) 2018;43(4):977–97.

Ultrasound of Renal Masses

Constantine M. Burgan, MD[a],*, Rupan Sanyal, MD[b], Mark E. Lockhart, MD[c]

KEYWORDS

- Contrast-enhanced ultrasound • Ultrasound of renal masses • Renal cyst ultrasound

KEY POINTS

- Ultrasound is a widely available, radiation-free, and inexpensive modality that can readily characterize many renal lesions.
- Grayscale sonography reliably differentiates between solid and cystic lesions, and can characterize complexity of cysts.
- Contrast-enhanced ultrasound adds to the diagnostic utility of grayscale ultrasound, and can not only determine the presence of enhancement but the pattern of enhancement.

Focal renal masses are commonly identified on imaging studies. Although the most commonly encountered etiology is a benign cyst, a significant subset of renal masses may represent malignant or inflammatory etiologies. Because of the possibility of more sinister etiologies, each renal lesion encountered on imaging needs to be characterized regarding its malignant potential. Ultrasound is a widely available, radiation-free, and relatively inexpensive modality that plays an important role in characterizing focal renal masses. It is used to differentiate benign cysts from solid renal neoplasms, characterize the degree of complexity of renal cysts, and identify features to help differentiate the etiologies of various lesions. In addition, the increasingly widespread availability of contrast-enhanced ultrasound (CEUS) has now provided us the ability to study the enhancement characteristics of renal lesions.

SOLID VERSUS CYSTIC RENAL LESIONS

When assessing a renal lesion, the first question that a radiologist needs to address is whether it is solid or cystic. The underlying reason for this bifurcation point is that most solid lesions are malignant and treated accordingly. On the other hand, all simple cysts and even most complex cysts are benign. As simple cysts far outnumber all other focal renal lesions, confident characterization of a lesion as a simple cyst can stop any further need for workup in most lesions.

The ability to differentiate cysts from solid renal lesions is one of the most important strengths of ultrasound. On ultrasound, renal cysts present as spherical or ovoid anechoic lesions with thin, smooth, or imperceptible walls and posterior acoustic enhancement. The ultrasound waves traverse the fluid within the cyst exceptionally well, resulting in the anechoic appearance of the cyst. Solid lesions, such as lymphoma and renal cell carcinoma (RCC), are sometimes quite hypoechoic but not completely anechoic.

Posterior acoustic enhancement is another feature of cysts (and other fluid-filled structures). After traversing the cyst, the relatively unattenuated sound beam results in increased brightness just posterior to the cyst.

Disclosures: C.M. Burgan: No disclosures. R. Sanyal: No disclosures. M.E. Lockhart: Book royalties, Oxford Publishing, Salary, deputy editor *Journal of Ultrasound in Medicine*.

[a] Department of Radiology, University of Alabama-Birmingham, 625 19th Street South, Birmingham, AL 35233, USA; [b] Department of Radiology, University of Alabama-Birmingham, 625 19th Street South, Birmingham, AL 35233, USA; [c] Department of Radiology, University of Alabama-Birmingham, 625 19th Street South, Birmingham, AL 35233, USA
* Corresponding author.
E-mail address: cburgan@uabmc.edu

Radiol Clin N Am 57 (2019) 585–600
https://doi.org/10.1016/j.rcl.2019.01.009
0033-8389/19/© 2019 Elsevier Inc. All rights reserved.

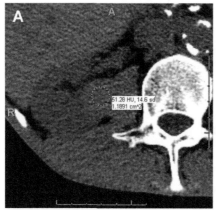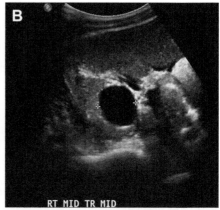

Fig. 1. Hyperdense renal cyst. Unenhanced CT (A) shows an incidental well-defined, homogeneous, hyperdense right renal lesion measuring 51 HU. Ultrasound (B) shows a well-defined, round, anechoic lesion with posterior acoustic enhancement consistent with a benign simple cyst. No further evaluation is needed.

In some cases, demonstration of vascularity within a lesion using Doppler can help differentiate hypoechoic solid lesions from renal cysts. CEUS, which is discussed separately, is also used to differentiate cysts from solid lesions by demonstrating presence or absence of enhancement.

IMAGE OPTIMIZATION TO CHARACTERIZE RENAL CYSTS

Optimization of the ultrasound technique may be necessary to clear internal echoes from a hypoechoic renal lesion to conclusively demonstrate it as a simple cyst. Depending on the body habitus and location of the renal cyst, it may be necessary to change the position of the patient to obtain an adequate acoustic window. Bowel gas may interfere, particularly in the evaluation of the left kidney, and decubitus positioning is usually required. The highest possible frequency setting should be

chosen, and the focal zone should be centered over the region of interest. Tissue harmonic imaging is particularly useful in identifying small renal lesions and clearing low-level internal echoes within cysts.[1,2]

ROLE OF ULTRASOUND IN CHARACTERIZATION OF HYPERDENSE RENAL LESIONS ON COMPUTED TOMOGRAPHY

Well-defined, homogeneous, hyperdense renal lesions are commonly encountered on computed tomography (CT). If such lesions have attenuation of 20 to 70 HU on unenhanced CT or greater than 20 HU on single-phase enhanced CT, they are considered indeterminate (**Fig. 1**). These lesions often represent benign hemorrhagic/proteinaceous cysts, although enhancing solid renal neoplasms can sometimes have this appearance (**Fig. 2**). Because of the possibility of malignancy,

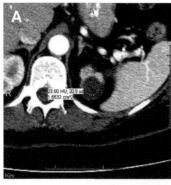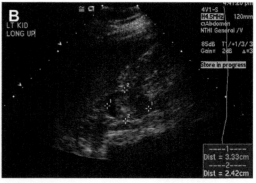

Fig. 2. Papillary RCC. Contrast-enhanced CT (A) shows a homogeneous left renal upper pole lesion measuring just above water attenuation (23 HU). Ultrasound (B) shows that the left renal upper pole lesion is actually a solid neoplasm. Pathology revealed papillary RCC. Papillary RCC can sometimes be homogeneous with only mild enhancement mimicking renal cysts on CT.

further imaging characterization with multiphasic CT, MR imaging, or ultrasound is usually recommended.

Although any of the 3 imaging modalities may be used for further characterization, ultrasound has some inherent advantages. Ultrasound is less expensive, widely available, radiation-free, and particularly good at identifying cysts as anechoic lesions. In 2017, Siddaiah and colleagues[3] showed that ultrasound can characterize most hyperdense cysts presenting as indeterminate hyperdense renal lesions on CT. This study, in combination with older studies performed in the 1980s by Zirinsky and colleagues[4] and Foster and colleagues,[5] suggest that ultrasound should be the next imaging examination for characterization of indeterminate homogeneously hyperdense renal lesions encountered on CT.

SIMPLE AND COMPLEX RENAL CYSTS

Simple cysts are defined as ovoid or spherical anechoic structures with posterior acoustic enhancement and imperceptible walls. Simple cysts are benign and do not require follow-up. Presence of wall thickening, septations, calcifications, and/or nodularity are all markers of complexity. The Bosniak classification is used to classify renal cysts based on their complexity. It was initially described for contrast-enhanced CT and uses presence of measurable enhancement as an important marker for possible malignancy. Because of this, the Bosniak classification cannot be directly used for conventional grayscale ultrasound, and ultrasound may overestimate its classification of a lesion due to increased sensitivity for small nodules or septations. On ultrasound, renal cysts with few thin (<1 mm) septae and small thin calcifications are likely benign, whereas cysts with multiple septae, thickening, or nodularity

require further characterization with a contrast-enhanced study.

RENAL CYSTIC NEOPLASMS
Cystic Nephroma/Mixed Epithelial and Stromal Tumor

Cystic nephroma and mixed epithelial and stromal tumor (MEST) represent a spectrum of the same entity.[6] These are benign, mixed solid and cystic renal tumors that occur more often in women in the 40 to 60 years age group. On ultrasound these appear as complex renal cysts with thick septae (**Fig. 3**). Enhancement is noted after contrast administration. These lesions may herniate into the renal pelvis.[7] On imaging, these are indistinguishable from cystic RCC and are therefore treated surgically.

Cystic Clear Cell Renal Cell Carcinoma

Although most clear cell renal cell carcinomas are solid, a cystic pattern is seen in 4% to 15% of all RCCs.[8] Ultrasound of cystic clear cell RCCs demonstrate cystic lesions with thick, irregular septae and thickened walls (**Fig. 4**). Nodular components are often present arising from the septae/walls. Calcification may be present.[9] Doppler examination may be able to demonstrate vascularity within the septa or nodular components, but flow is better detected as enhancement present after contrast administration. Nephron-sparing surgery is the treatment of choice. Cystic RCCs (including cystic clear cell RCC, multilocular cystic RCC, and papillary cystic RCC) show indolent growth with low metastatic potential and have excellent prognosis after successful surgery.[10,11]

Multilocular Cystic Renal Cell Carcinoma

Multilocular cystic RCC is a rare entity that is distinct from cystic clear cell RCC. These are

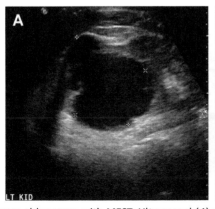
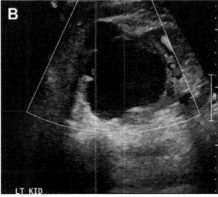

Fig. 3. 45-year-old woman with MEST. Ultrasound (A) shows a complex left renal cystic lesion with thick septae and wall thickening. Color Doppler (B) did not show vascularity within the lesion.

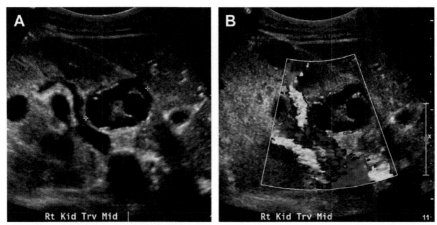

Fig. 4. 59-year-old woman with cystic clear cell RCC. Ultrasound (*A*) shows a complex right renal cyst (calipers). Irregular thick septae as well as a nodular component arising from a septum are noted. Doppler flow (*B*) is noted in the central nodular component as well as septae. These two features are highly concerning for malignancy.

very low-grade tumors with an excellent prognosis. The imaging appearance can vary from mildly complex renal cyst with thin septations in a significant number of patients or less commonly a much more complex cyst with wall nodularity. In a series of 23 patients with multilocular cystic RCC described by Hindman and colleagues,[12] 7 were classified on imaging as Bosniak IIF, 13 Bosniak III, and 3 Bosniak IV by CT or MR imaging.

Tubulocystic Renal Cell Carcinoma

Tubulocystic RCC is a recently described subtype of RCC. Cornelis and colleagues[13] described the distinct ultrasound appearance of this entity. Tubulocystic RCC is composed of very small cystic spaces separated by multiple thin septae (almost like a sponge). In 11 of 15 cases, this spongelike architecture resulted in an ultrasound

appearance that was markedly hyperechoic (like a solid tumor). Posterior acoustic enhancement was present in 8 of 15 cases, which is an important clue to its actual cystic nature (**Fig. 5**). Tubulocystic RCC must be considered in the differential of hyperechoic renal lesions.[13]

Calyceal Diverticulum

Calyceal diverticula are focal outpouchings arising from the collecting system. On ultrasound, they appear as simple or complex (usually due to hemorrhage or superinfection) cystic renal lesions. It is difficult to establish the diagnosis of calyceal diverticulum on ultrasound. Communication with the collecting system typically needs to be demonstrated by either excretory phase CT/MR or retrograde ureteroscopy to establish the diagnosis (**Fig. 6**).

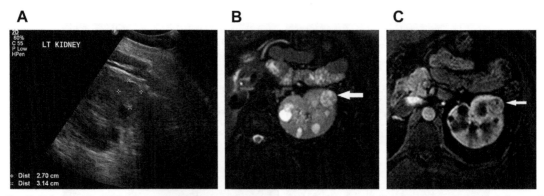

Fig. 5. Tubulocystic RCC. Ultrasound (*A*) in a 51-year-old man shows a well demarcated, echogenic left renal lesion with posterior acoustic enhancement. T2-weighted MR (*B*) shows a hyperintense cystic lesion with numerous septae corresponding to the echogenic lesion seen on ultrasound (*arrow*). Contrast-enhanced MR (*C*) shows enhancement within the lesion (*arrow*).

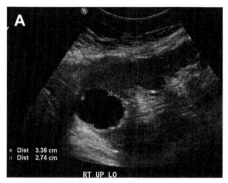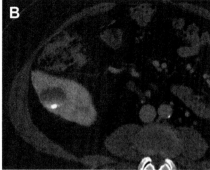

Fig. 6. Calyceal diverticulum. Ultrasound (A) shows a cystic lesion in a transplant kidney with mild wall thickening. Excretory phase CT (B) shows layering of excreted contrast within the cystic lesion confirming the diagnosis of a calyceal diverticulum. A dependent calculus is also noted.

Renal Abscess

On ultrasound, renal abscesses appear as complex cystic lesions. Knowing the patient's clinical presentation is key to reaching the correct diagnosis. Internal debris and increased adjacent parenchymal vascularity are indicators to the underlying etiology. Perinephric inflammatory fat stranding seen on CT is not usually appreciable on ultrasound.

SOLID RENAL MASSES

Once a renal lesion has been determined to be solid rather than cystic, a number of demographic, symptomatic, and sonographic characteristics can help further differentiate the lesion type. The most common situation in which a renal mass is diagnosed is as an incidental finding on a study performed for unrelated indications. Grayscale ultrasound with Doppler is an excellent initial imaging modality for detecting and preliminarily evaluating solid renal lesions. The presence or absence of Doppler flow can be a prognostic factor. Doppler also potentially has the ability to assess the pattern of flow within a solid lesion.

Renal Cell Carcinoma

RCC is commonly solid and represents the most common malignant renal lesion, potentially accounting for 80% to 90% of all malignant renal tumors. This accounts for approximately 4% of all cancers in adults. In the United States, at least 65,000 new cases are seen each year with 15,000 deaths. Patients tend to be older, between 50 and 70 (median age 64) with a 2:1 male predominance; 65% of patients have localized disease at initial presentation. Risk factors include cigarette smoking, hypertension, obesity, acquired cystic disease of the kidney, occupational exposures, certain chemotherapy agents, and use of nonsteroidal anti-inflammatory drugs. Genetic syndromes are also associated with RCC development.[14]

There are a variety of subtypes of RCC (Table 1), the most common of which is clear cell. Clear cell carcinoma has a worse prognosis than what is typically seen with other subtypes, such as chromophobe or papillary RCC. Statistically, larger resected tumors tend to be clear cell whereas smaller (<2 cm) lesions tend to be more likely to have papillary histology.[15] Accordingly, trials have shown better survival with papillary and chromophobe histology.[15] Two different subtypes of papillary RCCs have been demonstrated, with type 2 histology a significantly worse prognostic factor in a series from Pignot and colleagues.[16]

If presenting clinically, the most common presentation tends to be macroscopic hematuria, although flank pain and palpable mass may also

Table 1	
Histologic subtypes of renal cell carcinomas	
Subtype	**Percentage of Renal Cell Carcinomas**
Clear cell	75–85
Papillary	10–15
Chromophobe	5–10
Oncocytic	3–7
Unclassified	<5
Collecting (Bellini) duct	Rare, unclear

Data from Atkins MB, Choueiri TK. Epidemiology, pathology and pathogenesis of renal cell carcinoma. In: Richie JP, Vora SR, editors. UpToDate. Waltham, MA: UpToDate Inc. Available at: http://www.uptodate.com. Accessed July 31, 2018.

A **B**

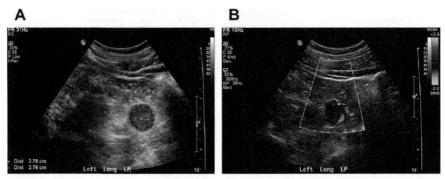

Fig. 7. RCC. A hypoechoic, solid mass (*A*) is present in the left renal lower pole. Color Doppler flow (*B*) is seen within this lesion.

occur. However, the combination of these findings are seen in only 10% to 15% of patients. Paraneoplastic syndromes are also seen with RCC in approximately 25% of patients.

The sonographic appearance of RCC can vary. It is typically a solid lesion, but may have cystic components, sometimes making up a large proportion of the lesion (as noted earlier). The solid lesions are typically isoechoic or hypoechoic to the background parenchyma (**Fig. 7**). Histologically, some RCCs can contain fat, and thus some of these tumors may have a hyperechoic appearance, although it does not need a fat component to appear mildly hyperechoic. A pseudocapsule may be visualized; if seen on grayscale sonography, it appears as a hypoechoic halo. The sensitivity for detection may be increased by the use of harmonic imaging.

Close attention should be paid if one suspicious renal lesion is found, as RCC, especially clear cell, may be multicentric.[17] Any renal lesion with Doppler flow should be assumed to be a RCC until proven otherwise. This includes any cystic lesion with measurable blood flow.

Examination of the renal vein should be performed in any patient with a suspected RCC. Color Doppler patency can reliably exclude presence of a renal vein thrombus, a finding seen in 4% to 10% of renal tumors.[18] Bland thrombus is also possible, but if a filling defect is observed, careful assessment within the thrombus for measurable arterial blood flow is necessary, as arterial flow is diagnostic of tumor (**Fig. 8**). In addition, if thrombus is seen, it should be followed as far centrally as is technically possible, as clot can extend potentially as far as the right atrium (**Fig. 9**). These findings are best evaluated by MR imaging if inferior vena cava (IVC) involvement is suspected; however, ultrasound can detect venous involvement at the time of initial evaluation and will make a significant difference for surgical planning.

Urothelial Carcinoma

Urothelial carcinoma is another possible etiology for a solid mass found associated with the kidney. These involve older patients, are more common in men with a 2:1 ratio,[8] and many may be secondary to industrial exposures. Risk factors include smoking, dye exposure, cyclophosphamide, and other factors.[19] Urothelial carcinomas may comprise up to 15% of all renal tumors. Synchronous lesions are seen in up to 24%, and 11% have metachronous involvement.[20,21] The 5-year survival is approximately 73% for upper tract tumors, and no known difference in survival is seen between primary pelvic versus primary ureteral tumors.[22–25]

Unlike RCC, which involves the cortex, upper tract urothelial carcinomas involve either the renal pelvis or proximal ureter. Both are much less common than urothelial neoplasms involving the bladder; however, renal pelvic origin is 2 to 3 times more common than the ureter. As these tumors involve the collecting system, they present most

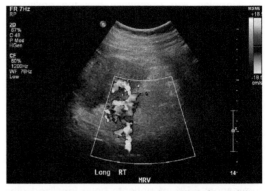

Fig. 8. Renal vein tumor thrombus. Ill-defined filling defect in the right renal vein, demonstrating vascularized color Doppler flow, diagnostic for tumor thrombus rather than bland thrombus.

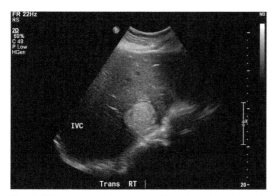

Fig. 9. Tumor thrombus extending into intrahepatic IVC. Echogenic, expansile filling defect is noted.

frequently with hematuria, but could cause flank pain and renal colic as well.

Sonographically, these lesions are solid and typically hypoechoic in appearance. They can appear slightly hyperechoic to the renal cortex[19] but typically more hypoechoic than the renal sinus fat (Fig. 10). They may arise from the central pelvis or a renal calyx, and could potentially be mistaken for hydronephrosis. Urothelial carcinomas may be focal or infiltrative, the latter more difficult to detect by sonography.

Lymphoma

Lymphoma involving the kidneys is primarily a manifestation of non-Hodgkin lymphoma (NHL) and can be seen in up to 50% of patients with NHL on autopsy. Most of renal lymphoma presents as multiple masses (Fig. 11). Lymphoma also can present as solitary lesions in 10% to 20% of patients. Adenopathy may or may not be seen in these cases. The perinephric space may also be preferentially involved, or the kidneys may be diffusely infiltrated and enlarged[20] (Fig. 12). This can be particularly difficult to detect by sonography.

Most renal lymphoma cases are secondarily involved, with primary renal lymphoma making up fewer than 1% of all extranodal lymphomas.[17] Lymphoma also may mimic RCC or urothelial carcinoma, making sonographic imaging differentiation nearly impossible in these cases; however, differentiating factors can include the lack of renal vein invasion, which is atypical for lymphoma. Renal lymphoma also can present in the renal sinus or as hilar adenopathy.

Metastases

Metastasis to the kidney is uncommon, with variable incidence being reported (2%–20% per Mittal and Sureka,[17] and <1% on clinicopathological studies).[20] Lung cancer is the most common metastatic source to the kidney, aside from lymphoma, although renal metastases have occurred in patients with breast, gynecologic, head and neck, colon, and prostate cancer. Renal metastases are difficult to differentiate from primary tumors on sonography, but are usually small, and can be multiple and bilateral[20] (Fig. 13). The imaging features are nonspecific, and clinical history or tissue sampling is necessary to suggest the diagnosis.

Angiomyolipoma

Angiomyolipoma (AML) is the most common benign solid renal neoplasm. This is considered a PEComa, a tumor in the spectrum of perivascular epithelioid cell differentiation. AML can be either sporadic or associated with syndromes such as tuberous sclerosis (TS) and lymphangioleiomyomatosis (LAM). There are numerous subtypes, but the most important for imaging differentiation are classic, fat-containing AMLs and lipid-poor AMLs. These lesions are at risk for intralesional hemorrhage, with significantly increased risk once the lesion measures beyond 4 cm.

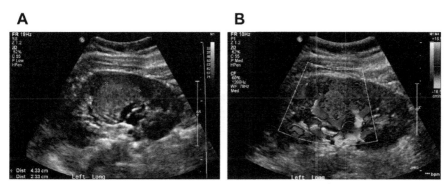

Fig. 10. Urothelial carcinoma. Slightly hyperechoic mass (A, B) is present in the renal pelvis, with associated vascularity and splaying of the renal pelvic vasculature.

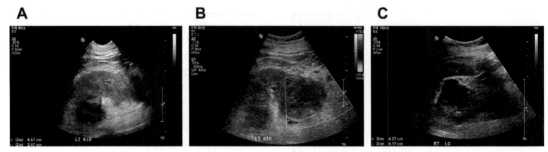

Fig. 11. Renal lymphoma. Bilateral, ill-defined masses (*A–C*) are demonstrated. Note the relative hypovascularity of the masses (*B*).

Syndromic AMLs can be seen in up to 75% to 90% of cases of TS.[17,20] TS-associated AMLs are more likely to be large and hemorrhagic, more commonly bilateral than those associated with LAM. Most AMLs will be considered for embolization or surgical treatment over the 4-cm threshold due to risk of bleeding from small lesional pseudoaneurysms.

Classic AML is a lipid-rich tumor but contains other vascular and soft tissue elements, any of which can be absent or predominate histologically.[26] Thus, these lesions are hyperechoic on ultrasound (**Fig. 14**). There is an overlap with RCC, which can also appear hyperechoic.[20] Similar features as seen in RCC may be seen in classic AML, including hypo/anechoic rim, cystic foci, and acoustic shadowing. Aneurysms, enlarged/bridging vessels, and perinephric hematoma can be seen in AML.[17]

Lipid-poor AML is another variant, which appears essentially isoechoic to renal parenchyma on ultrasound. These are essentially impossible to differentiate from RCC based on grayscale sonography alone. MR imaging is the most accurate means of identifying a lipid-poor AML. Other AML variants can show less fat, including the epithelial cystic variant.

Epithelioid AML is a rare subtype, which presents with large masses with cystic component, showing hemorrhage and necrosis. This always has an epithelioid cell component, but of a variable percentage (10%–100%).[26] This variant is potentially malignant and can metastasize.

Oncocytoma

Oncocytomas are benign epithelial neoplasms. In fact, they represent the most common benign solid renal mass without fat, up to 7% of renal cortical neoplasms. A characteristic central scar is sometimes seen, mostly in larger lesions, with 33% overall showing scar.[20] Oncocytomas are also characteristically very difficult to differentiate from RCC, and often go to surgery given the indistinguishable appearance (**Figs. 15** and **16**). Oncocytoma and RCC also can be difficult to distinguish histologically.[14] Oncocytoma also can demonstrate cystic change and hemorrhage, as well as calcification, although this is less common and mostly seen in the associated scar (**Fig. 17**). Subtypes of oncocytoma are known, with the telangiectatic variant demonstrating cystic spaces and internal hemorrhage.[17]

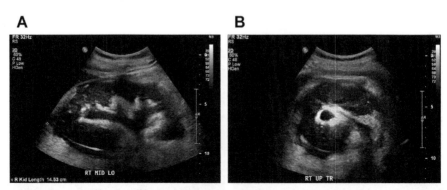

Fig. 12. Renal lymphoma. Diffusely infiltrated capsulelike thickening surrounding the right kidney (*A, B*). Mild hydronephrosis is noted, less than would be expected in other infiltrative soft tissue processes (eg, retroperitoneal fibrosis).

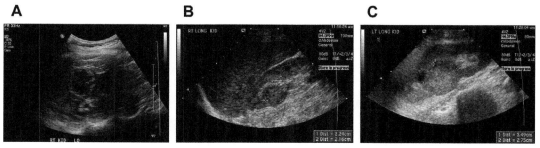

Fig. 13. Renal metastasis. (*A*) Grayscale image demonstrates a heterogeneous mass in a patient with a history of lung cancer. (*B, C*) In a patient with breast cancer, grayscale ultrasound demonstrates bilateral masses, slightly hypoechoic on the right, and slightly hyperechoic on the left.

Patients with oncocytoma can have a coexisting RCC in up to 10% to 32%[14,17] in either kidney, or in some instances as a hybrid tumor. However, presence of metachronous renal tumors is low, with subsequent tumors seen in 4%.[14] Oncocytoma also can be seen presenting multifocally or bilaterally (up to 16% and 12% of cases, respectively), related to Birt-Hogg-Dube syndrome, TS, or sporadic cases. Oncocytosis is a process in which the renal parenchyma is replaced by a variety of oncocytic tumors. Single-photon emission CT (SPECT)/CT can be a useful adjunct if oncocytoma is strongly considered clinically to differentiate from other renal pathology.[27]

CONTRAST-ENHANCED ULTRASOUND OF RENAL MASSES

Dynamic CEUS is a technique used for assessment of lesions seen on ultrasound, which can be used to replace contrast-enhanced MR imaging and CT examinations in the proper patient population. Given the excellent safety profile, these agents can be chosen for patients who have renal insufficiency when administration of other intravenous (IV) contrast agents is undesirable, or can often be helpful in small lesions in which pseudoenhancement may be more evident on other modalities. Typically, microbubble contrast is used to establish enhancement (and the pattern of enhancement), differentiate between solid masses and pseudotumors (**Fig. 18**), and evaluate complex cystic lesions.

Microbubble agents are enclosed in polymers, lipids, or proteins, approximately 1 to 10 μm in size.[28] These agents stay within the circulation and are considered purely blood pool agents. The microbubbles expand and contract with oscillation in response to the ultrasound waves and produce returning harmonic signals, allowing for the detection of enhancement. After a short period, the bubbles break down and are exhaled, while the enclosures are metabolized, typically by the liver. Given the size of these agents and accentuated reflectivity, they can facilitate visualization of much smaller vessels than typically assessed by color and spectral Doppler.

Technique

At our institution, the patient is brought to the ultrasound department and a careful history is taken to

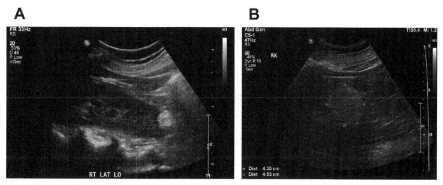

Fig. 14. Lipid-rich AML. Ultrasound (*A, B*) demonstrates hyperechoic renal lesions in 2 different patients. Both lesions contained fat on CT imaging (not shown).

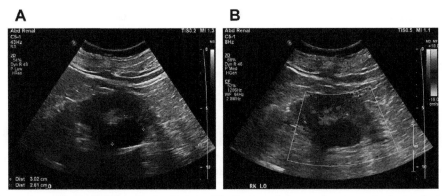

Fig. 15. Oncocytoma. Grayscale (*A*) and color Doppler (*B*) ultrasound shows a hypovascular, hypoechoic exophytic mass. Although eventually diagnosed as oncocytoma, the appearance is also compatible with RCC.

establish a history of prior contrast allergy or history of prior intracardiac shunt. IV access is established, and the examination is typically performed with a curved abdominal probe. The lesion in question is visualized to ensure that it does not appear purely cystic and is easily reproducible. A maximum dose of microbubble contrast is calculated using a weight-based protocol. The dose is split between 2 and 3 injections, with dose dependent on the agent used. The maximal total volume is frequently divided into fewer, larger boluses for larger patients and deep kidneys. Following this, the lesion is maintained in view, typically with split screen in real time and contrast is injected, followed by a saline flush. The contrast is injected in straight line with nonkinked tubing to reduce bubble breakage, and the flush is injected through the side port of a 3-way connector. Between injections, additional time or increased mechanical power pulses are used to clear any residual contrast agent, but consideration should be given to the potential for bioeffects of bubble fragmentation.

In the kidney, we are able to directly visualize the structures in the arterial, venous, and more

delayed phases. Contrast-specific imaging with color-encoded images is typically used to accentuate visualization of the lesion and its enhancement. Images are taken under a low mechanical index setting to limit destruction of microbubbles and intermittent imaging may be used at later time points after the first minute to preserve as many bubbles as possible. Arterial/corticomedullary phase images are obtained in an initial cine clip with more intermittent images/clips taken following in the venous/nephrographic phase.

Renal Cell Carcinoma

RCC, more specifically the clear cell subtype, will show strong contrast uptake in the arterial phase and typically will have slightly less bubble retention relative to the parenchyma on the venous and more delayed phases, termed "washout" (**Fig. 19**). A chromophobe RCC may demonstrate a "spoke-wheel" microbubble enhancement pattern and may demonstrate central scar. Chromophobe tumors have also shown heterogeneous isoenhancement in the cortical phase. Less

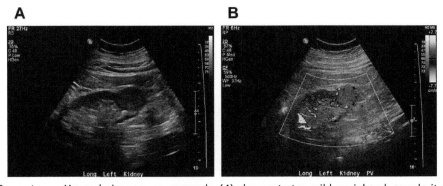

Fig. 16. Oncocytoma. Hypoechoic mass on grayscale (*A*) demonstrates mild peripheral vascularity on color Doppler (*B*). This was biopsy proven to be oncocytoma.

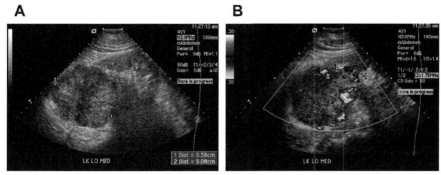

Fig. 17. Oncocytoma. Grayscale ultrasound (*A*) shows a heterogeneous, exophytic mass with slightly hypoechoic central scar. On color Doppler (*B*), extensive vascularity is present. This was interpreted as RCC by imaging, with the diagnosis made at pathology.

vascular lesions, such as papillary RCC, may have subtle enhancement that is difficult to appreciate (**Fig. 20**). Papillary tumors show less early enhancement and demonstrate a more heterogeneous cortical phase as well.

In RCC, microbubble arterial phase hyperenhancement also may be seen within renal vein/IVC, indicating tumor thrombus. Rapid washin/washout is common in malignancy. Larger lesions are more likely to be heterogeneous.[29] Chromophobe and papillary carcinomas commonly display slower to washin than the more aggressive variants. However, subtyping between papillary variants is difficult on CEUS, with some characteristics currently better defined on MDCT.[30–33]

CEUS also has been shown to be excellent in classifying previously indeterminate lesions on CT. On a recent series, CEUS was definitive in assessing the large majority (>95%) of cases referred from CT, including more than 94% of equivocal enhancement CT cases.[34] Many lesions became definitively surgical or nonsurgical based on CEUS results. CEUS was specifically useful in

small papillary RCCs that did not clearly enhance on CT.

Urothelial Carcinoma

CEUS detects 94% of renal pelvic tumors based on a series from Xue and colleagues,[35] as compared with approximately 79% by conventional sonography. Approximately three-fourths of lesions enhanced slowly relative to the renal cortex, whereas one-fourth were similarly enhancing to cortex. Most (78%) lesions overall hypoenhance compared with background parenchyma. The large majority also homogeneously enhanced, with the minority more heterogeneously enhancing (**Fig. 21**), typically associated with necrosis and hemorrhage. Nearly all lesions demonstrated rapid washout, although slower washout was seen in a few lesions. This series also demonstrated enhancement in approximately 73% of lesions misdiagnosed by conventional sonography, including smaller tumors, some of which were subcentimeter in size.

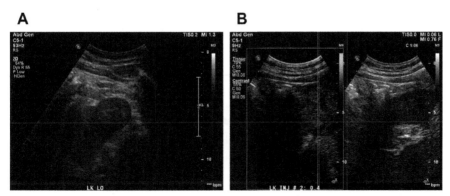

Fig. 18. Column of Bertin on CEUS. (*A*) This slightly prominent area of cortex was suspected to not represent a renal mass, but prompted subsequent contrast ultrasound. (*B*) Uniform enhancement similar to the adjacent regions of the cortex was noted, with no discrete mass seen, consistent with a column of Bertin.

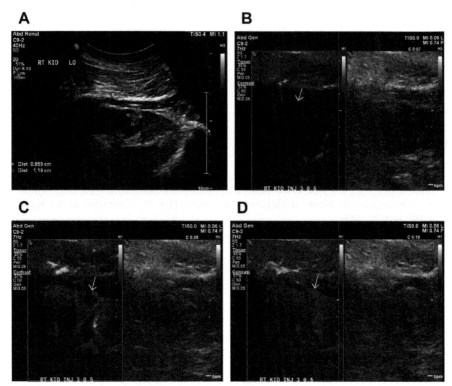

Fig. 19. RCC. (A) Grayscale ultrasound shows a small, hyperechoic mass in the right kidney (calipers). (B–D) After microbubble injection, the lesion demonstrates heterogeneous enhancement, with rapid wash in progression from time points 7 to 19 seconds after flush (arrows). Despite hyperechoic appearance, this was found to be a small RCC at surgery. Note that up to 30% of small RCCs may be echogenic, even in the absence of intralesional fat.

Benign Lesions: Angiomyolipoma and Oncocytoma

Benign lesions demonstrate a typically slow washin and washout pattern.[29] Enhancement patterns of angiomyolipomas are variable, as the portions containing vasculature and musculature are what typically enhances and can vary significantly based on the composition of the lesion. Enhancement may be difficult to see in a lipid-rich angiomyolipoma given the hyperechoic parenchyma. Angiomyolipoma, when enhancing, tends to either hyperenhance or isoenhance relative to the background, often starting peripherally[36] (Fig. 22). Oncocytomas can have the "spoke-wheel" classic enhancement pattern, as in chromophobe RCC, but also may demonstrate nonspecific enhancement patterns, including early enhancement with

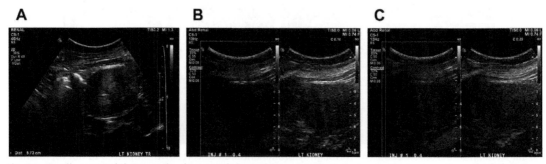

Fig. 20. Papillary RCC. (A) Grayscale ultrasound shows large, exophytic heterogeneous mass from the left kidney. (B, C) The microbubble enhancement of this lesion was uniform, but fairly mild with slow fill-in.

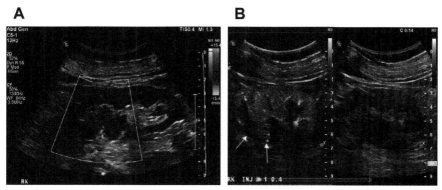

Fig. 21. Urothelial carcinoma. (A) Color Doppler shows a hypoechoic, infiltrative lesion in the right renal pelvis. (B) This mass heterogeneously enhanced with microbubble contrast (arrows).

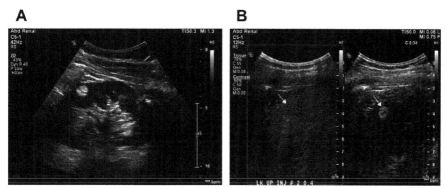

Fig. 22. AML. (A) Characteristic appearance of classic AML with hyperechoic appearance on grayscale. (B) After injection of microbubbles, this uniformly enhances, with slow washin (arrows).

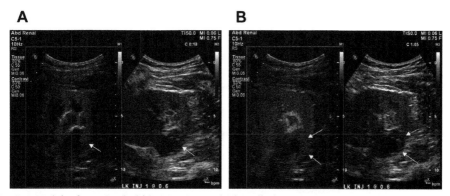

Fig. 23. Cystic RCC. (A) After microbubble injection, a thick-walled cyst is seen in the posterior left kidney, which enhances on early post-contrast images (arrow). (B) After approximately 65 seconds, this lesion enhanced more uniformly with progressive fill-in (arrow). This is classified as a Bosniak III cyst, and diagnosis of RCC was confirmed at surgery.

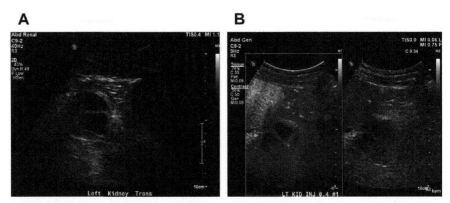

Fig. 24. Cystic RCC. (*A*) On grayscale, a thickly septated cyst is present. (*B*) On CEUS, enhancement is clearly seen within the septations. This also would be considered a Bosniak III lesion.

washout. Other lesions are nonspecific, with appearance similar to renal lymphoma and renal metastases.

Cystic Lesions

Although differentiation of solid renal lesions can be performed with CEUS, the most common use in our practice is to evaluate for enhancement in cystic lesions. Echogenic internal material, septations, wall thickening, nodules, and calcifications all may be assessed by CEUS. CEUS shows very good agreement with the reference standard of CT, with sensitivity and negative predictive values at 100% in one study,[37] and higher than CT for subtle vascularity in low-vascularity lesions in another study.[28] Volume averaging is also not a limiting factor on CEUS, as seen on CT in smaller lesions.

Characteristics of the Bosniak classification system may also be applied with CEUS, with similar distributions of risk of malignancy found on CEUS series.[28] When early or late enhancement is seen within thickened septations, the cyst wall, or a nodule within a cyst, the lesion is suspicious for neoplasm and may be classified as Bosniak III (**Figs. 23** and **24**).

Posttreatment Patients

In patients who have had previous ablations or prior surgery, CEUS can be used to detect residual enhancement suggestive of residual or recurrent tumor in the ablation or postoperative site (**Fig. 25**). This can be particularly useful, as the patient population that may be poor surgical candidates and require ablation or partial resection have a higher propensity for renal disease or other contraindications for CT/MR contrast administration. Postablation enhancement of AMLs may also be evaluated in this fashion.

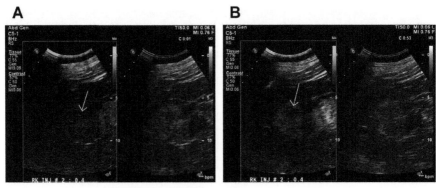

Fig. 25. AML with persistent enhancement postablation. (*A*) A hyperechoic mass is noted in the right kidney. (*B*) CEUS demonstrates mild, heterogeneous enhancement despite embolization (*arrows*). Given the persistent vascularity and size, this patient returned for repeat embolization.

SUMMARY

Ultrasound is an excellent modality for characterization of renal lesions. With the rise of CEUS, many renal lesions are now able to be completely characterized in the ultrasound suite without the need for iodinated contrast or gadolinium, which is beneficial in the case of allergy or renal dysfunction. Ultrasound should be considered the first-line modality for evaluation of an incidentally found renal lesion. Simple or minimally complex cysts are easily diagnosed. In addition, if there is concern for renal infection, ultrasound may demonstrate a drainable abscess and facilitate treatment. Solid lesions also are well characterized and differentiated with grayscale and CEUS. Neoplasms with benign-appearing features can be readily followed sonographically, whereas those with more worrisome appearance and enhancement can rapidly be referred for surgical management or ablation. If findings remain poorly characterized, referral for CT or preferably MR imaging may help make a final diagnosis.

REFERENCES

1. Schmidt T, Hohl C, Haage P, et al. Diagnostic accuracy of phase-inversion tissue harmonic imaging versus fundamental B-mode sonography in the evaluation of focal lesions of the kidney. AJR Am J Roentgenol 2003;180:1639–17.
2. Anvari A, Forsberg F, Samir AE. A primer on the physical principles of tissue harmonic imaging. Radiographics 2015;35:1955–64.
3. Siddaiah M, Krishna S, McInnes MDF, et al. Is ultrasound useful for further evaluation of homogeneously hyperattenuating renal lesions detected on CT? AJR Am J Roentgenol 2017;209: 604–10.
4. Zirinsky K, Auh YH, Rubenstein WA, et al. CT of the hyperdense renal cyst: sonographic correlation. AJR Am J Roentgenol 1984;143:151–6.
5. Foster WL, Roberts L, Halvorsen RA, et al. Sonography of small renal masses with indeterminant density characteristics on computed tomography. Urol Radiol 1988;10:59–67.
6. Jevremovic D, Lager DJ, Lewin M. Cystic nephroma (multilocular cyst) and mixed epithelial and stromal tumor of the kidney: a spectrum of the same entity? Ann Diagn Pathol 2006;10:77–82.
7. Chu LC, Hruban RH, Horton KM, et al. Mixed epithelial and stromal tumor of the kidney: radiologic-pathologic correlation. Radiographics 2010;30: 1541–51.
8. Hartman DS, Davis CJ, Johns T, et al. Cystic renal cell carcinoma. Urology 1986;28:145–53.

9. Zhang J, Liu B, Song N, et al. Diagnosis and treatment of cystic renal cell carcinoma. World J Surg Oncol 2013;11:158.
10. Jhaveri K, Gupta P, Elmi A, et al. Cystic renal cell carcinomas: do they grow, metastasize, or recur? AJR Am J Roentgenol 2013;201:W292–6.
11. Winters BR, Gore JL, Holt SK, et al. Cystic renal cell carcinoma carries an excellent prognosis regardless of tumor size. Urol Oncol 2015;33: 505.e9-13.
12. Hindman NM, Bosniak MA, Rosenkrantz AB, et al. Multilocular cystic renal cell carcinoma: comparison of imaging and pathologic findings. AJR Am J Roentgenol 2012;198:W20–6.
13. Cornelis F, Hélénon O, Correas JM, et al. Tubulocystic renal cell carcinoma: a new radiological entity. Eur Radiol 2016;26:1108–15.
14. Atkins MD, Choueiri TK. Epidemiology, pathology and pathogenesis of renal cell carcinoma. In: Richie JP, Vora SR, editors. UpToDate. Waltham, (MA): UpToDate Inc. Available at: http://www.uptodate.com. Accessed July 31, 2018.
15. Kang SK, Huang WC, Pandharipande PV, et al. Solid renal masses: what the numbers tell us. AJR Am J Roentgenol 2014;202(6):1196–206.
16. Pignot G, Elie C, Conquy S, et al. Survival analysis of 130 patients with papillary renal cell carcinoma: prognostic utility of type 1 and type 2 subclassification. Urology 2007;69(2):230–5.
17. Mittal MK, Sureka B. Solid renal masses in adults. Indian J Radiol Imaging 2016;26(4):429–42.
18. Nouh MAA-M, Inui M, Kakchi Y. Renal cell carcinoma with IVC thrombi; current concepts and future perspectives. Clin Med Oncol 2008;2:247–56.
19. Raman JD, Messer J, Sielatycki JA, et al. Incidence and survival of patients with carcinoma of the ureter and renal pelvis in the USA, 1973-2005. BJU Int 2011;107(7):1059.
20. Kay FU, Pedrosa I. Imaging of solid renal masses. Radiol Clin North Am 2017;55(2):243–58.
21. Browne RF, Meehan CP, Colville J, et al. Transitional cell carcinoma of the upper urinary tract: spectrum of imaging findings. Radiographics 2005;25(6): 1609–27.
22. Margulis V, Shariat SF, Matin SF, et al, The Upper Tract Urothelial Carcinoma Collaboration. Outcomes of radical nephroureterectomy: a series from the Upper Tract Urothelial Carcinoma Collaboration. Cancer 2009;115(6):1224.
23. Lughezzani G, Jeldres C, Isbarn H, et al. Nephroureterectomy and segmental ureterectomy in the treatment of invasive upper tract urothelial carcinoma: a population-based study of 2299 patients. Eur J Cancer 2009;45(18):3291.
24. Jeldres C, Sun M, Lughezzani G, et al. Highly predictive survival nomogram after upper urinary tract urothelial carcinoma. Cancer 2010;116(16):3774.

25. Raman JD, Ng CK, Scherr DS, et al. Impact of tumor location on prognosis for patients with upper tract urothelial carcinoma managed by radical nephroureterectomy. Eur Urol 2010;57(6):1072.

26. Aydin H, Magi-Galluzzi C, Lane BR, et al. Renal angiomyolipoma: clinicopathologic study of 194 cases with emphasis on the epithelioid histology and tuberous sclerosis association. Am J Surg Pathol 2009; 33(2):289–97.

27. Gorin MA, Rowe SP, Baras AS, et al. Prospective evaluation of (99m)Tc-sestamibi SPECT/CT for the diagnosis of renal oncocytomas and hybrid oncocytic/chromophobe tumors. Eur Urol 2016;69(3): 413–6.

28. Cokkinos DD, Antypa EG, Skilakaki M, et al. Contrast enhanced ultrasound of the kidneys: what is it capable of? Biomed Res Int 2013;2013:595873.

29. Li X, Liang P, Guo M, et al. Real-time contrast-enhanced ultrasound in diagnosis of solid renal lesions. Discov Med 2013;16(86):15–25.

30. Young JR, Coy H, Douek M, et al. Type 1 papillary renal cell carcinoma: differentiation from Type 2 papillary RCC on multiphasic MDCT. Abdom Radiol (NY) 2017;42(7):1911–8.

31. Barr RG. Is there a need to modify the Bosniak renal mass classification with the addition of contrast-enhanced sonography? J Ultrasound Med 2017; 36(5):865–8.

32. Barr RG, Peterson C, Hindi A. Evaluation of indeterminate renal masses with contrast-enhanced US: a diagnostic performance study. Radiology 2014; 271(1):133–42.

33. Atri M, Tabatabaeifar L, Jang HJ, et al. Accuracy of contrast-enhanced US for differentiating benign from malignant solid small renal masses. Radiology 2015;276(3):900–8.

34. Zarzour JG, Lockhart ME, West J, et al. Contrast-enhanced ultrasound classification of previously indeterminate renal lesions. J Ultrasound Med 2017;36(9):1819–27.

35. Xue LY, Lu Q, Huang BJ, et al. Evaluation of renal urothelial carcinoma by contrast-enhanced ultrasonography. Eur J Radiol 2013;82(4):e151–7.

36. Malhi H, Grant EG, Duddalwar V. Contrast-enhanced ultrasound of the liver and kidney. Radiol Clin North Am 2014;52(6):1177–90.

37. Sanz E, Hevia V, Gómez V, et al. Renal complex cystic masses: usefulness of contrast-enhanced ultrasound (CEUS) in their assessment and its agreement with computed tomography. Curr Urol Rep 2016;17(12):89.

Ultrasound of Pelvic Pain in the Nonpregnant Woman

Maitray D. Patel, MD*, Scott W. Young, MD,
Nirvikar Dahiya, MD

KEYWORDS

• Ultrasound • Sonography • Pelvic pain • Ovary • Uterus • Non-gynecologic

KEY POINTS

- Sonographic findings effectively distinguish between ovarian hemorrhage, ovarian torsion, and pelvic inflammatory disease in women as a cause of acute pelvic pain; among these entities, color Doppler imaging is least useful for suspected torsion.
- Endometriosis is a common cause of chronic or episodic pelvic pain; in addition to identification of endometriomas, cognizant sonologists can detect clinically important imaging manifestations of deeply infiltrating endometriosis.
- A variety of other gynecologic and non-gynecologic conditions can cause pain in the nonpregnant woman, and the effective sonologist will be aware of these possibilities and use special techniques and observations to facilitate proper diagnosis when needed.

INTRODUCTION

Pelvic pain is a common symptom in nonpregnant women; it can be characterized as acute, chronic, or recurrent.[1] *Acute pelvic pain* is usually defined as pain that is new and present for less than 3 months, and *chronic pelvic pain* is usually defined as symptoms that are non-cyclical and lasting for at least 6 months.[2] As this timeline is arbitrary, it helps to have the third category of patients with *recurrent pelvic pain*, encompassing those who have recurrent cyclic or episodic pelvic pain. Pelvic pain is a common presenting symptom for women seeking care in the emergency department or at their physician's office. Whereas there is a broad range of gynecologic and non-gynecologic causes of pelvic pain in the nonpregnant woman, and the choice of imaging work-up depends greatly on the clinical scenario, pelvic imaging with endovaginal ultrasound (EVUS) is often the imaging test of choice in the initial evaluation of these patients.[3] This article considers the sonographic findings and diagnostic considerations in 3 subgroups of nonpregnant women presenting with pelvic pain: (1) women without chronic symptoms who present with acute pain, and in whom pelvic ultrasound identifies adnexal findings of concern for ovarian hemorrhage, ovarian torsion, or pelvic inflammatory disease; (2) women with chronic or recurrent pelvic pain, in whom pelvic ultrasound identifies evidence of endometriosis and/or adenomyosis; and (3) women with acute, chronic, or recurrent pelvic pain with alternative considerations.

WOMEN WITHOUT CHRONIC SYMPTOMS WHO PRESENT WITH ACUTE PAIN
Ovarian Hemorrhage

Bleeding into a corpus luteum at the time of ovulation results in an intraovarian mass called a hemorrhagic ovarian cyst (HOC). If the hemorrhage is contained within the corpus luteum, the resultant expansion of the cyst causes acute pain due to

Disclosures: None.
Department of Radiology, Mayo Clinic Arizona, Phoenix, AZ 85054, USA
* Corresponding author.
E-mail address: patel.maitray@mayo.edu

mass effect. If the cyst ruptures, irritation of the peritoneal lining by hemorrhage surrounding the ovary can also contribute to acute pain. Given that ovarian cyst development and ovulation are inherent physiologic processes in premenopausal women, it is no surprise that HOC is a common cause of acute pelvic pain in women.

The sonographic features of an acute HOC can be characteristic, although some features can be confusing.[4] Acutely, hemorrhage into a cyst can lead to a pattern of diffuse low-level echoes that mimics the appearance of an endometrioma, but usually there are coexisting fibrin strands, which manifest as a lace-like or fishnet reticular pattern of echogenic lines superimposed on the low-level echoes[5] (**Fig. 1**). The presence of these fibrin strands intermixed with the low-level echoes makes the diagnosis of an acute HOC very likely, although some endometriomas with acute hemorrhage can appear similar.[6]

As the blood in the cyst settles and organizes, one may see the "retracting clot" sign (**Fig. 2**), which is highly specific for an acute HOC—this particular feature is considered pathognomonic of HOCs not seen in other entities that can contain internal hemorrhage, such as endometriomas.[5] The key feature of the retracting clot sign is the concavity or straight-line geometry of the interface of the suspected clot with the adjacent anechoic fluid. It is imperative that sonographers evaluate suspected areas of clot with color Doppler, as clots should not have any demonstrable internal flow.[7] Whereas peripheral flow along the margin of the cyst may be readily demonstrable, reflecting

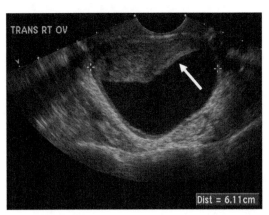

Fig. 2. Hemorrhagic ovarian cyst with retracting clot. EVUS demonstrates a clot along the wall of the cyst, recognized by the concave interface (*arrow*) with the adjacent fluid.

the fact that the hemorrhagic cyst arose from the corpus luteum, there should be no flow in the clot itself; the demonstration of peripheral flow is further evidence that the cyst is an acute HOC arising in the corpus luteum[7] (see **Fig. 1**).

When an HOC ruptures, the sonographic appearance can be confusing, especially if the HOC largely deflates and there is substantial clot around the ovary (**Fig. 3**). A clot around the ovary leads to apparent ovarian enlargement with indistinct margins, and it can be difficult to distinguish ovarian parenchyma from the clot. In this regard, looking for the distribution of follicles can be of assistance, because they would define the ovarian parenchyma. Furthermore, color Doppler evaluation will sometimes show readily demonstrable flow in the ovarian parenchyma, sometimes centrally located in the "adnexal mass" with absence of flow in the clot around the ovary. The circumferential flow along the margin of the ruptured corpus luteum can be a helpful clue to recognize the deflated HOC. Usually there is coexisting fluid with echoes in the cul-de-sac, reflecting dependent accumulation of hemoperitoneum.

Ovarian Torsion

Ovarian torsion is a gynecologic surgical emergency that can occur in women of all ages, with the highest prevalence in postmenarcheal premenopausal women. Whereas the pain associated with ovarian torsion is often sharp, intense, and severe, symptoms usually do not sufficiently distinguish torsion from the more common ovarian hemorrhage. The twisted ovary initially has compromised venous and lymphatic outflow, usually with sustained arterial inflow, resulting in edematous enlargement that stretches the ovarian

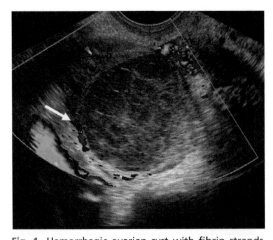

Fig. 1. Hemorrhagic ovarian cyst with fibrin strands. Endovaginal ultrasound (EVUS) shows a hemorrhagic ovarian cyst with fibrin strands superimposed on a background of low-level echoes. Note the circumferential flow at the edge of the cyst (*arrow*), a commonly identified feature of corpus luteal cysts.

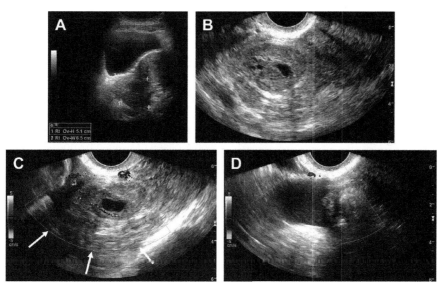

Fig. 3. Ruptured or leaking hemorrhagic cyst with extraovarian clot. Transabdominal ultrasound (*A*) shows an abnormal collection or mass in the right adnexa, denoted with electronic calipers. EVUS without color Doppler (*B*) does not clearly differentiate the clot from ovarian parenchyma. EVUS with color Doppler shows an avascular clot (*C, arrows*) along the margin of the vascularized ovary, with circumferential flow at the margin of the hemorrhagic corpus luteum and fluid (*D*), with low-level echoes representing unclotted blood - adjacent to the clot.

capsule, causing pain.[8] This enlargement of the ovary is the hallmark of imaging findings in ovarian torsion; a morphologically normal-appearing ovary effectively excludes torsion as a diagnostic possibility.[9,10]

Indeed, the morphologic findings of a twisted ovary are the most important clues to the diagnosis, because arterial and/or venous flow is demonstrable with color and spectral Doppler in more than 50% of cases, although usually not completely "normal."[11] The biggest misunderstanding about the role of sonographic and Doppler imaging is the misconception that Doppler findings are important in making or excluding the diagnosis of ovarian torsion. Because a morphologically abnormal twisted ovary can show normal arterial and venous Doppler flow, it follows that Doppler cannot be used to exclude torsion as a diagnostic possibility. Because an atrophic ovary may not show arterial or venous flow,[7] it follows that Doppler cannot be used to make the diagnosis of torsion in the absence of morphologically suspicious findings. The diagnosis of ovarian torsion is made based on the morphologic features of the ovary, not the Doppler features.

Fortunately, the morphologic features of the twisted ovary can be highly suggestive of the diagnosis.[8,9] The ovarian stromal edema can lead to a "hazy" or "ground glass" appearance of the ovarian parenchyma, with follicles pushed to the margins of the ovary by the central stromal edema (Fig. 4). In many cases, the ovarian twist occurs due to the presence of an eccentric mass in the ovary, often a cyst (HOC, cystic teratoma, or cystadenoma). In these cases, the cyst often has a thickened wall (Fig. 5), and may be deformed along the ovarian capsule by the increased parenchymal pressure from edema. Another useful morphologic finding is the identification of the twisted vascular pedicle.[12] When imaged along the short axis, this can be seen as a heterogeneously echogenic round or beaked "mass" along the margin of the enlarged ovary (Fig. 6). Doppler demonstration of the coiled vessels has been termed as the whirlpool sign.[13]

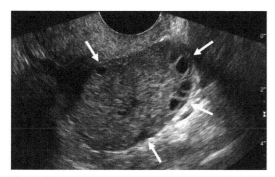

Fig. 4. Edematous ovary due to ovarian torsion. The ovary is enlarged with a "hazy" or "ground glass" appearance of the ovarian parenchyma centrally, and with follicles pushed to the margins of the ovary (*arrows*) by the central stromal edema.

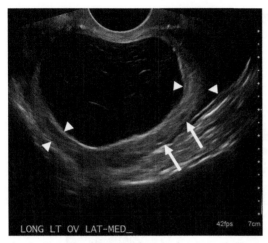

LONG LT OV LAT-MED_   42fps   7cm

Fig. 5. Ovarian torsion with cystadenoma. A 6.5-cm cyst in the left ovary has a thickened wall (*arrowheads*) due to ovarian parenchymal edema. Note visualization of deformed follicles at the edge of the ovary (*arrows*). The cyst proved to be a cystadenoma at pathology.

Pelvic Inflammatory Disease

The clinical presentation of pelvic inflammatory disease (PID) is variable and can mimic other causes of acute pelvic pain. Systemic signs of infection, such as fever and elevated white blood cell count, and pertinent physical examination findings, such as mucopurulent cervical discharge, leukorrhea, and cervical motion tenderness, can help to raise PID as a diagnostic consideration, but these features are not always present or reliable.[14] Pelvic ultrasound is not needed to make the diagnosis, but is often used when the clinical diagnosis is uncertain. Although transvaginal ultrasound has limited ability to diagnose acute PID,[15] the sonographic features of PID are important to recognize.[16]

The sonographic findings associated with the fallopian tubes are the most important features of

PID that help to distinguish this condition from ovarian hemorrhage and ovarian torsion. As the tube and mesosalpinx become increasingly inflamed, they become edematous and hyperemic with thickening of the endosalpingeal folds. This tubal and mesosalpingeal edema may initially be distinct from the ovary, and hyperemia shown with color Doppler imaging distinguishes this tissue from a paraovarian clot that may be seen in some cases of ovarian hemorrhage with a leaking corpus luteum (**Fig. 7**). If the tube fills with fluid, it often has echoes, which can make the presence of the fluid subtle (see **Fig. 7**); when recognized, it often has a characteristic tubular configuration that may exhibit incomplete "septi" (thickened folds seen in the long axis) and the "cog wheel sign" (thickened folds in cross-section)[17] (**Fig. 8**).

With progression, the inflammation involves the ovary, such that the margin of the ovary is no longer distinguishable from the tube and mesosalpinx (**Fig. 9**). At this stage, the sonographic findings become more confusing, indistinguishable on imaging from an ovarian malignancy, appearing as an adnexal mass with poorly identified margins, usually with locules of fluid containing echoes. The terminology for the adnexal inflammatory process is confusing.[18–20] Some reserve the term "tuboovarian abscess" for the case where an encapsulated collection of pus is evident, but others point out that these inflammatory collections are often multiloculated. The term "tuboovarian complex" was coined to convey the heterogeneous nature of the inflammatory process when a clearly defined pus collection is not evident, but others reserve that term for when the inflammation does not involve the ovary. In most cases, "tuboovarian phlegmon" would probably more accurately convey the heterogeneity of the composition of the inflamed tissue, but historically this term has not been used. In practice, not all tuboovarian "abscesses" require percutaneous or surgical drainage, as these can respond to antibiotic treatment.

WOMEN WITH RECURRENT OR CHRONIC SYMPTOMS
Endometriosis, Endometriomas, and Deeply Infiltrating Endometriosis

Endometriosis, the proliferation of endometrial tissue outside the uterus, is a common condition affecting up to 45% of women and is found in as many as 80% of women with chronic pelvic pain at laparoscopy.[21–23] Because the definitive diagnosis of endometriosis is made at laparoscopy, the delay between the onset of symptoms and the diagnosis is typically 7 years or longer.[24–26]

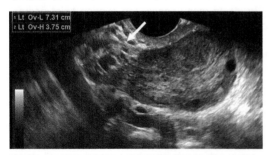

1 Lt Ov-L 7.31 cm
2 Lt Ov-H 3.75 cm

Fig. 6. Ovarian torsion with twisted vascular pedicle. The heterogeneously echogenic round "mass" (*arrow*) along the margin of the enlarged ovary is the twisted vascular pedicle.

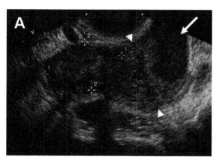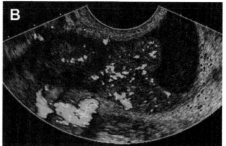

Fig. 7. Tuboovarian complex in a patient with pelvic inflammatory disease. EVUS (A) shows an adnexal abnormality in which the ovary (calipers) is still distinguishable from the adjacent inflamed tube and mesosalpinx (arrowheads). The arrow points to a collection of fluid with echoes in the fallopian tube. Color Doppler ultrasound of the mass (B) shows hyperemia in the inflamed tube and mesosalpinx.

There are no highly specific imaging markers of superficial endometriosis. However, the presence of ovarian endometriomas or deeply invasive endometriosis (DIE) implants allow confident imaging diagnosis. Defined as endometriosis invading 5 mm or deeper into the peritoneal surface, DIE is associated with more severe pelvic pain.[27,28]

Endometriomas typically present as cystic structures that are occasionally multilocular and contain homogeneous, low-level (ground glass) internal echoes. When multiple cysts or multiple loculations of a cyst are noted, one can expect some variation in the overall level of echogenicity between the cysts.[29] Color or power Doppler flow should be used to demonstrate absence of flow within the cystic components. Echogenic wall foci are sometimes observed, and their presence increases the specificity of the ultrasound diagnosis.

Occasionally, tumefactive debris within an endometrioma may mimic the appearance of solid, nodular components (Fig. 10).[29] Lack of Doppler signal in solid components may suggest the correct diagnosis of endometrioma, provided that Doppler settings are adjusted to their most sensitive (color gain increased and scale decreased). One should view any solid-appearing areas with suspicion, because there is small chance of malignant change, particularly to endometrioid or clear-cell ovarian carcinoma.[30] Rarely, solid areas adjacent to the wall representing nodular fibrosis can simulate neoplasm with color flow in the solid area (Fig. 11). In addition, flow is detected between loculations in some multiloculated endometriomas with extensive adhesions or prior rupture.[29]

Overlap with the appearance of functional hemorrhagic cyst can occur. Follow-up imaging, usually after 8 weeks, can demonstrate the persistence of endometrioma. The presence of an endometrioma should prompt a search for DIE, with particular attention to the uterosacral ligaments and rectosigmoid colon because implants in these areas are commonly associated.[31,32]

Cystic ovarian neoplasms, especially benign mucinous cystadenoma, can occasionally

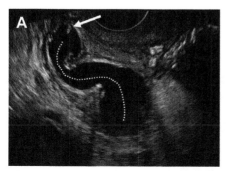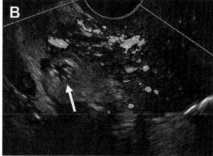

Fig. 8. Pyosalpinx. The thick-walled fallopian tube (A) in this patient has accumulated fluid, leading to a characteristic tubular configuration (dotted line), and allowing for demonstration of thickened endosalpingeal folds, which appear as incomplete septations (arrow) when imaged in longitudinal plane. When the thick-walled fallopian tube in this patient is imaged in cross-section (B), the presence of fluid in the tube allows for visualization of the "cog wheel" sign (arrow). Note the hyperemia of the mesosalpinx with color Doppler imaging.

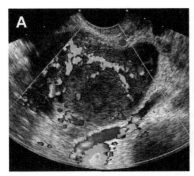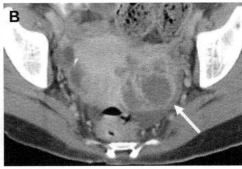

Fig. 9. Tuboovarian abscess. The advanced inflammatory process involving the left fallopian tube and ovary in this patient results in loss of definition of structural margins, such that the ovary and tube are indistinguishable on this color Doppler EVUS (*A*). Computed tomographic imaging (*B*) shows the inflamed enlarged adnexal tissue with avascular locules of fluid (*arrow*).

simulate the appearance of endometrioma with low-level echoes. In addition, a complex appearance can be seen in endometriomas that undergo decidualization during pregnancy. These may present as a growing cystic mass with nodular, vascularized papillations, simulating a neoplasm.[33] Knowledge of this diagnosis, along with MR observation of solid tissue closely following the signal characteristics of decidualized endometrium, may allow observation and obviate unnecessary surgical intervention in these cases.[34]

The ultrasound diagnosis of DIE is well established. Unfortunately, American College of Radiology and American Institute of Ultrasound in Medicine guidelines do not include compulsory images of the most common locations for DIE. Transvaginal sonography demonstrates very good accuracy for the detection of DIE in the pelvis, even with modest training.[35–40] Deeply invasive endometriosis presents as solid, typically nodular hypoechoic tissue involving the bowel, most commonly the rectosigmoid colon and uterosacral ligaments.[41] The surrounding fibrotic response frequently creates irregularity and spiculation of DIE masses. The fibrotic response, which may or may not show glandular elements at histology, is often not as hypoechoic as bowel wall nodules (**Fig. 12**). Tapering ends are commonly observed in bowel wall lesions (**Fig. 13**).[42] Occasional bright echoes are also typical (see **Figs. 12** and **19**).[43] Unlike endometriomas, these echogenic foci are not limited to the periphery of the lesion.

Masses involving the rectum show thickening of the anterior bowel wall. An hourglass configuration is observed when the bowel lesion has adjacent infiltration and fibrosis, commonly the retrocervical area (**Fig. 14**). The bowel may be curved and tethered inward into a C-shape or ε-shape (**Fig. 15**). This is the sonographic equivalent of the

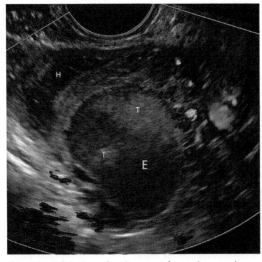

Fig. 10. Color Doppler image of ovarian endometrioma (E) with tumefactive debris (T). A collapsing hemorrhagic cyst is also present (H).

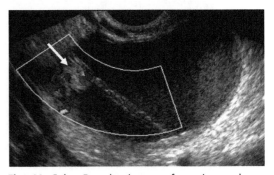

Fig. 11. Color Doppler image of ovarian endometrioma with nodule and septation demonstrating internal flow (*arrow*). These nodules can be fibrotic or related to deformed adjacent ovarian parenchyma.

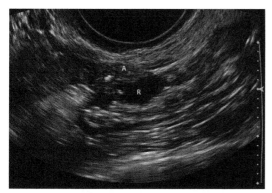

Fig. 12. Endovaginal image of rectal wall DIE (R) with fibrotic endometriotic adhesion (A). Both areas demonstrate hyperechoic internal foci (*red arrows*). The rectal wall component is more hypoechoic.

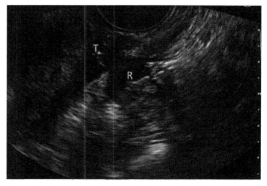

Fig. 14. Hourglass-shaped DIE nodule with torus uterinus/uterosacral ligament component (T) and rectal wall component (R). These are bound by an adhesive isthmus (*red arrows*).

mushroom cap sign on MR imaging. The depth of bowel wall invasion can be predicted by observing the inner and outer layers of the hypoechoic muscularis propria. Disruption of the echogenic connective tissue band between the layers is taken as evidence of invasion to the inner muscularis propria. Irregularity of the interface between the inner muscularis propria and the echogenic submucosa is evidence of submucosal invasion.[44] Mucosal invasion is rare; therefore, most bowel involvement is occult on endoscopy.[45]

The size and extent of DIE lesions significantly change surgical management. Sonographic reporting should include an estimation of the length of the segment or segments involved, length of any skip segments, degree of luminal stenosis, and the percentage of the circumference of the bowel loop involved.[46] When the bowel is curved by a DIE mass, it is appropriate to use a curved measurement tool for the length, in order not to underestimate the true length of bowel involved (**Fig. 16**).

Tenderness directed scanning can aid the detection of DIE lesions.[47] Other less-common but important DIE sites include the urinary bladder and other bowel segments, especially the ileum and appendix, rectovaginal septum, and vagina.[41] Vaginal lesions may be better observed by instillation of 20 mL or more of ultrasound gel into the posterior vaginal fornix before insertion of the endovaginal transducer (**Fig. 17**).[48]

Although most superficial endometriosis is not sonographically visualized with adequate sensitivity, markers for endometriosis may suggest the presence of adhesions caused by superficial endometriosis or DIE, even if implants are not directly imaged. Peritoneal implants with adhesions are thought to be more prevalent than endometriomas.[49] Gentle ballottement using the endovaginal transducer on the cervix in the anterior vaginal fornix elicits the uterine sliding sign. Free sliding of rectosigmoid colon and surrounding adipose tissue with respect to the posterior

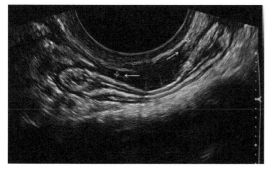

Fig. 13. Rectal wall DIE shows tapering ends (*yellow arrows*) and smooth interface with the submucosa (*red arrows*), indicating absence of submucosal invasion.

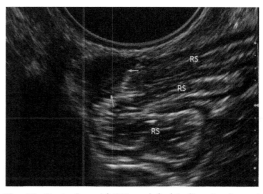

Fig. 15. Rectosigmoid DIE nodule binding 3 adjacent segments of the rectosigmoid colon (RS) into a ε-shape.

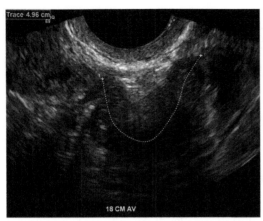

Fig. 16. Curved measurement tool more accurately estimates the length of the sigmoid colon affected by DIE. Lengths exceeding 3 cm often require segmental surgical resection.

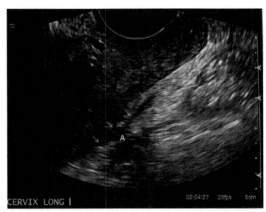

Fig. 18. Image from a cine clip performed to elicit the uterine sliding sign, which was negative, indicating cul-de-sac obliteration. The transducer tip is in the anterior vaginal fornix and attention is focused on the retrocervical (torus uterinus) region. Green arrows depict endometriotic plaque with adhesion (*A*) to a rectal DIE mass (*red arrows*).

uterine serosa is expected in the absence of adhesions. Attention is focused on the serosal interface, primarily near the cervicouterine junction (**Fig. 18**).[50,51] The torus uterinus, located near the posterior cervicouterine junction, where the uterosacral ligaments meet in the midline, should be imaged for nodular or plaque-like endometriotic implants.[43]

Lack of free motion (negative uterine sliding sign) indicates obliteration of the posterior cul-de-sac and should prompt further sonographic or MR interrogation of the rectosigmoid colon and uterosacral ligaments. In addition, manual suprapubic pressure with the non-scanning hand can elicit the sliding sign. Similar ballottement can

elucidate adhesions in other areas, including the uterine fundus, and posterior and trigone areas of the urinary bladder and adnexa.[52] Sometimes adhesions can be directly observed as variable echogenicity bars or bands of tissue tethering segments of the bowel or the bladder to adjacent structures. Adhesive bands may bind the ovaries together low in the posterior cul-de-sac (kissing ovaries) or may occur between the ovaries and the uterus, pelvic sidewall, or adjacent bowel segments (**Fig. 19**). Hypoechoic bars of tissue may be observed between the anterior uterine serosa and posterior bladder wall. The presence of adhesions, particularly in patients with pelvic pain and no history of PID or abdominopelvic surgery, should prompt further clinical, imaging, or surgical investigation of endometriosis.

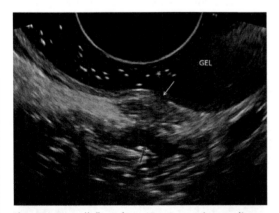

Fig. 17. A small (less than 15 mm maximum dimension) rectovaginal septum recurrence of DIE with extension to the vaginal mucosa (*yellow arrow*) is only depicted with copious gel in the vagina (GEL). The lesion had been occult on MR and routine EVUS, which the patient tolerated poorly because of severe pain on probe insertion.

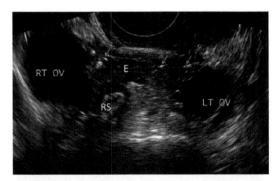

Fig. 19. Transverse image of right and left ovaries, bound together low in the posterior cul-de-sac by a fibrotic endometriotic adhesion (*E*). Several bright foci are noted (*green arrows*). An adjacent cross-section of the rectosigmoid colon (RS) is also tethered.

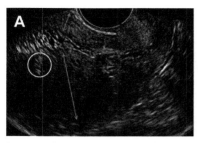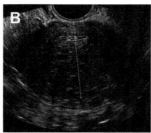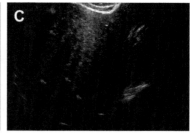

Fig. 20. Adenomyosis. Longitudinal image of the uterus (*A*) demonstrates asymmetric thickening of the posterior myometrium (*blue arrows*). There is an echogenic island of adenomyosis (*yellow circle*) but discrete, anechoic cysts (*red arrows*) clinch the diagnosis. An incidental endometrial polyp (P) is also present. Transverse image (*B*) showing asymmetric posterior myometrial thickening (*blue arrows*). Longitudinal image (*C*) demonstrates alternating, radiating hyperechoic and hypoechoic striations (*red arrows*).

Adenomyosis

Adenomyosis represents the abnormal proliferation of endometrial glandular and stromal elements within the uterine myometrium, resulting in hypertrophy and hyperplasia in the surrounding myometrium. Adenomyosis is associated with abnormal menstrual and intermenstrual bleeding and may present with pelvic pain, particularly dysmenorrhea and chronic pelvic pain. It is present in 20% to 35% of hysterectomy specimens following surgical removal for benign conditions.[53,54]

The ultrasound diagnosis can present a challenge. The sonographic appearance of focal, nodular adenomyosis (adenomyoma) may be similar to uterine leiomyoma and the definitive diagnosis is only made at hysterectomy. Fortunately, endovaginal sonography can still make the diagnosis with good sensitivity and specificity.[55]

Adenomyosis infiltrating the uterus may create globular enlargement or asymmetric thickening of the anterior or posterior myometrium. Isolated or clustered small anechoic cysts are highly specific (**Fig. 20**). Alternating, radiating striations of hyperechogenicity and hypoechogenicity simulating light streaming through a Venetian blind may be observed (see **Fig. 20**). This criterion should be applied only when a distinct mass is not visible, because leiomyomas also may create a striated appearance. In addition, this appearance can be mimicked by enlarged arcuate vessels, but color imaging of vascular flow and the anatomic distribution of vessels in the mid myometrium should easily distinguish vessels from cystic changes.

Hyperechoic islets in the myometrium are occasionally observed (see **Fig. 20**). Echogenic lines and buds may be seen in the junctional zone.[56] These should not be confused with very bright echoes in the immediate subendometrium, which are not typically of clinical relevance and may be seen with prior instrumentation.[57] Adenomyosis may result in irregularity, thickening, or ill-definition of the junctional zone. Thickening of the junctional myometrium greater than 8 mm or excessive variation in the thickness greater than 4 mm, detected on 3D ultrasound, have also been proposed as criteria.[58] Fixed retroflexion of the uterus is also strongly associated with adenomyosis.[59]

Leiomyomas are benign tumors in which smooth muscle elements proliferate, pushing on the normal myometrium and creating a

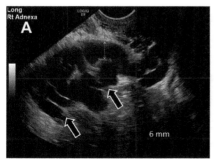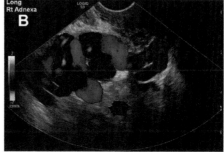

Fig. 21. Pelvic venous congestion: dilated serpiginous venous channels (*A, arrows*) in the adnexa are consistent with dilated veins. Color Doppler (*B*) shows reflux within the veins on Valsalva.

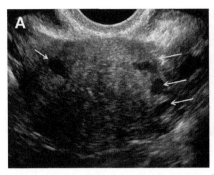
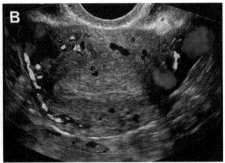

Fig. 22. Pelvic venous congestion. Transverse image of the uterus (*A*) show anechoic peripherally placed dilated arcuate veins (*arrows*) in a patient with pelvic congestion. Color Doppler (*B*) confirms the vascular nature of the anechoic areas.

pseudocapsule. They demonstrate a well-defined border and peripheral color flow, whereas adenomyomas demonstrate less mass effect and are ill defined, with diffuse and central color flow, owing to the interspersion of glandular elements within the myometrium.[55] Therefore, the addition of color flow imaging can improve the discrimination of adenomyoma from leiomyoma.[60] The differentiation is important, because it may affect the surgical approach. When the diagnosis of adenomyoma is in doubt, or when adenomyosis and leiomyomas are suspected to coexist, MR correlation may be helpful to distinguish these entities.[61] When reporting the presence of adenomyosis, it is useful to the surgeon to describe whether the involvement is diffuse or focal, its location and size or thickness, as well as its relationship to the uterine cavity.

WOMEN WITH PELVIC PAIN WITH ALTERNATIVE CONSIDERATIONS
Pelvic Congestion Syndrome

Pelvic congestion syndrome (PCS) has remained a challenging diagnosis by ultrasound, and usually one of exclusion. Pelvic congestion syndrome is defined as a condition in which pelvic varicosities cause chronic pelvic pain in women, postulated by way of mass effect on adjacent nerves or episodes of thrombosis and associated inflammatory changes. Sonographers often obtain images of dilated adnexal veins, but these images do not usually have all the needed information to suggest the diagnosis. When physicians cognizant of PCS participate in sonographic imaging, the likelihood of making the diagnosis is higher.

There are some predisposing factors for PCS. A history of multiple pregnancies is associated with PCS, likely secondary to venous distention during pregnancy with valve dysfunction.[62] Anatomic variations such as retro aortic left renal vein can also be a contributing cause. The compression of left

renal vein between the aorta and the superior mesenteric artery (nutcracker syndrome) can lead to engorgement of ovarian veins and cause the syndrome. Compression of the left common iliac vein between the right common iliac artery and the pelvic brim/spine (May-Thurner syndrome) is a known cause of pelvic varices. In rare cases, a renal malignancy that has invaded the renal vein can cause left pelvic varices.

When clinically suspected, endovaginal ultrasound evaluation of the pelvis is performed as an initial imaging test, in part to first exclude other causes of pelvic pain. The following criteria have been used for the diagnosis of PCS by ultrasound[63–66]:

1. Tortuous parametrial/adnexal pelvic veins with diameter more than 4 mm (**Fig. 21**)

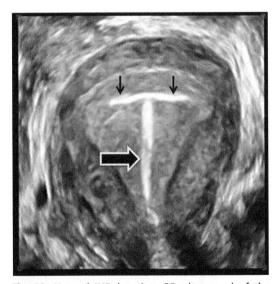

Fig. 23. Normal IUD location: 3D ultrasound of the uterus with rendering of the coronal plane on a normally located IUD within the endometrial cavity. The vertical shaft (*block arrow*) and the horizontal limbs (*small arrows*) are well visualized.

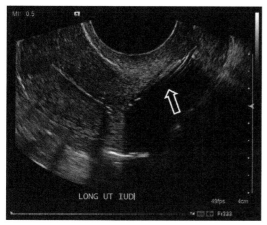

Fig. 24. Malposition of an IUD. Sagittal image of the uterus shows the IUD (*arrow*) in lower uterine segment.

2. Tortuous and dilated arcuate veins in myometrium that communicate with the varicose veins in the adnexa (**Fig. 22**)
3. Slow blood flow (>3 cm/s) or reversal of blood flow in the left ovarian vein, with/without Valsalva maneuver
4. Fifty percent of women have clusters of cysts in ovaries. This polycystic appearance of ovaries is not associated with hirsutism or amenorrhea.

Attention to endovaginal ultrasound technique when evaluating for adnexal varices is important because pressure from the transducer can compress the varicosities and mask the sonographic findings. Color Doppler must be used to differentiate dilated venous channels from non-

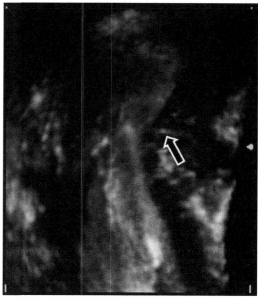

Fig. 26. Malposition of an IUD. Coronal plane of 3D ultrasound shows the horizontal limb of the IUD embedded in the myometrium (*arrow*).

vascular similar appearing structures such as dilated fallopian tubes, the ureter, or elongated cysts. Once ultrasound suggests the diagnosis, MR imaging is often a preferred additional test used by the interventional radiologist who wants to evaluate the morphology of the veins to determine treatment choices.[67]

Malposition of an Intrauterine Contraceptive Device

An intrauterine contraceptive device (IUD) is a common form of contraception around the world. Once an IUD has been inserted, one usually can

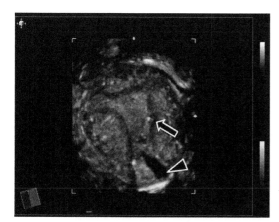

Fig. 25. Malposition of an IUD. Coronal plane of 3D ultrasound shows one of the horizontal limbs of the IUD extending beyond the endometrial cavity penetrating the myometrium. The vertical limb of the IUD is rendered as a dark shadow (*arrowhead*) in the cervical area of the uterus.

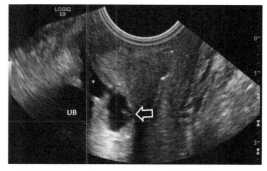

Fig. 27. Urethral diverticulum: voiding introital ultrasound shows urine in the bladder (UB) and in the urethra (*asterisk*). The arrow shows the outpouching behind the urethra that represents the urethral diverticulum.

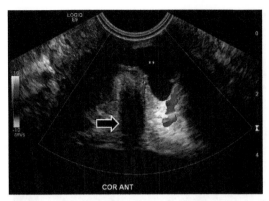

Fig. 28. Urethral diverticulum: coronal 2D image of the urethra (*arrow*) shows a diverticulum (*double asterisk*) posteriorly.

visualize the retrieval string protruding from the external os of the cervix on physical inspection. Non-visualization of the string is a common indication to use ultrasound to check the position of the IUD. Pelvic pain or dyspareunia is another important indication for evaluating the position of the IUD and its configuration.

A normally placed IUD is relatively easy to demonstrate on ultrasound, although the newer levonorgestrel-releasing IUDs are less readily apparent than the older copper-containing IUDs.[68] The straight stem of the IUD is identified along the length of the endometrial cavity. The horizontal limbs extending toward the cornua are better demonstrated using 3D ultrasound in the coronal plane, but can be traced from the IUD shaft on cine clip images.

Most of the IUD should be located in the fundus and body of the uterus (**Fig. 23**). The retrieval string can sometimes be demonstrated extending through the cervical canal. If the IUD stem is centered in the lower uterine segment or in the cervix, it is clearly malpositioned (**Fig. 24**). Demonstrating malposition of an IUD has become significantly easier following widespread use of

3D ultrasound. Reformatting the uterus in the coronal plane helps to evaluate the position of the IUD and the relationship of the shaft and the horizontal limbs of the IUD to the endometrial cavity. These 3D images also facilitate visualization of embedment of the IUD arms or stem into the myometrium (**Figs. 25** and **26**).

A displaced IUD may be asymptomatic; however, if any part of the IUD is embedded in the myometrium, the likelihood of pain or bleeding increases. In a study by Benacerraf and colleagues,[69] of the 21 patients with an abnormally located IUD who presented with pelvic pain or bleeding, 20 reported improvement in symptoms following removal of the IUD. This clearly indicates the importance of making the diagnosis of a malpositioned IUD or where components of the IUD are embedded in the myometrium.

Non-gynecologic Causes of Pain

There are many non-gynecological conditions that can present with pelvic pain.[70,71] Some of these are related to intraperitoneal structures, but abdominal wall and musculoskeletal conditions can also present with pelvic pain. A short list of non-gynecological causes for pelvic pain would include:

1. Urinary tract infection (may or may not be associated with urethral diverticulum)
2. Acute appendicitis
3. Acute ileitis/colitis/diverticulitis
4. Distal ureteric calculus
5. Hernia
6. Intestinal Obstruction
7. Musculoskeletal causes

Although one could easily devote a chapter to each of these possible causes of pelvic pain, a limited discussion follows.

Urinary tract infection, especially interstitial cystitis, can present with acute or episodic pelvic

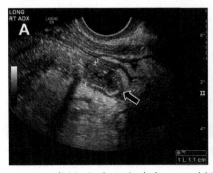
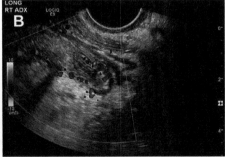

Fig. 29. Acute appendicitis. Endovaginal ultrasound (*A*) shows a thickened appendix of more than 6 mm in anteroposterior dimension (between cursors). Note the blind ending tubal shape (*arrow*) of the appendix. Doppler (*B*) shows increased vascularity within the walls of the thickened appendix.

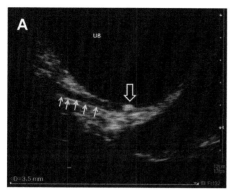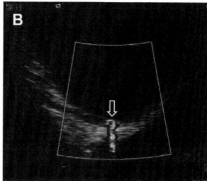

Fig. 30. Ureteral calculus: oblique transabdominal ultrasound (*A*) through the urinary bladder (UB) shows a small hyperechoic calculus impacted at the ureterovesical junction (*block arrow*) with a dilated ureter (*small arrows*) more proximally. Doppler (*B*) demonstrates twinkle artifact.

pain. Recurrent cystitis can also be secondary to a urethral or urinary diverticulum. Whereas bladder diverticula are easily detected as outpouchings from the bladder wall, urethral diverticula are more difficult to detect and require special techniques. Usually the female urethra can be sonographically evaluated with the endovaginal transducer placed at the introitus and angled anteriorly to lay out the urethra as a hypoechoic linear structure. A urethral diverticulum is seen as a fluid-filled structure adjacent to the urethra that may or may not show an obvious connection to the urethra (**Figs. 27** and **28**). Sometimes a voiding examination is performed to better identify the diverticulum.[72]

Acute appendicitis is one of the most common causes of acute right lower quadrant pain. Whereas computed tomography is very sensitive in detecting acute appendicitis, transabdominal ultrasound using graded compression is favored by many experts when imaging children and premenopausal women of thin body habitus. In rare cases, a more medially located inflamed appendix may be better visualized using endovaginal ultrasound (**Fig. 29**).

Urolithiasis can be overlooked as a cause of acute pelvic pain in women initially sent for pelvic ultrasound. A calculus in the distal ureter at or near the ureterovesical junction can be seen on both endovaginal examination and transabdominal pelvic ultrasound with a distended bladder. Identification of a distal ureteral calculus is facilitated when the ureter is dilated proximal to the impacted calculus (**Fig. 30**). Color Doppler can be used to look for "twinkling" artifact.

Bowel inflammation secondary to any cause (Crohn's disease, ulcerative colitis, and other gastrointestinal inflammatory processes) can present with acute or episodic pelvic pain. Usually a bowel segment with hypoechoic thickened walls

is noted with increased vascularity. Complicated diverticulitis can lead to abscess formation that involves the adnexal structures, and this may be the initial finding on a pelvic ultrasound (**Fig. 31**).

Abdominal and inguinal hernias can be small and subtle, and should remain in the differential diagnosis of pelvic pain in women. Musculoskeletal causes of pelvic pain can include inguinal strain, muscle or tendon inflammation or tear, sports pubalgia, and, rarely, stress fracture of the pubis. It is important to differentiate superficial causes of pelvic pain from deep causes, and a diligent history can help narrow the area of concern. Linear, high-frequency ultrasound probes are necessary to examine superficial structures. An abnormal fluid collection within a muscle may be a hematoma with an underlying muscle tear. A muscle or tendon tear usually presents as an ill-defined hypoechoic area (**Fig. 32**). Chronic inflammation of adductor tendon (tendinosis) at its insertion on pubic bone can also manifest as chronic pelvic pain.[73]

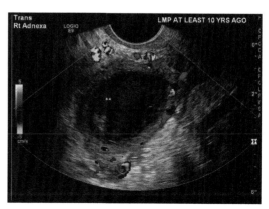

Fig. 31. Adnexal abscess: endovaginal ultrasound demonstrates a collection of fluid (*double asterisk*) with internal echoes consistent with adnexal abscess.

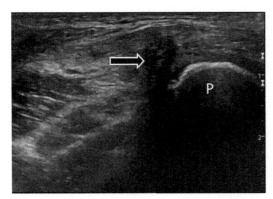

Fig. 32. Tendon tear: small hypoechoic intrasubstance tear (*arrow*) within the adductor tendon at its insertion on the pubic (P) bone.

SUMMARY

Ultrasound plays an important diagnostic role in the evaluation of nonpregnant women with pelvic pain. When the pain is acute, the leading consideration is ovarian hemorrhage, with ovarian torsion and PID as important alternative possibilities. When the pain is episodic, endometriosis and adenomyosis are common considerations, and sonologists play an important role in making these diagnoses, especially in suspecting and diagnosing deeply infiltrating endometriosis. Finally, there are a large variety of other causes of acute or chronic pelvic pain, so when the common gynecologic causes of pain are not identified on sonographic evaluation, careful consideration of other gynecologic and non-gynecologic conditions is important.

REFERENCES

1. Howard FM, Perry P, Carter J, et al. Pelvic pain: diagnosis & management. Philadelphia: Lippincott Williams & Wilkins; 2000.
2. Ahangari A. Prevalence of chronic pelvic pain among women: an updated review. Pain Physician 2014;17(2):E141–7.
3. Bhosale PR, Javitt MC, Atri M, et al. ACR appropriateness criteria® acute pelvic pain in the reproductive age group. Ultrasound Q 2016;32(2):108–15.
4. Patel MD. Practical approach to the adnexal mass. Radiol Clin North Am 2006;44(6):879–99.
5. Patel MD, Feldstein VA, Filly RA. The likelihood ratio of sonographic findings for the diagnosis of hemorrhagic ovarian cysts. J Ultrasound Med 2005;24(5):607–14 [quiz: 15].
6. Patel MD, Feldstein VA, Chen DC, et al. Endometriomas: diagnostic performance of us. Radiology 1999;210(3):739–45.
7. Patel MD. Pitfalls in the sonographic evaluation of adnexal masses. Ultrasound Q 2012;28(1):29–40.
8. Chang HC, Bhatt S, Dogra VS. Pearls and pitfalls in diagnosis of ovarian torsion. Radiographics 2008;28(5):1355–68.
9. Bronstein ME, Pandya S, Snyder CW, et al. A meta-analysis of B-mode ultrasound, Doppler ultrasound, and computed tomography to diagnose pediatric ovarian torsion. Eur J Pediatr Surg 2015;25(1):82–6.
10. Lam A, Nayyar M, Helmy M, et al. Assessing the clinical utility of color Doppler ultrasound for ovarian torsion in the setting of a negative contrast-enhanced CT scan of the abdomen and pelvis. Abdom Imaging 2015;40(8):3206–13.
11. Albayram F, Hamper UM. Ovarian and adnexal torsion: spectrum of sonographic findings with pathologic correlation. J Ultrasound Med 2001;20(10):1083–9.
12. Lee EJ, Kwon HC, Joo HJ, et al. Diagnosis of ovarian torsion with color Doppler sonography: depiction of twisted vascular pedicle. J Ultrasound Med 1998;17(2):83–9.
13. Vijayaraghavan SB. Sonographic whirlpool sign in ovarian torsion. J Ultrasound Med 2004;23(12):1643–9 [quiz: 1650–1].
14. Mitchell C, Prabhu M. Pelvic inflammatory disease: current concepts in pathogenesis, diagnosis and treatment. Infect Dis Clin North Am 2013;27(4):793–809.
15. Romosan G, Valentin L. The sensitivity and specificity of transvaginal ultrasound with regard to acute pelvic inflammatory disease: a review of the literature. Arch Gynecol Obstet 2014;289(4):705–14.
16. Horrow MM. Ultrasound of pelvic inflammatory disease. Ultrasound Q 2004;20(4):171–9.
17. Timor-Tritsch IE, Lerner JP, Monteagudo A, et al. Transvaginal sonographic markers of tubal inflammatory disease. Ultrasound Obstet Gynecol 1998;12(1):56–66.
18. Amstey MS. Definition of pelvic abscess. Am J Obstet Gynecol 1993;168(2):740–1.
19. Monif GR, Osborne NG. Tuboovarian complex versus tuboovarian abscesses. Am J Obstet Gynecol 1993;169(3):751.
20. Nelson GH. Definition of pelvic abscess. Am J Obstet Gynecol 1994;170(1 Pt 1):257.
21. Giudice LC, Kao LC. Endometriosis. Lancet 2004;364(9447):1789–99.
22. Nnoaham KE, Hummelshoj L, Webster P, et al. Impact of endometriosis on quality of life and work productivity: a multicenter study across ten countries. Fertil Steril 2011;96(2):366–73.e8.
23. Rawson JM. Prevalence of endometriosis in asymptomatic women. J Reprod Med 1991;36(7):513–5.
24. Ballard K, Lowton K, Wright J. What's the delay? A qualitative study of women's experiences of reaching a diagnosis of endometriosis. Fertil Steril 2006;86(5):1296–301.

25. Hadfield R, Mardon H, Barlow D, et al. Delay in the diagnosis of endometriosis: a survey of women from the USA and the UK. Hum Reprod 1996; 11(4):878–80.

26. Husby GK, Haugen RS, Moen MH. Diagnostic delay in women with pain and endometriosis. Acta Obstet Gynecol Scand 2003;82(7):649–53.

27. Chapron C, Fauconnier A, Dubuisson JB, et al. Deep infiltrating endometriosis: relation between severity of dysmenorrhoea and extent of disease. Hum Reprod 2003;18(4):760–6.

28. Koninckx PR, Martin D. Treatment of deeply infiltrating endometriosis. Curr Opin Obstet Gynecol 1994;6(3):231–41.

29. Asch E, Levine D. Variations in appearance of endometriomas. J Ultrasound Med 2007;26(8): 993–1002.

00. Krawczyk N, Danys-Paluchowski M, Schmidt D, et al. Endometriosis-associated malignancy. Geburtshilfe Frauenheilkd 2016;76(2):176–81.

31. Kondo W, Ribeiro R, Trippia CH, et al. Association between ovarian endometrioma and deep infiltrating endometriosis. Rev Bras Ginecol Obstet 2012;34(9): 420–4 [in Portuguese].

32. Lazzeri L, Di Giovanni A, Exacoustos C, et al. Preoperative and postoperative clinical and transvaginal ultrasound findings of adenomyosis in patients with deep infiltrating endometriosis. Reprod Sci 2014; 21(8):1027–33.

33. Bailleux M, Bernard JP, Benachi A, et al. Ovarian endometriosis during pregnancy: a series of 53 endometriomas. Eur J Obstet Gynecol Reprod Biol 2017;209:100–4.

34. Poder L, Coakley FV, Rabban JT, et al. Decidualized endometrioma during pregnancy: recognizing an imaging mimic of ovarian malignancy. J Comput Assist Tomogr 2008;32(4):555–8.

35. Guerriero S, Ajossa S, Minguez JA, et al. Accuracy of transvaginal ultrasound for diagnosis of deep endometriosis in uterosacral ligaments, rectovaginal septum, vagina and bladder: systematic review and meta-analysis. Ultrasound Obstet Gynecol 2015; 46(5):534–45.

36. Guerriero S, Ajossa S, Orozco R, et al. Accuracy of transvaginal ultrasound for diagnosis of deep endometriosis in the rectosigmoid: systematic review and meta-analysis. Ultrasound Obstet Gynecol 2016; 47(3):281–9.

37. Hudelist G, English J, Thomas AE, et al. Diagnostic accuracy of transvaginal ultrasound for non-invasive diagnosis of bowel endometriosis: systematic review and meta-analysis. Ultrasound Obstet Gynecol 2011;37(3):257–63.

38. Tammaa A, Fritzer N, Lozano P, et al. Interobserver agreement and accuracy of non-invasive diagnosis of endometriosis by transvaginal sonography. Ultrasound Obstet Gynecol 2015;46(6):737–40.

39. Tammaa A, Fritzer N, Strunk G, et al. Learning curve for the detection of pouch of Douglas obliteration and deep infiltrating endometriosis of the rectum. Hum Reprod 2014;29(6):1199–204.

40. Young SW, Dahiya N, Patel MD, et al. Initial accuracy of and learning curve for transvaginal ultrasound with bowel preparation for deep endometriosis in a US tertiary care center. J Minim Invasive Gynecol 2017;24(7):1170–6.

41. Chapron C, Fauconnier A, Vieira M, et al. Anatomical distribution of deeply infiltrating endometriosis: surgical implications and proposition for a classification. Hum Reprod 2003;18(1):157–61.

42. Benacerraf BR, Groszmann Y, Hornstein MD, et al. Deep infiltrating endometriosis of the bowel wall: the comet sign. J Ultrasound Med 2015;34(3): 537–42.

43. Young SW, Saphier NB, Dahiya N, et al. Sonographic evaluation of deep endometriosis: protocol for a US radiology practice. Abdom Radiol (NY) 2016;41(12): 2364–79.

44. Goncalves MO, Podgaec S, Dias JA Jr, et al. Transvaginal ultrasonography with bowel preparation is able to predict the number of lesions and rectosigmoid layers affected in cases of deep endometriosis, defining surgical strategy. Hum Reprod 2010; 25(3):665–71.

45. Wolthuis AM, Meuleman C, Tomassetti C, et al. Bowel endometriosis: colorectal surgeon's perspective in a multidisciplinary surgical team. World J Gastroenterol 2014;20(42):15616–23.

46. Abrao MS, Petraglia F, Falcone T, et al. Deep endometriosis infiltrating the recto-sigmoid: critical factors to consider before management. Hum Reprod Update 2015;21(3):329–39.

47. Guerriero S, Ajossa S, Gerada M, et al. Diagnostic value of transvaginal 'tenderness-guided' ultrasonography for the prediction of location of deep endometriosis. Hum Reprod 2008;23(11):2452–7.

48. Reid S, Lu C, Hardy N, et al. Office gel sonovaginography for the prediction of posterior deep infiltrating endometriosis: a multicenter prospective observational study. Ultrasound Obstet Gynecol 2014; 44(6):710–8.

49. Redwine DB. Ovarian endometriosis: a marker for more extensive pelvic and intestinal disease. Fertil Steril 1999;72(2):310–5.

50. Hudelist G, Fritzer N, Staettner S, et al. Uterine sliding sign: a simple sonographic predictor for presence of deep infiltrating endometriosis of the rectum. Ultrasound Obstet Gynecol 2013;41(6): 692–5.

51. Reid S, Lu C, Casikar I, et al. Prediction of pouch of Douglas obliteration in women with suspected endometriosis using a new real-time dynamic transvaginal ultrasound technique: the sliding sign. Ultrasound Obstet Gynecol 2013;41(6):685–91.

52. Timor-Tritsch IE. Sliding organs sign in gynecological ultrasound. Ultrasound Obstet Gynecol 2015; 46(1):125–6.

53. Azziz R. Adenomyosis: current perspectives. Obstet Gynecol Clin North Am 1989;16(1):221–35.

54. Devlieger R, D'Hooghe T, Timmerman D. Uterine adenomyosis in the infertility clinic. Hum Reprod Update 2003;9(2):139–47.

55. Chiang CH, Chang MY, Hsu JJ, et al. Tumor vascular pattern and blood flow impedance in the differential diagnosis of leiomyoma and adenomyosis by color Doppler sonography. J Assist Reprod Genet 1999; 16(5):268–75.

56. Van den Bosch T, Dueholm M, Leone FP, et al. Terms, definitions and measurements to describe sonographic features of myometrium and uterine masses: a consensus opinion from the morphological uterus sonographic assessment (MUSA) group. Ultrasound Obstet Gynecol 2015;46(3):284–98.

57. Burks DD, Stainken BF, Burkhard TK, et al. Uterine inner myometrial echogenic foci. Relationship to prior dilatation and curettage and endocervical biopsy. J Ultrasound Med 1991;10(9):487–92.

58. Exacoustos C, Brienza L, Di Giovanni A, et al. Adenomyosis: three-dimensional sonographic findings of the junctional zone and correlation with histology. Ultrasound Obstet Gynecol 2011;37(4):471–9.

59. Di Donato N, Bertoldo V, Montanari G, et al. Question mark form of uterus: a simple sonographic sign associated with the presence of adenomyosis. Ultrasound Obstet Gynecol 2015;46(1):126–7.

60. Sharma K, Bora MK, Venkatesh BP, et al. Role of 3D ultrasound and Doppler in differentiating clinically suspected cases of leiomyoma and adenomyosis of uterus. J Clin Diagn Res 2015;9(4):Qc08–12.

61. Bazot M, Cortez A, Darai E, et al. Ultrasonography compared with magnetic resonance imaging for the diagnosis of adenomyosis: correlation with histopathology. Hum Reprod 2001;16(11):2427–33.

62. Stones RW. Pelvic vascular congestion-half a century later. Clin Obstet Gynecol 2003;46(4):831–6.

63. Beard RW, Highman JH, Pearce S, et al. Diagnosis of pelvic varicosities in women with chronic pelvic pain. Lancet 1984;2(8409):946–9.

64. Coakley FV, Varghese SL, Hricak H. CT and MRI of pelvic varices in women. J Comput Assist Tomogr 1999;23(3):429–34.

65. Osman MW, Nikolopoulos I, Jayaprakasan K, et al. Pelvic congestion syndrome. Obstet Gynaecol 2013;15:151–7.

66. Park SJ, Lim JW, Ko YT, et al. Diagnosis of pelvic congestion syndrome using transabdominal and transvaginal sonography. AJR Am J Roentgenol 2004;182(3):683–8.

67. Ignacio EA, Dua R, Sarin S, et al. Pelvic congestion syndrome: diagnosis and treatment. Semin Intervent Radiol 2008;25(1):361–8.

68. Boortz HE, Margolis DJ, Ragavendra N, et al. Migration of intrauterine devices: radiologic findings and implications for patient care. Radiographics 2012; 32(2):335–52.

69. Benacerraf BR, Shipp TD, Bromley B. Three-dimensional ultrasound detection of abnormally located intrauterine contraceptive devices which are a source of pelvic pain and abnormal bleeding. Ultrasound Obstet Gynecol 2009;34(1):110–5.

70. Karnath BM, Breitkopf DM. Acute and chronic pelvic pain in women. Hosp Physician 2007;43(7):41–8.

71. Shaaban AM, Rezvani M, Olpin JD, et al. Nongynecologic findings seen at pelvic US. Radiographics 2017;37(7):2045–62.

72. Singla P, Long SS, Long CM, et al. Imaging of the female urethral diverticulum. Clin Radiol 2013;68(7): e418–25.

73. Pesquer L, Reboul G, Silvestre A, et al. Imaging of adductor-related groin pain. Diagn Interv Imaging 2015;96(9):861–9.

Ultrasound of the First Trimester

Peter S. Wang, MD*, Shuchi K. Rodgers, MD, Mindy M. Horrow, MD

KEYWORDS

- Ultrasound • Pregnancy • First trimester • Ectopic pregnancy

KEY POINTS

- After the diagnosis of pregnancy via a positive β-hCG, TVUS is the imaging modality of choice in the first trimester to characterize the implantation location and viability of the gestation as well as to evaluate complications such as retained products or molar pregnancy.
- High-quality imaging in experienced hands will result in the highest rate of visualized EP and IUP and the lowest rates of PUL. Interpreting physicians should use clear terminology in their interpretations to avoid misunderstandings with their clinical colleagues.

 Video content accompanies this article at http://www.radiologic.theclinics.com.

INTRODUCTION

Serum beta human chorionic gonadotropin (β-hCG) is the most sensitive pregnancy test, becoming positive 6 to 12 days after ovulation. However, a single positive β-hCG value assesses neither the location nor the morphology and potential outcome of the pregnancy. Ultrasound (US) is the imaging study of choice for detection and full characterization of early pregnancies based on its accuracy, low cost, safety profile, and abundant availability. This article reviews the goals and utility of first-trimester ultrasound in gestation localization, viability determination, and abnormal pregnancies, including ectopic implantation, retained products, and molar pregnancy.

NORMAL INTRAUTERINE PREGNANCY

Sonographic confirmation of an early first-trimester intrauterine pregnancy (IUP) is based on the detection of an intrauterine gestational sac. The gestational sac typically appears as a small round or ovoid fluid collection within a decidualized endometrium and is visible on ultrasound as early as 4 to 5 weeks of gestation.[1] Two sonographic appearances have been used to confirm that a small intrauterine fluid collection corresponds to a gestational sac, the double sac sign and the intradecidual sign. The double sac sign appears as 2 concentric echogenic rings around a small fluid collection corresponding to the outer decidua parietalis and inner decidua capsularis surrounding the gestational sac (**Fig. 1**).[2] Before the development of the decidua parietalis and capsularis, the gestational sac can be seen eccentrically located on one side of the uterine cavity in a decidualized endometrium, adjacent to the collapsed endometrial cavity. This corresponds to the intradecidual sign on ultrasound (**Fig. 2**).[3] However, both signs have poor interobserver agreement and the signs are often absent when early pregnancies are detected with modern sonographic equipment.[2] In fact, more than 99% of small intrauterine endometrial fluid collections in pregnant women result in IUPs, regardless of the presence or absence of either sign (**Fig. 3**).[2]

The yolk sac functions in maternal-fetal exchange, is the first structure to develop in the

Department of Radiology, Einstein Medical Center, 5501 Old York Road, Philadelphia, PA 19141, USA
* Corresponding author.
E-mail address: wangp@einstein.edu

Radiol Clin N Am 57 (2019) 617–633
https://doi.org/10.1016/j.rcl.2019.01.006
0033-8389/19/© 2019 Elsevier Inc. All rights reserved.

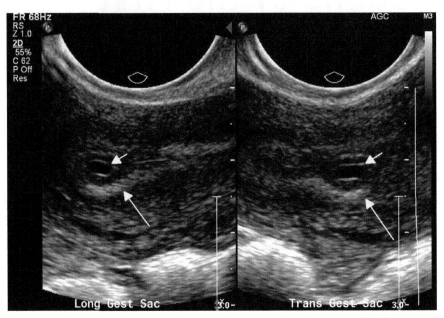

Fig. 1. Double sac sign. Sagittal and transverse images of the uterus showing a gestational sac surrounded by inner (*short arrows*) and outer echogenic rims (*long arrows*) corresponding to the decidua capsularis and parietalis, respectively.

gestational sac, and its visualization definitively confirms a pregnancy. On ultrasound, the yolk sac can be seen at 5.5 weeks of gestation as a round cystic structure with a thin echogenic rim located eccentrically in the gestational sac (**Fig. 4**A).[1] In early pregnancy, the rim is often incompletely visualized and only the anterior and posterior walls are visible as parallel echogenic lines (**Fig. 4**B). The embryo usually becomes visible on ultrasound at 6 weeks of gestation and typically appears as a featureless ovoid echogenic structure adjacent to the yolk sac (**Fig. 5**).[1]

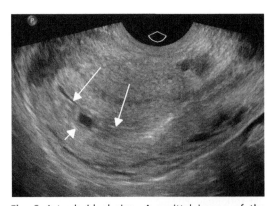

Fig. 2. Intradecidual sign. A sagittal image of the uterus demonstrating a gestational sac with a single echogenic rim (*short arrow*) located eccentrically from the collapsed endometrial cavity (*long arrows*).

After 7 weeks, a thin faintly echogenic amniotic membrane may be visible around the embryo (**Fig. 6**). The embryo, amniotic sac, and gestational sac grow proportionally until 10 weeks of gestation when the amniotic sac enlarges faster because of fetal urine production.[4] Cardiac activity may be seen when the embryo is visible with crown-rump lengths (CRLs) as small as 1 to 2 mm, but the lack of detectable cardiac activity with CRLs less than 7 mm may be due to differences in equipment and imaging techniques (Video 1).[5] At 7 to 8 weeks, the spine can be visualized, and, at approximately 8 weeks, the head becomes a distinct structure and the limb buds are visible (**Fig. 7**).[5,6] At 8 to 10 weeks, an anechoic round structure develops in the head representing the rhombencephalon as the developing hindbrain (see **Fig. 7**).[7]

During the first trimester, the most accurate measurement for gestational age determination is the CRL, which is the length of the embryo from the head to the buttocks. In the absence of an embryo, the mean sac diameter (MSD) may be used as a substitute for gestational age calculation. The gestational age obtained from ultrasound is calculated from the first day of the patient's last menstrual period and differs from the histologic gestational age, which is based on conception that occurs 2 weeks after the last menstrual period.

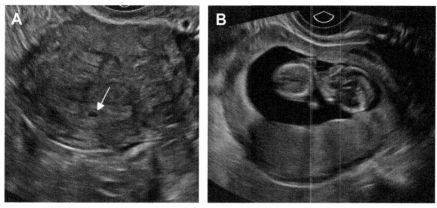

Fig. 3. (*A*) Transverse image of the uterus demonstrating a small round empty fluid-filled structure, which is most likely an early gestational sac (*arrow*) and should not be considered a "pseudogestational sac." (B) Follow-up ultrasound 2 months later shows a developing embryo.

Determination of chorionicity and amnionicity in multiple gestations is important for risk stratification and is best performed with transvaginal ultrasound (TVUS) in the first trimester. Chorionicity is easily and accurately assessed because the number of chorions is equal to the number of gestational sacs.[8,9] Amnionicity determination for monochorionic twins is crucial because mortality rates for monoamniotic pregnancies are as high as 64%.[9] The older literature concluded that the number of yolk sacs equaled the number of amnions.[10] Because a more recent analysis of 97 pregnancies found that the number of yolk sacs did not correlate with the number of amnions in 9.3% of monochorionic pregnancies, conclusive determination of amnionicity should wait until the eighth week of pregnancy when the amniotic membranes are clearly visualized.[11,12]

ABNORMAL FIRST-TRIMESTER PREGNANCY
Intrauterine Pregnancy Failure

The sonographic appearance and visualization of early first-trimester structures in a normal IUP occur in a consistent, well-established order. Deviation from this sequence raises the possibility of a failing or failed pregnancy. Although several discriminatory values to indicate pregnancy failure were previously established, more recent studies have shown that these values may result in the false-positive diagnosis of pregnancy failure.[13,14] In 2012, the Society of Radiologists in Ultrasound consensus panel published more conservative criteria to establish thresholds at which pregnancy failure is an absolute certainty rather than a high probability, because incorrectly diagnosing a nonviable or failed pregnancy may result in

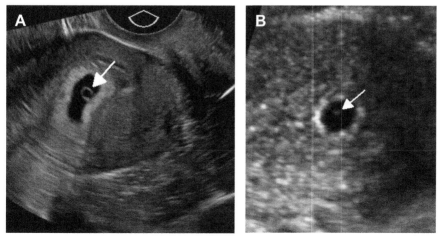

Fig. 4. (*A*) The yolk sac typically appears as a small round cystic structure with an echogenic rim (*arrow*). (*B*) Occasionally, the complete echogenic rim is not completely visible and only a portion of the wall is seen (*arrow*).

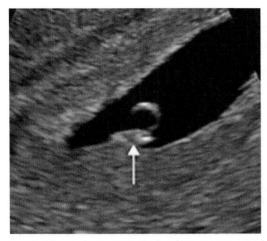

Fig. 5. The embryo (*arrow*) develops as an ovoid featureless echogenic structure adjacent to the yolk sac.

surgical or medical management that irreversibly harms an IUP.[15]

The consensus TVUS criteria diagnostic of pregnancy failure include:

- No cardiac activity when CRL is ≥7 mm
- No cardiac activity ≥2 weeks after demonstrating a gestational sac without a yolk sac
- No cardiac activity ≥11 days after demonstrating a gestational sac and a yolk sac
- No embryo when MSD is ≥25 mm

Consensus TVUS criteria for findings suspicious for pregnancy failure include (these findings should not be considered diagnostic of pregnancy failure):

- No cardiac activity when CRL is <7 mm
- No cardiac activity 7 to 13 days after demonstrating a gestational sac without a yolk sac

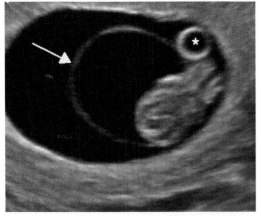

Fig. 6. The amniotic sac (*arrow*) appears as a thin round echogenic structure around the embryo and adjacent to the yolk sac (*asterisk*).

- No cardiac activity 7 to 10 days after demonstrating a gestational sac with a yolk sac
- No embryo when MSD is 16 to 24 mm
- No embryo ≥6 weeks after the last menstrual period
- Empty amnion
- Enlarged yolk sac (>7 mm)
- Discordant gestational sac and embryo sizes for gestational age (<5 mm difference between MSD and CRL)

In addition, the abnormal morphologic appearance of early first-trimester structures may also raise the possibility of a poor pregnancy outcome and include:[5]

- A gestational sac that has irregular contours and/or is low-lying in the uterus (**Fig. 8**)
- A calcified or large (>7 mm) yolk sac
- An empty or enlarged amnion (**Fig. 9**)
- An amorphous embryo
- Bradycardia (≤85 beats/min)
- Hydropic changes to the chorionic villi
- Large subchorionic hemorrhage (encircles ≥two-thirds of gestational sac) (**Fig. 10**)
- A "chorionic bump," which appears as a focal convexity of varying echogenicity bulging into the gestational sac[16,17]

As the most sensitive test for early pregnancy, serum β-hCG can be detected before an intrauterine gestational sac is visible on ultrasound. Studies without visualization of an intra- or extrauterine pregnancy or retained products of conception (RPOC) should be labeled pregnancy of unknown location (PUL), which has a differential diagnosis including early IUP, occult ectopic pregnancy (EP), and a spontaneous abortion. Although studies have tried to establish a threshold β-hCG above which an IUP should be visible, even above 3000 mIU/mL, there is still a small chance of a non-visualized viable IUP.[15,18,19] Therefore, although an EP is possible in PUL, in a hemodynamically stable patient, it is more prudent to confirm the diagnosis with serial β-hCG and follow-up ultrasound rather than treating a presumed failed or EP and risk irreparable harm to an IUP (**Table 1**).

Ectopic Pregnancy

The last 35 to 40 years have seen an increased incidence of EP matched by a parallel decrease in morbidity and mortality. The mortality ratio of deaths due to EP per 100,000 live births declined from 1.15 in 1980 to 1984 to 0.5 from 2003 to 2007.[18] Causes for the increased incidence of EP

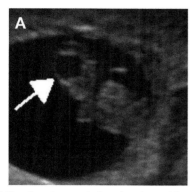
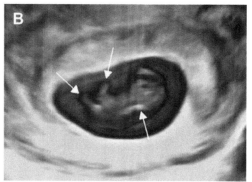

Fig. 7. (*A*) The rhombencephalon develops at 8 to 10 weeks and appears as a cystic structure in the head (*arrow*). (*B*) 3D reformat image of a 9-week embryo demonstrating limb buds (*arrows*).

include increased rates of pelvic inflammatory disease particularly *Chlamydia trachomatis* infection, assisted reproductive technologies and cesarean deliveries. However, nearly half of women with an EP still have no identifiable risk factors, placing EP in the differential diagnosis of any woman with early pregnancy and symptoms of pain and/or bleeding.[19]

In the modern era, the diagnosis of EP is made primarily by TVUS. Although the widespread use of TVUS contributes to the higher diagnostic rate of EP ranging between 1% and 2% of all pregnancies, it also allows for earlier and more patient-specific management. Because EP is diagnosed in 6%–16% of pregnant women presenting to an emergency room with bleeding and/or pain and remains the most common cause of maternal death in the first trimester, radiologists should aim for high-quality TVUS examinations

and interpretations using a standard lexicon. An equally important goal in the modern era is to avoid a false-positive TVUS diagnosis of EP and the inappropriate medical treatment of an early IUP.

Ectopic pregnancy is defined as any pregnancy implanted outside the endometrial cavity, the majority of which (93%–98%) are in the non-interstitial portion of the fallopian tube. The US diagnosis requires visualization of an extra-ovarian adnexal mass, not merely the absence of an IUP. The rate of visualization of EP using TVUS varies based primarily on the experience and quality of the imager, but is also affected by body habitus, patient cooperation, and the size and position of the uterus. A meta-analysis by Kirk and colleagues,[20] reported the sensitivity and specificity of TVUS for EP in experienced laboratories ranged

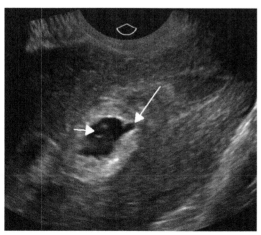

Fig. 8. The irregular contour (*long arrow*) of this gestational sac, which also contains a yolk sac (*short arrow*) raises the possibility of a poor prognosis for the pregnancy.

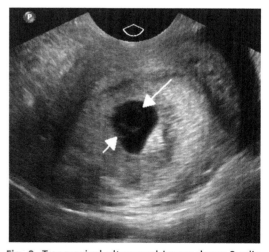

Fig. 9. Transvaginal ultrasound image shows 2 adjacent cystic structures within a gestational sac; the amnion is the larger structure (*long arrow*) and the yolk sac (*short arrow*) is the smaller one. The lack of an embryo in this setting is a poor prognostic sign.

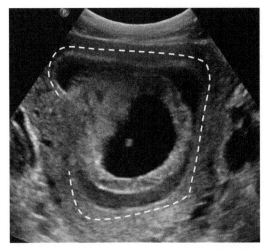

Fig. 10. A transabdominal image of a gestational sac depicts a large subchorionic hemorrhage (*dashed line*) as a rind of hypoechoic fluid with fine low-level echoes surrounding greater than two-thirds of the gestational sac.

Table 1 Differential diagnosis of first-trimester pregnancy and β-hCG levels	
Diagnosis	**Pearls for β-hCG Levels**
IUP and PUL	Do not use single threshold or discriminatory level for TVUS IUP detectability
	Even above 3000 mIU/mL, there is still a chance of viable IUP
	Serial levels in PUL may be helpful to distinguish normal vs abnormal pregnancy
	Normal IUPs have mean doubling time of 1.4–2.1 d
Ectopic pregnancy	EPs can be diagnosed even with levels <1000 mIU/mL
	Higher levels increase risk of nonresponse to medical therapy and may require multiple treatments
	EPs with yolk sac, embryo, or cardiac activity have higher levels
	Serial levels increase slower than normal IUPs, but this may also occur with failed IUPs
Retained products of conception	Limited role (RPOC still possible with normal or negative levels)
Gestational trophoblastic disease	Levels >100,000 mIU/mL occur in 50% of patients <10% of partial molar pregnancies are associated with elevated β-hCG level >100,000 mIU/mL

between 87%–99% and 94%–99%, respectively, with approximately 75% of EPs localized on the first scan.

The rate of PUL is conversely related to the rate of visualization of EP and ranges between 5% and 42%, with 6%–20% of PULs eventually diagnosed as EP. In most cases when the EP was not visualized until a follow-up scan, it was just too small to be appreciated on the initial study. Because the ultrasound appearance of classic EP is well appreciated, the goal of this review is to: (1) describe pitfalls in the diagnosis of EP, (2) understand which findings are important in determining management, (3) assist radiologists in the diagnosis of more unusual findings and EP locations, and (4) present a logical pathway and lexicon for interpreting these US studies.

Currently the most efficacious clinical workup for a suspected EP is TVUS after a positive urine pregnancy test. If the US is non-diagnostic and interpreted as a PUL the next step is a quantitative β-hCG. PUL is not a diagnosis but rather a "place holder" with the diagnosis pending further investigation. Modern data show that most EPs are diagnosed with a β-hCG less than 1000 mIU/mL. It must also be remembered that a β-hCG less than 2000 mIU/mL does not exclude a viable IUP. Thus, for a PUL in an asymptomatic and stable patient, the plan of action should be clinical monitoring with serial β-hCG rather than relying on a single value.

The most common ultrasound appearance of a tubal EP is either the "blob" (inhomogeneous adnexal mass) or "bagel" (extrauterine sac-like structure) sign consisting of a non-simple cystic adnexal mass separate from the ovary (**Fig. 11**). The mass may be round or tubular, the latter due to bleeding into the fallopian tube resulting in a hematosalpinx (Video 2). Some authors contend that this finding should be interpreted as "probable EP" reserving the "definitive EP" for visualization of an extrauterine gestational sac with or without a yolk sac or embryo.[21] More recently, Nadim et al. reported a positive predictive value of greater than 95% for the blob/bagel appearance and contend that such a finding when identified by experienced imagers should be considered a definitive or likely EP.[22] This distinction is most important when the EP will be treated medically as opposed to either surgical or expectant management. A false-positive diagnosis of EP

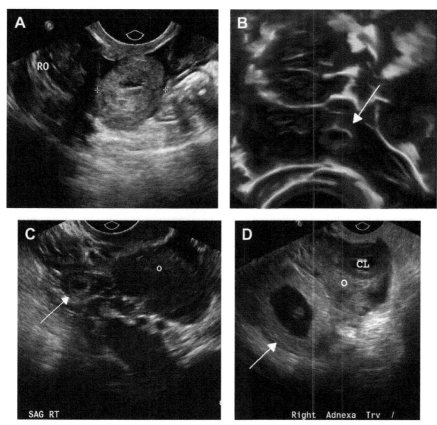

Fig. 11. Four different cases of EP with 4 different appearances. (*A*) Transverse image of the right ovary (RO) with separate echogenic "blob" measured by calipers corresponding to an EP. (*B*) Coronal 3D image of hematosalpinx containing a "bagel" (*arrow*) corresponding to an EP. (*C*) Sagittal image of the right adnexa with ovary (O) and adjacent EP (*arrow*) characterized by an echogenic chorion surrounding a fluid collection containing a yolk sac. (*D*) Transverse view of the right adnexa with live EP (*arrow*) medial to the right ovary (O), which contains a partially cystic corpus luteum (CL). The solid component of the CL is less echogenic than the chorion of the EP.

must be avoided when methotrexate would be administered to prevent termination of a desired pregnancy or congenital abnormalities in a surviving pregnancy.

Multiple pitfalls may be encountered in the US diagnosis of EP (Table 2). The most common is an exophytic corpus luteum. In such a situation, one should apply gentle pressure with the

Table 2
Pitfalls encountered in US diagnosis of ectopic pregnancy

Pitfalls	Features Favoring Ectopic Pregnancy	Features against Ectopic Pregnancy
Exophytic corpus luteum simulating tubal ectopic pregnancy	Movement separate from the ovary with TVUS pressure Tubal ring is more echogenic than ovarian stroma	Movement with the ovary with TVUS pressure Echogenicity similar to ovary
Adnexal cysts simulating ectopic pregnancy	Cystic masses with a thick echogenic rim similar to a gestational sac separate from the ovary	Simple cysts should not be considered an ectopic pregnancy
Color and spectral Doppler vascularity	Does not help to distinguish ectopic pregnancy from corpus luteum	

ultrasound probe to determine whether the putative EP moves with, or separately from, the ovary (Video 3). Caveats for this technique include adhesions that prohibit free movement and technically limited studies secondary to pain. The push technique on the uterus can also help exclude an exophytic myoma masquerading as an EP.

Another useful gray scale finding is the relative echogenicity of the peripheral ring of tissue. The chorionic tubal ring will be more echogenic than the ovarian stroma, whereas the solid component of a corpus luteum is similar (see **Fig. 11**D). Lastly, the diagnosis of EP should not be made if the adnexal mass is a simple cyst. Neither color nor spectral Doppler is considered of primary use because the findings of EP overlap with the corpus luteum (**Fig. 12**). Occasional misdiagnoses occur because of failure to recognize the true myometrium. A large focal myoma may be interpreted as the corpus of the uterus, with the IUP considered to be ectopic (**Fig. 13**), or a solid-appearing hematoma around an EP may be interpreted as a uterus containing an IUP (**Fig. 14**).

When EP is treated medically, the false-negative diagnosis of an IUP must be avoided. The recent literature is clear on this subject: when there is no extra-ovarian adnexal mass, a small indeterminant fluid collection in the central uterus is more likely to be an early IUP. The concept of visualizing a "pseudosac" as a way to diagnose an EP should be avoided. A small collection of complex fluid in the endometrial canal that is not an IUP is more likely to represent residual blood from a spontaneous abortion.[23] As eloquently articulated by Barnhart, even if the error rate is low for the US diagnosis of EP, the sheer number of patients undergoing TVUS early in pregnancy will result in significant absolute numbers of incorrectly interpreted scans.[21]

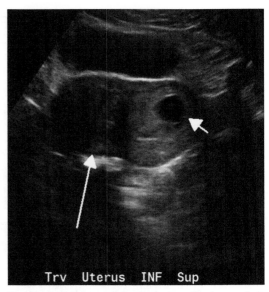

Fig. 13. In this transabdominal view, the hypoechoic myoma (*long arrow*) was initially interpreted as the body of the uterus with an adjacent EP that was actually an intrauterine pregnancy (*short arrow*).

The most common US finding leading to surgery is hemoperitoneum (**Table 3**). Whereas a small amount of free, complex fluid only in the cul-de-sac is common with a clinically stable EP, blood above the uterus or surrounding the adnexa is more likely to require laparoscopy. In this situation, transabdominal imaging should also be used because it provides a wider field of view. A brief look in the right upper quadrant in Morison's pouch is also important, because blood in this location suggests a significant volume of hemoperitoneum and makes surgery more likely (**Fig. 15**).[24] Important technical factors include appropriate gain settings to maximize visualization

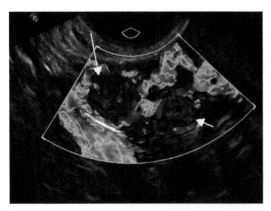

Fig. 12. Adjacent echogenic EP (*short arrow*) and more hypoechoic CL (*long arrow*) have identical peripheral color Doppler appearances.

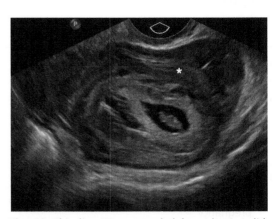

Fig. 14. This live EP surrounded by a large solid-appearing collection of blood (*asterisk*) was initially considered to be the uterus with an IUP.

Table 3
Findings leading to surgical management and pearls for US evaluation

Findings Leading to Surgical Management of Ectopic Pregnancies	Pearls
Hemoperitoneum	Transabdominal imaging provides wider field of view for blood above uterus and in adnexa Blood in Morison's pouch suggests larger volume Appropriate gain settings needed to maximize differentiation from bowel, uterus, liver, spleen
Failed methotrexate therapy	Interval growth of embryo or gestational sac Visualization of cardiac activity Interval development of hemoperitoneum Rising β-hCG levels

of low-level echoes and understanding the appearance of clotted blood, which may not be appreciated as distinct from bowel, uterus, liver, or spleen.

Because bleeding can occur from the fimbriated end of an intact tube, hemoperitoneum does not necessarily imply tubal rupture, although it is clinically unnecessary to make this distinction because surgery is required in either case.[25] Occasionally surgery will reveal a ruptured ovarian cyst as the source of hemoperitoneum in a patient with an early, non-visualized IUP, but this is considered to be an unavoidable outcome. Surgical management is the only treatment to preserve the IUP in a heterotopic pregnancy.[26] Surgery is also preferred when the EP is alive, because medical therapy is less successful. Lastly, surgery is usually necessary in patients in whom methotrexate fails because of increasing β-hCG levels, interval growth with a live IUP, or

hemoperitoneum. In the latter 2 situations, TVUS plays an important role.

Non-tubal EPs cause a disproportionate percentage of morbidity and mortality related to EP. Ultrasound diagnosis is important because surgery is more frequent in these situations. However, the US diagnosis is often more difficult because their appearance can overlap with both tubal EP and abnormal IUP, and is confounded by their relative rarity. Among non-tubal EPs, the interstitial EP is most common, accounting for 2% to 4% of all EPs, with a morbidity 7 times higher than for all EPs.[26] An interstitial EP is defined by an empty uterine cavity with an eccentrically located gestational sac 1 cm from the uterine wall with less than 5 mm of surrounding myometrium (**Fig. 16**).[27] Also useful is visualization of the "interstitial line" of either the collapsed endometrial cavity or the inner portion of the interstitial tube leading to the EP.[28] A more advanced interstitial

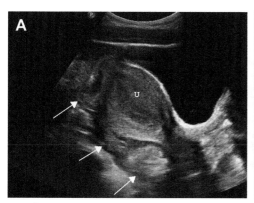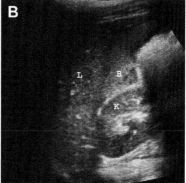

Fig. 15. A case of surgically proven ruptured EP with hemoperitoneum in pelvis and right upper quadrant. (*A*) A transabdominal sagittal view of the uterus (U) with a significant amount of surrounding echogenic blood (*arrows*). (*B*) A transverse view of the right upper quadrant with echogenic blood (B) between liver (L) and right kidney (K).

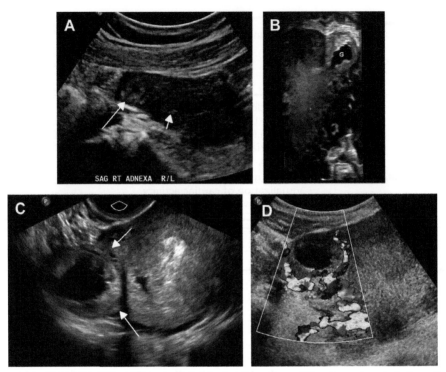

Fig. 16. Examples of interstitial EPs. (*A*) A transabdominal oblique view of the uterus demonstrates a 5-mm gestational sac surrounded by a thin rim of myometrium (*long arrow*) and separate from the collapsed endometrial cavity (*short arrow*) suspicious for an interstitial EP. Because of the early stage and possibility that the sac might be in an angular location, the pregnancy was followed carefully and was proven to be in an interstitial location. (*B*) A coronal reformat of an interstitial EP shows the gestational sac (G) in the expected location of the interstitial portion of the fallopian tube with adjacent myometrium. (*C*) Transvaginal grayscale and (*D*) transabdominal color Doppler images of an interstitial EP show the myometrial mantle sign (*arrows*) separating the gestational sac from the endometrium, and exuberant vascularity fed by uterine vessels.

EP may initially appear to be extrauterine, but careful scanning should demonstrate a "claw" or "myometrial mantle" of partially surrounding uterine tissue (see **Fig. 16**C).[29] Gentle pressure with the probe will not show movement of the EP independently from the uterus. Because of their better blood supply, interstitial EPs have a greater likelihood of bleeding.

The differential diagnosis of interstitial EP includes an angular location of an IUP and a tubular EP. Angular pregnancy is an IUP implanted eccentrically in the lateral fundus of the uterine cavity, but remains completely in the endometrium (**Fig. 17**); whereas an interstitial EP is separated from the endometrial cavity by a rim of myometrium. An angular IUP is associated with a higher spontaneous abortion rate than standard IUP implantations, and requires observation. We have found 2D and 3D coronal reformats extremely useful in differentiating angular IUP from interstitial EP.

Other, rarer non-tubal EPs include cervical, cesarean scar, ovarian rudimentary horn, and abdominal locations (**Table 4**). Both cervical and cesarean scar implantation sites may be mistaken for the more common spontaneous abortion in progress (**Figs. 18** and **19**). Key diagnostic tools include color Doppler to determine the site of implantation based on trophoblastic blood flow and a lack of "sliding sign" of the gestational sac within the lower uterus or cervix, indicating an inability to displace the sac from its implantation site. In both the cervical and scar EPs, the gestational sac will usually be round and cause bulging of the lower uterus or cervix and often demonstrates embryonic cardiac activity. In contrast, a gestational sac undergoing spontaneous abortion is usually flattened or ovoid and though it may contain an embryo, cardiac activity is unlikely.

Ovarian EP is a challenging diagnosis, frequently missed on TVUS and interpreted as a corpus luteum or other ovarian cyst. The US diagnosis is suggested when a sac-like structure with a rim more echogenic than ovarian stroma is visualized within or on the surface of the ovary. Abdominal pregnancy is extremely rare. It can occur anywhere on the peritoneal surface or on multiple

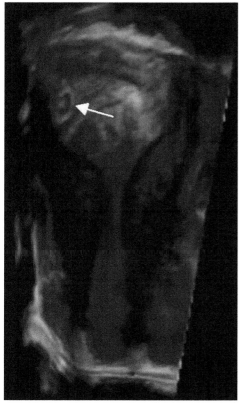

Fig. 17. A coronal 3D reformat of a 5-week intrauterine gestational sac in an angular location, which is in the lateral fundus of the uterus, but remains completely within the endometrium (*arrow*). The eventual outcome was a spontaneous abortion.

Table 4 Non-tubal ectopic pregnancies	
Types of Non-tubal Ectopic Pregnancies	**Pearls**
Cervical and cesarean scar	May be mistaken for abortion in progress Color Doppler may reveal trophoblastic flow in ectopic implantation Lack of "sliding sign" or inability to displace sac from implantation site Cardiac activity usually indicates ectopic implantation Rounded shape causing bulging of uterus/cervix suggests ectopic
Ovarian	Frequently misinterpreted as corpus luteum or ovarian cyst Sac-like structure with rim more echogenic than ovarian stroma on the ovarian surface is suggestive of ectopic
Abdominal	Extremely rare May occur anywhere on peritoneal surface or visceral organ

visceral organs. Pre-operative imaging diagnoses are often difficult. False-positive diagnoses can occur with uterine fibroids.[30] Most ovarian and abdominal EPs are probably due to extrusion of an EP from the fallopian tube or other ectopic implantation site.

Heterotopic pregnancy is also a challenging diagnosis. An analysis of 82 reported cases from 2005 to 2010 found 71% of patients had at least 1 risk factor, with 61% who had some type of assisted reproductive technology.[31] Histories also included pelvic inflammatory disease and pelvic surgery. However, 29% had no identifiable risk factors. The median gestational age at diagnosis was 7 weeks with two-thirds of cases diagnosed

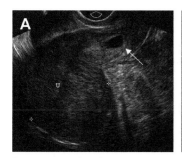 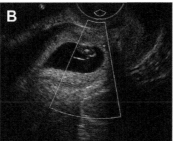 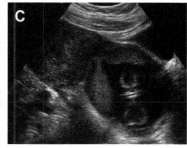

Fig. 18. Example of a cervical EP. (*A*) A sagittal TV image of the entire uterus (U) in a patient with a prior history of cesarean delivery demonstrates a gestational sac (*arrow*) in the cervix. (*B*) A color Doppler image from the same study shows a live 7-week embryo within the gestational sac. The interpretation was a spontaneous abortion in progress. (*C*) The patient returned 6 weeks later with increasing hCG and pelvic pain. A transabdominal sagittal view of the uterus shows interval growth of the cervical EP with a live 13-week fetus.

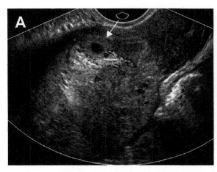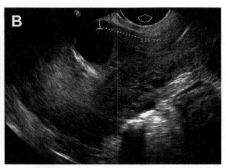

Fig. 19. A cesarean section scar EP that failed systemic methotrexate requiring surgical excision. (*A*) A sagittal view of the uterus in a patient with a history of one prior cesarean section demonstrates a 5.5-week intrauterine gestational sac (*arrow*) in a low position in the uterus. Color Doppler shows trophoblastic flow confirming the implantation at the cesarean section scar site. The patient was treated with systemic methotrexate. (*B*) Repeat imaging 1 week later shows interval growth of the pregnancy with a 4-mm measurement of the overlying myometrium. Surgical excision was required for definitive treatment.

using US. However, a third of women presented with hemodynamic instability, attesting to the difficulty of this diagnosis.

Does the β-hCG level matter? The threshold to perform TVUS is merely a positive urine pregnancy test since there is no specific β-hCG value below which visualization of an EP or even ruptured EP is unlikely. On the other hand, once an EP is detected, the quantitative β-hCG may predict the outcome of medical therapy. Non-responders to systemic methotrexate tended to have higher β-hCG levels and often more vascularity on color Doppler.[32] If the β-hCG level is > 5000 mIU/mL, multiple courses of methotrexate may be required for successful medical treatment.[33] Patients with a definitive EP on TVUS (yolk sac, embryo/cardiac activity) had higher quantitative β-hCG levels compared to those with a blob or bagel. Serial β-hCG values are used in evaluating IUPs which usually have a mean doubling time of 1.4 to 2.1 days in early pregnancy or an increase of 66% every 2 days.[25] While most EPs have a slower rise of β-hCG, rates that rise too slowly, plateau or decline may also occur with failed IUPs.[34] Lastly, recent evidence is compelling against the use of a specific discriminatory ßhCG (1000 – 2000 mIU/mL) for a viable IUP particularly because of multiple gestations and the occasional normal viable singleton pregnancy not visualized until the ßhCG was > 3000 mIU/mL.[35,36]

Retained Products of Conception

Retained products of conception is a common post-pregnancy complication and refers to intrauterine tissue containing chorionic villi, and most frequently presents with vaginal bleeding and pelvic pain. Although RPOC may occur after any trimester pregnancy or mode of delivery (vaginal or cesarean section) and following any type of abortion (medical, spontaneous, or surgical), the incidence of RPOC depends on the gestational age of the pregnancy. Retained products of conception in the first trimester of pregnancy is particularly common after a medical or spontaneous abortion; however, the highest incidence occurs after second-trimester pregnancy.[37] A full list of incidence rates of RPOC is listed in **Table 5**.

Ultrasound is the first-line imaging test to evaluate for potential RPOC. The grayscale US finding of a thickened endometrium measuring greater than 10 mm results in an 80% sensitivity, but a low 20% specificity, the latter secondary to overlap with blood clot.[37,38] An additional grayscale US finding for RPOC is an endometrial mass, which has a reported sensitivity ranging between 29% and 79%.[39,40] However, the diagnostic accuracy of RPOC dramatically increases with the addition of color Doppler, because the presence of color Doppler flow extending from the myometrium to the endometrium increases the positive predictive value of RPOC to 96% (**Fig. 20**).[38] If vascularity is isolated to the myometrium, an alternative diagnosis such as arteriovenous malformation (AVM) or gestational trophoblastic neoplasia (GTN) is more likely (see subsequent section).

In RPOC, the degree of vascularity of the endometrial component compared with the myometrium can vary greatly and range from no detectable vascularity, despite using sensitive

Table 5 Incidence of RPOC based on pregnancy trimester	
Incidence (Percentage)	**Pregnancy Trimester**
2.7	3rd trimester
40	2nd trimester
17	1st trimester

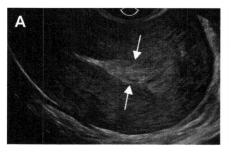
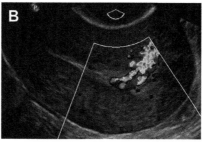
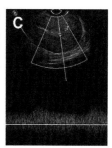

Fig. 20. Retained products of conception in a patient status post D&C 1 month earlier, β-hCG 335 mIU/mL. Sagittal grayscale transvaginal image (*A*) shows a focally thickened endometrium slightly greater than 1 cm (*arrows*). The color Doppler image (*B*) shows color Doppler flow extending from the myometrium to the endometrium, and is low-resistance arterial flow on the (*C*) spectral Doppler image.

color Doppler settings, to marked vascularity mimicking an AVM (**Fig. 21**). Spectral Doppler analysis reveals peak systolic velocities ranging from 10 to 108 cm/s with low-resistance arterial waveforms, noting that higher velocities cannot be distinguished from AVM.[38]

A patient's β-hCG level has a limited role in the diagnosis for RPOC, and can be normal to mildly elevated. In a retrospective review of 35 patients who underwent pathologic evaluation for RPOC, of whom 28 had RPOC and the remaining 7 did not, there was no statistically significant difference in the β-hCG levels between the 2 groups.[38] In the proper clinical setting and in conjunction with typical ultrasound findings, patients with low and/or negative β-hCG levels can still have RPOC.

The imaging appearance of RPOC overlaps with blood clot, endometritis, AVM, endometrial polyp, intracavitary fibroid, partial molar pregnancy, and invasive molar pregnancy.[37] AVM typically occurs after a dilatation and curettage (D&C) or surgical procedure, and presents with myometrial vascularity and none to minimal endometrial vascularity on color Doppler. However, markedly vascular RPOC with enhanced myometrial vascularity mimics AVM and may benefit from pre-operative embolization to minimize bleeding if the patient

undergoes D&C. A summary of RPOC mimics and imaging findings is listed in **Table 6**. RPOC treatment options include conservative management, D&C, uterotonic medications such as prostaglandin E1 analogs, and angiographic embolization. Patients presenting immediately after medical and spontaneous abortion of first trimester pregnancy may require additional time for involution of endometrial vascularity and eventual passage of blood clot/chorionic villi. In a retrospective review of 176 patients sonographically evaluated for RPOC, patients with thicker endometrial stripes, marked endometrial vascularity, and lower serum hemoglobin were predictors for surgical management.[41]

Gestational Trophoblastic Disease

Gestational trophoblastic disease (GTD) encompasses a variety of tumors that arise from the placental trophoblasts, which in turn arises from the fertilized ovum. Gestational trophoblastic disease is divided into molar pregnancy and GTN. Two types of molar pregnancy exist, complete hydatidiform mole or partial hydatidiform mole. Gestational trophoblastic neoplasia includes invasive molar pregnancy, choriocarcinoma, placental

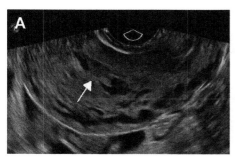
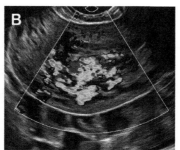
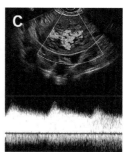

Fig. 21. Highly vascular RPOC mimicking AVM in a patient status post D&C of a 12-week pregnancy, 3 weeks earlier; β-hCG of 568 mIU/mL. Sagittal grayscale transvaginal image (*A*) shows a thickened endometrium (*arrow*). (*B*) Color Doppler image shows marked vascularity extending from the myometrium to the endometrium. (*C*) Spectral Doppler shows low-resistance arterial flow.

Table 6
Ultrasound imaging findings of retained products of conception and mimics

Diagnosis	Ultrasound Imaging Findings	Clinical Pearls
Retained products of conception	Thickened endometrium with varying degrees of bridging myometrial to endometrial vascularity on color Doppler Marked vascular RPOC mimics AVM	β-hCG levels can be normal (negative) Markedly vascular RPOC may require angiographic embolization before D&C
Blood clot	Thickened endometrium, no color Doppler flow	Indistinguishable from avascular RPOC
Endometritis	Thickened endometrium with foci of gas	Fever, elevated WBC
Arteriovenous malformation	Predominant myometrial vascularity	History of surgical procedure or D&C
Endometrial polyp/ intracavitary fibroid	Echogenic or hypoechoic endometrial mass	Evaluate for presence on prior imaging studies, may be indistinguishable from RPOC
Partial molar pregnancy	Gestational sac containing fetal parts, thickened placenta containing cystic spaces	Persistent or rising β-hCG levels
Complete molar pregnancy	Cluster of anechoic cystic spaces in endometrium invading the myometrium; "cluster of grapes"	Markedly elevated β-hCG levels, often >100,000 mIU/mL
Invasive molar pregnancy	Myometrial mass with variable endometrial component	Follows a molar pregnancy, persistent or rising β-hCG levels

site trophoblastic tumor, and epithelioid trophoblastic tumor, and is beyond the scope of this review.

A complete molar pregnancy occurs when an empty ovum devoid of maternal chromosomes is fertilized by 1 sperm, which then duplicates its own DNA, occurring in 90% of cases. In the remaining 10% of cases, an empty ovum is fertilized by 2 sperm.[42] Many patients with complete molar pregnancy are asymptomatic in the first trimester, but when symptoms occur, they include vaginal bleeding, large uterine size for dates, and hyperemesis. In contrast to RPOC, serum β-hCG level play an important role in diagnosing GTD, because levels greater than 100,000 mIU/mL occur in 50% of patients. In contradistinction, abnormal pregnancies or miscarriages are associated with normal or declining β-hCG. Progression to GTN occurs in 15% to 20% of patients. Partial molar pregnancies arise from the fertilization of a normal ovum by 2 sperm (triploidy) and patients present with vaginal bleeding.

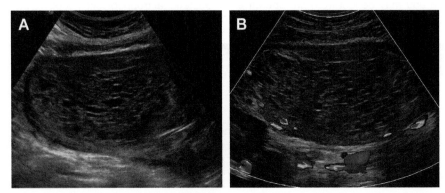

Fig. 22. Classic complete molar pregnancy in a patient with markedly elevated β-hCG of 940,000 mIU/mL. Sagittal grayscale transabdominal image (A) shows an expanded endometrial cavity containing an echogenic mass with tiny cystic spaces. Color Doppler image (B) shows avascularity of the endometrial cavity. Enlarged ovaries because of theca lutein cysts were present (not shown).

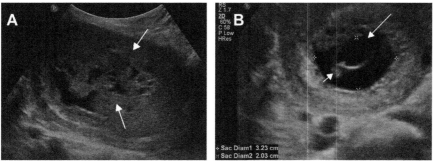

Fig. 23. Partial molar pregnancy in a patient with β-hCG of 382,815 mIU/mL. Sagittal grayscale transabdominal image (*A*) shows an expanded endometrial cavity secondary to an echogenic mass (*arrows*) containing small cystic spaces. A grayscale image of a different area of the uterus (*B*) shows a small irregular gestational sac containing an amorphous embryo (*short arrow*) and an abnormal yolk sac (*long arrow*).

Progression to GTN occurs in less than 5% of patients.[42]

Complete molar pregnancies appear as a cluster of anechoic cystic spaces expanding the endometrial cavity without invading the myometrium, and are described as a "cluster of grapes."[42,43] Color Doppler images show decreased vascularity (**Fig. 22**). Enlarged ovaries secondary to theca lutein cysts result from hyperstimulation because of elevated β-hCG levels, occurring in less than 20% of patients.[42]

The ultrasound appearance of a partial molar pregnancy is much less classic than complete molar pregnancy and is more often diagnosed on histology rather than imaging due to overlap in appearance with a nonviable pregnancy,

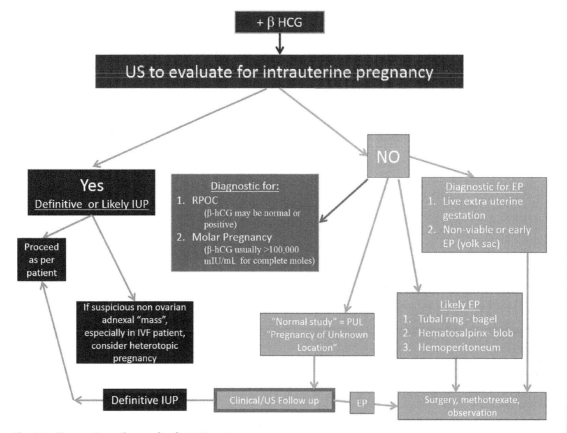

Fig. 24. Diagnostic pathways for first trimester pregnancy.

miscarriage, or RPOC.[44] Ultrasound appearance of a partial molar pregnancy includes a large empty gestational sac, a large sac containing fetal parts, fetal demise with anomalies or growth retardation, oligohydramnios, and enlarged placenta relative to the uterine size with hydropic placental change (**Fig. 23**).[42,43] The sensitivity, specificity, positive predictive value, and negative predictive value for detection of all types of molar pregnancies on pre-D&C US is 44%, 74%, 88%, and 23%, respectively.[45] Treatment for complete and partial molar pregnancy is suction D&C. After D&C or miscarriage, β-hCG levels should be followed to ensure normalization to exclude the possibility of GTD.

SUMMARY

After the diagnosis of pregnancy via a positive β-hCG, TVUS is the imaging modality of choice in the first trimester to characterize the implantation location and viability of the gestation as well as to evaluate complications such as retained products or molar pregnancy. The possible diagnostic pathways are shown in **Fig. 24**. High-quality imaging in experienced hands will result in the highest rate of visualized EP and IUP and the lowest rates of PUL. Interpreting physicians should use clear terminology in their interpretations to avoid misunderstandings with their clinical colleagues.

SUPPLEMENTARY DATA

Supplementary video related to this article can be found at https://doi.org/10.1016/j.rcl.2019.01.006.

REFERENCES

1. Bree RL, Edwards M, Böhm-Vélez M, et al. Transvaginal sonography in the evaluation of normal early pregnancy: correlation with HCG level. AJR Am J Roentgenol 1989;153(1):75–9.
2. Doubilet PM, Benson CB. Double sac sign and intradecidual sign in early pregnancy. J Ultrasound Med 2013;32(7):1207–14.
3. Yeh HC, Goodman JD, Carr L, et al. Intradecidual sign: a US criterion of early intrauterine pregnancy. Radiology 1986;161(2):463–7.
4. Yeh HC, Rabinowitz JG. Amniotic sac development: ultrasound features of early pregnancy–the double bleb sign. Radiology 1988;166(1 Pt 1):97–103.
5. Rodgers SK, Chang C, DeBardeleben JT, et al. Normal and abnormal US findings in early first-trimester pregnancy: review of the society of radiologists in ultrasound 2012 consensus panel recommendations. Radiographics 2015;35(7):2135–48.
6. Doubilet PM. Ultrasound evaluation of the first trimester. Radiol Clin North Am 2014;52(6):1191–9.
7. Cyr DR, Mack LA, Nyberg DA, et al. Fetal rhombencephalon: normal US findings. Radiology 1988;166(3):691–2.
8. Carroll SGM, Soothill PW, Abdel-Fattah SA, et al. Prediction of chorionicity in twin pregnancies at 10–14 weeks of gestation. BJOG 2002;109(2):182–6.
9. Glanc P, Nyberg DA, Khati NJ, et al. ACR appropriateness criteria® multiple gestations. J Am Coll Radiol 2017;14(11, Supplement):S476–89.
10. Bromley B, Benacerraf B. Using the number of yolk sacs to determine amnionicity in early first trimester monochorionic twins. J Ultrasound Med 1995;14(6):415–9.
11. Park SY, Chung JH, Han YJ, et al. Prediction of amnionicity using the number of yolk sacs in monochorionic multifetal pregnancy. J Korean Med Sci 2017;32(12):2016–20.
12. Shen O, Samueloff A, Beller U, et al. Number of yolk sacs does not predict amnionicity in early first-trimester monochorionic multiple gestations. Ultrasound Obstet Gynecol 2006;27(1):53–5.
13. Rowling SE, Coleman BG, Langer JE, et al. First-trimester US parameters of failed pregnancy. Radiology 1997;203(1):211–7.
14. Abdallah Y, Daemen A, Kirk E, et al. Limitations of current definitions of miscarriage using mean gestational sac diameter and crown-rump length measurements: a multicenter observational study. Ultrasound Obstet Gynecol 2011;38(5):497–502.
15. Doubilet PM, Benson CB, Bourne T, et al. Diagnostic criteria for nonviable pregnancy early in the first trimester. N Engl J Med 2013;369(15):1443–51.
16. Harris RD, Couto C, Karpovsky C, et al. The chorionic bump. J Ultrasound Med 2006;25(6):757–63.
17. Sana Y, Appiah A, Davison A, et al. Clinical significance of first-trimester chorionic bumps: a matched case–control study. Ultrasound Obstet Gynecol 2013;42(5):585–9.
18. Creanga AA, Shapiro-Mendoza CK, Bish CL, et al. Trends in ectopic pregnancy mortality in the United States: 1980–2007. Obstet Gynecol 2011;117(4):837–43.
19. Berry J, Davey M, Hon M-S, et al. Optimising the diagnosis of ectopic pregnancy. J Obstet Gynaecol 2016;36(4):437–9.
20. Kirk E, Bottomley C, Bourne T. Diagnosing ectopic pregnancy and current concepts in the management of pregnancy of unknown location. Hum Reprod Update 2014;20(2):250–61.
21. Barnhart KT. Early pregnancy failure: beware of the pitfalls of modern management. Fertil Steril 2012;98(5):1061–5.
22. Nadim B, Infante F, Lu C, et al. Morphological ultrasound types known as "blob" and "bagel" signs

should be reclassified from suggesting probable to indicating definite tubal ectopic pregnancy. Ultrasound Obstet Gynecol 2018;51(4):543–9.

23. Doubilet PM, Benson CB. First, do no harm... To early pregnancies. J Ultrasound Med 2010;29(5): 685–9.

24. Moore C, Todd WM, O'Brien E, et al. Free fluid in Morison's pouch on bedside ultrasound predicts need for operative intervention in suspected ectopic pregnancy. Acad Emerg Med 2007;14(8): 755–8.

25. Frates MC, Doubilet PM, Peters HE, et al. Adnexal sonographic findings in ectopic pregnancy and their correlation with tubal rupture and human chorionic gonadotropin levels. J Ultrasound Med 2014;33(4): 697–703.

26. Moawad NS, Mahajan ST, Moniz MH, et al. Current diagnosis and treatment of interstitial pregnancy. Am J Obstet Gynecol 2010;202(1):15–29.

27. Timor-Tritsch IE, Monteagudo A, Matera C, et al. Sonographic evolution of cornual pregnancies treated without surgery. Obstet Gynecol 1992; 79(6):1044–9.

28. Ackerman TE, Levi CS, Dashefsky SM, et al. Interstitial line: sonographic finding in interstitial (cornual) ectopic pregnancy. Radiology 1993;189(1):83–7.

29. Araujo Júnior E, Zanforlin Filho SM, Pires CR, et al. Three-dimensional transvaginal sonographic diagnosis of early and asymptomatic interstitial pregnancy. Arch Gynecol Obstet 2007;275(3):207–10.

30. Alalade AO, Smith FJE, Kendall CE, et al. Evidence-based management of non tubal ectopic pregnancies. J Obstet Gynaecol 2017;37(8):982–91.

31. Talbot K, Simpson R, Price N, et al. Heterotopic pregnancy. J Obstet Gynaecol 2011;31(1):7–12.

32. Desai A, Fleischer AC, Wahab SA, et al. Sonography of responsive versus nonresponsive ectopic pregnancies. J Ultrasound Med 2016;35(6):1341–7.

33. Menon S, Colins J, Barnhart KT. Establishing a human chorionic gonadotropin cutoff to guide methotrexate treatment of ectopic pregnancy: a systematic review. Fertil Steril 2007;87(3):481–4.

34. Visconti K, Zite N. hCG in ectopic pregnancy. Clin Obstet Gynecol 2012;55(2):410–7.

35. Doubilet PM, Benson CB. Further evidence against the reliability of the human chorionic gonadotropin discriminatory level. J Ultrasound Med Off J Am Inst Ultrasound Med 2011;30(12):1637–42.

36. Ko JKY, Cheung VYT. Time to revisit the human chorionic gonadotropin discriminatory level in the management of pregnancy of unknown location. J Ultrasound Med Off J Am Inst Ultrasound Med 2014;33(3):465–71.

37. Sellmyer MA, Desser TS, Maturen KE, et al. Physiologic, histologic, and imaging features of retained products of conception. Radiographics 2013;33(3): 781–96.

38. Kamaya A, Petrovitch I, Chen B, et al. Retained products of conception: spectrum of color Doppler findings. J Ultrasound Med 2009;28(8):1031–41.

39. Durfee SM, Frates MC, Luong A, et al. The sonographic and color Doppler features of retained products of conception. J Ultrasound Med 2005; 24(9):1181–6 [quiz: 1188–9].

40. Alcázar JL, Baldonado C, Laparte C. The reliability of transvaginal ultrasonography to detect retained tissue after spontaneous first-trimester abortion, clinically thought to be complete. Ultrasound Obstet Gynecol 1995;6(2):126–9.

41. Kamaya A, Krishnarao PM, Nayak N, et al. Clinical and imaging predictors of management in retained products of conception. Abdom Radiol (NY) 2016; 41(12):2429–34.

42. Shaaban AM, Rezvani M, Haroun RR, et al. Gestational trophoblastic disease: clinical and imaging features. Radiographics 2017;37(2):681–700.

43. Fowler DJ, Lindsay I, Seckl MJ, et al. Routine pre-evacuation ultrasound diagnosis of hydatidiform mole: experience of more than 1000 cases from a regional referral center. Ultrasound Obstet Gynecol 2006;27(1):56–60.

44. Savage JL, Maturen KE, Mowers EL, et al. Sonographic diagnosis of partial versus complete molar pregnancy: A reappraisal. J Clin Ultrasound 2017; 45(2):72–8.

45. Zhou Q, Lei X-Y, Xie Q, et al. Sonographic and Doppler imaging in the diagnosis and treatment of gestational trophoblastic disease: a 12-year experience. J Ultrasound Med 2005; 24(1):15–24.

Scrotal Ultrasound

Kristin Rebik, DO[a],*, Jason M. Wagner, MD[a], William Middleton, MD[b]

KEYWORDS

- Scrotum • Testis • Testicular cancer • Testicular trauma • Epididymis • Ultrasound

KEY POINTS

- Ultrasound is the imaging modality of choice to evaluate the scrotum.
- Urologic emergencies that require prompt diagnosis and intervention include testicular torsion, testicular rupture, and Fournier gangrene.
- A palpable scrotal lesion can be characterized by location (intratesticular or extratesticular), composition (cystic or solid), and vascularity with sonography.
- Most solid intratesticular lesions are malignant.

INTRODUCTION

Ultrasound is the imaging modality of choice to evaluate the scrotum because of its high resolution, Doppler capabilities, availability, and lack of ionizing radiation.[1] Real-time grayscale and color Doppler images provide a comprehensive assessment of the scrotum, including the testis, epididymis, spermatic cord, and inguinal canal. Common causes of acute scrotal pain include testicular torsion, epididymo-orchitis, and testicular trauma, all of which require different treatment. It is critical to determine the location and composition of a palpable scrotal lesion, given that the vast majority of solid intratesticular lesions are malignant.[2]

This article reviews the scrotal anatomy and scanning technique. The etiology and ultrasonographic appearance of acute scrotal processes and lesions within the testis, epididymis, and scrotal wall are discussed.

SCROTAL ANATOMY

The scrotum is divided into right and left compartments by the scrotal septum, each containing a testis, epididymis, and spermatic cord. The normal scrotal wall thickness is 8 mm or less. The scrotal wall lymphatics drain into the adjacent inguinal lymph nodes.[3]

The tunica vaginalis originates from the peritoneum and descends into the scrotum at approximately 8 weeks gestational age (Fig. 1).[3] The peripheral parietal layer covers the inner aspect of the scrotal wall. The central visceral layer envelopes the greater part the testis and epididymis.[4]

The fibrous connective tissue surrounding the testis is the tunica albuginea (see Fig. 1). The testicular mediastinum is an incomplete septum formed by infolding of the posterior surface of the tunica albuginea into the testis, producing a curvilinear echogenic band coursing parallel to the long axis of the testis (Fig. 2D).[4,5]

Each testis is composed of numerous lobules containing seminiferous tubules.[6] At the testicular mediastinum, the tubules merge to form the rete testis (see Fig. 2).[7]

The testicular arteries originate from the infrarenal abdominal aorta. In the testis, the testicular artery forms the capsular arteries,

Disclosures: None.
[a] Department of Radiological Sciences, University of Oklahoma Health Sciences Center, Garrison Tower, Suite 4G4250, Oklahoma City, OK 73104, USA; [b] Mallinckrodt Institute of Radiology, Washington University School of Medicine, 510 South Kingshighway Boulevard, St Louis, MO 63110, USA
* Corresponding author.
E-mail address: kristin-rebik@ouhsc.edu

Radiol Clin N Am 57 (2019) 635–648
https://doi.org/10.1016/j.rcl.2019.01.007

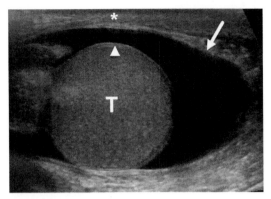

Fig. 1. Scrotal anatomy. Transverse view of a hemiscrotum demonstrates the layers of the scrotum (from superficial to deep): skin and musculature (*asterisk*), the tunica vaginalis (*arrow*), and the tunica albuginea (*arrowhead*). The layers of the wall are best visualized when a hydrocele is present. The testis (T) is located centrally.

which are located in the tunica vasculosa, immediately beneath the tunica albuginea.[4,7] The capsular arteries supply centripetal arteries that enter the testis directed toward the mediastinum. Before reaching the mediastinum, the centripetal arteries branch into recurrent rami that curve back away from the mediastinum. In 50% of men, one or more large arteries pass through the mediastinum and travel to the opposite side of the testis. These transmediastinal arteries are accompanied by a transmediastinal vein.[8,9]

The testis and epididymis are drained by the pampiniform plexus, a network formed by approximately 10 veins.[10] The veins converge in the inguinal canal to form the testicular veins. The right testicular vein drains into the inferior vena cava and the left testicular vein drains into the left renal vein.[4,7] The lymphatic drainage of the testes is to the para-aortic and paracaval lymph nodes at the level of the renal hila.[11]

The epididymis is an elongated structure that functions in sperm maturation and transportation. It overlies the posterolateral testis, usually near the mediastinum, and is divided into 3 segments: the head, body, and tail. Relative to the testicular parenchyma, the epididymal head is isoechoic and the body and tail are hypoechoic (**Fig. 3**).[4,7]

ULTRASOUND TECHNIQUE

The ultrasound examination is typically performed in the supine position. A towel placed between the thighs will elevate the scrotum. Warm gel is recommended to decrease the cremasteric reflex.[7] A linear high frequency transducer is preferred.

If the scrotal ultrasound scan is to evaluate scrotal pain, the examination should begin on the asymptomatic side. This allows for optimization of grayscale and color Doppler parameters. A transverse image of both testes ("buddy" view) is important to document that there are 2 testes and to compare size, echogenicity, and vascularity.

Grayscale images of the testes and epididymides are obtained in the longitudinal and transverse planes. Color and spectral Doppler images with high-sensitivity Doppler settings are used to evaluate perfusion. Images of the inguinal canal and spermatic cord can be obtained in the upright position during Valsalva maneuver to evaluate for inguinal hernias and varicoceles, respectively.[1,4]

ACUTE SCROTUM
Vascular Emergencies

Testicular torsion
Testicular torsion is a surgical emergency, which is most common in adolescents. Twisting of the

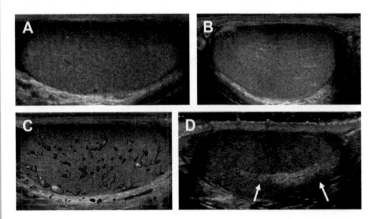

Fig. 2. Normal testis. (*A*) Longitudinal and (*B*) transverse views of the testis demonstrate a homogeneous intermediate echogenicity. (*C*) On color Doppler, there is flow throughout the parenchyma. (*D*) The testicular mediastinum is seen as a hyperechoic band (*arrows*).

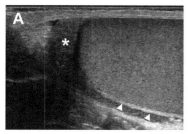
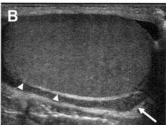

Fig. 3. Normal epididymis. Longitudinal views of the epididymis (*A*, *B*) show the head (*asterisk*), body (*arrowheads*), and tail (*arrow*).

spermatic cord results in venous and then arterial obstruction. A predisposing factor is the "bell-clapper" deformlty whereby the tunica vaginalis completely envelopes the testis, epididymis, and distal spermatic cord.[1] The deformity is frequently bilateral. In normal cases, there is a bare area on the testis where the tunica vaginalis does not attach, which stops the testis from rotating.[12] Patients present with acute pain, nausea, and vomiting.

Testicular torsion is a spectrum ranging from partial to complete. In partial torsion, twisting of the spermatic cord is incomplete and there is asymmetric decreased flow to the affected testis. On spectral Doppler, the arterial waveforms in the torsed testis are abnormal, and may demonstrate absent or reversed diastolic flow or tardus parvus waveforms (**Fig. 4**).[4] In complete torsion, there is absence of flow to the testis (**Fig. 5**).

In the early stages of testicular torsion, the affected testis may have a normal grayscale appearance. As the duration of torsion increases, the testis will become enlarged and hypoechoic. After 24 hours ("missed torsion"), the testis develops hemorrhage and necrosis resulting in a heterogeneous echogenicity (**Fig. 6**).[4,12] In the setting of torsion, abnormal testicular echogenicity indicates infarction and a very low likelihood that the testis will be salvageable. Alternatively, if the testis is normal in echogenicity it is almost always viable.[13] If intervention occurs within 6 hours of symptom onset, the testicular salvage rate is as high as 80% to 100%. After 12 hours, the salvage rate is less than 20%.[14] If the testis is viable at the time of surgery, detorsion and orchidopexy is performed; otherwise orchiectomy is performed.

Torsion of the testicular appendages
The testicular appendages are remnants of embryonic tissue. Torsion of the testicular appendage typically occurs in prepubertal boys, who present with focal scrotal pain over the superior aspect of the testis. Physical examination may demonstrate a superior paratesticular nodule with blue discoloration of the overlying skin ("blue dot" sign).[15]

On the ultrasound scan there are extratesticular avascular nodules of variable echogenicity (**Fig. 7**).

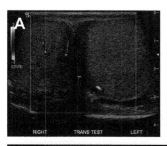
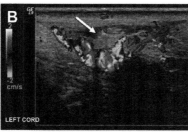
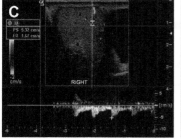
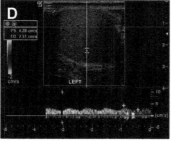

Fig. 4. Partial testicular torsion. (*A*) Color Doppler image of both testes shows asymmetric decreased flow in the left testis. (*B*) The left spermatic cord is twisted with an area of avascularity (*arrow*). (*C*) Spectral Doppler of the right testis shows a normal arterial waveform. (*D*) Spectral Doppler of the left testis shows an abnormal tardus parvus waveform.

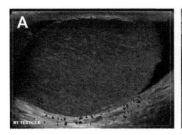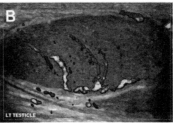

Fig. 5. Complete testicular torsion. (*A*) The right testis lacks internal flow on color Doppler, compatible with torsion. (*B*) Flow is maintained in the left testis.

A reactive hydrocele and overlying scrotal wall thickening are commonly present. Patients are treated conservatively and the pain resolves in several days. Some speculate that a torsed appendage may detach and calcify to become a scrotolith (scrotal pearl).[15]

Infectious Emergencies

A retrograde bacterial infection is frequently the source of epididymo-orchitis.[1] *Escherichia coli* and *Proteus* are common infections in young boys and the elderly. Sexually transmitted infections (ie, *Chlamydia trachomatis* and *Neisseria gonorrhoeae*) are frequent in adolescents and young men. The most vascularized portion of the epididymis is the tail, which is often the first site of infection.[16] Extension of the infection into the testis (orchitis) occurs in 20% to 40%. Isolated orchitis is rare and should raise concern for mumps.[4] In acute cases, the epididymis is enlarged, hypoechoic, and hypervascular on the ultrasound scan. If the testis is involved it is enlarged, heterogeneous, and hyperemic (**Fig. 8**).[17] Complications include abscess, ischemia, chronic epididymitis, or infertility.[16] An abscess is a hypoechoic avascular collection with internal debris, often with indistinct or irregular margins and peripheral hyperemia (**Fig. 9**).[4,18]

Traumatic Emergencies

Intratesticular hematoma

Intratesticular hematomas have a variable appearance related to the time between injury and imaging. In the acute setting, a hematoma may be isoechoic to the testicular parenchyma or heterogeneous in echogenicity (**Fig. 10**). Chronic hematomas are hypoechoic or anechoic secondary to liquefaction. On color Doppler, a hematoma is avascular. Follow-up ultrasound is recommended to document resolution and exclude an underlying lesion. Potential complications include abscess or necrosis.[4,5]

Testicular rupture

The key feature of testicular rupture is disruption of the tunica albuginea, resulting in an irregular testicular contour and possible extrusion of seminiferous tubules (**Fig. 11**). In most cases, a discrete disruption in the tunica albuginea is not seen and the diagnosis is suspected based on an abnormally shaped testis. Additional signs of testicular rupture include heterogeneous internal echogenicity and regions of avascularity. If a large hematoma is present, it may be difficult

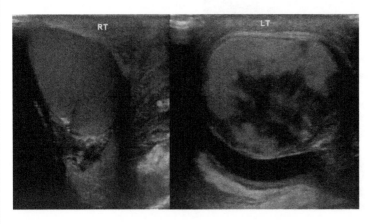

Fig. 6. Missed testicular torsion. This patient was a 14-year-old boy with 12 days of left scrotal pain. The left testis is enlarged and heterogeneous in echogenicity. Orchiectomy demonstrated hemorrhagic necrosis of the left testis.

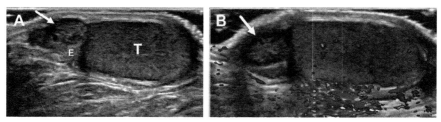

Fig. 7. Torsion of a testicular appendage. (A) Longitudinal view of the scrotum shows a heterogeneously hypo-echoic nodule (*arrow*), separate from the testis (T) and adjacent to the epididymis (E). (B) On color Doppler, there is no flow within the nodule.

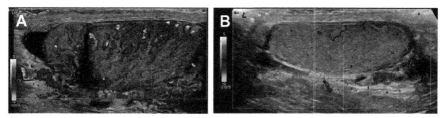

Fig. 8. Epididymo-orchitis. (A) The right testis and epididymis are enlarged and hyperemic. (B) There is normal vascularity of the left testis and epididymis.

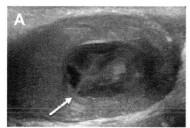
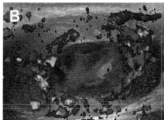

Fig. 9. Testicular abscess. (A) Gray-scale image of a testis shows a heterogeneous intratesticular lesion (*arrow*). (B) On color Doppler, there is hyperemia within the adjacent testis and no flow in the lesion.

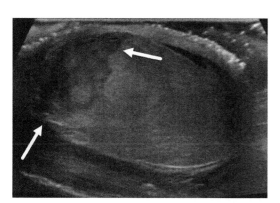

Fig. 10. Intratesticular hematoma. Longitudinal view of a testis demonstrates a heterogeneous, predomi-nantly hypoechoic region in the superior pole of the testis (*arrows*).

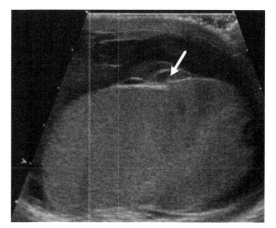

Fig. 11. Testicular rupture. Longitudinal view of the testis demonstrates focal disruption of the tunica al-buginea (*arrow*) with extrusion of adjacent seminifer-ous tubules.

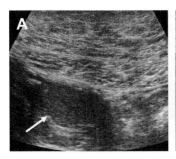
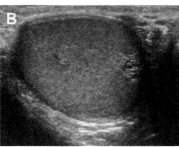

Fig. 12. Unilateral undescended testis. (*A*) The small hypoechoic undescended right testis is located in inguinal canal (*arrow*). (*B*) There is a normal testis in the left hemiscrotum.

to evaluate the integrity of the tunica albuginea. Prompt diagnosis and treatment is required. If surgical repair is performed within 72 hours of injury, the testicular salvage rate is greater than 80%.[5]

TESTICULAR PROCESSES
Undescended Testis (Cryptorchidism)

Cryptorchidism is the incomplete descent of a testis into the scrotum. Initially, the testes are located in the retroperitoneum near the fetal kidney.[15] In most cases, the testes descend to the deep internal ring by 22 to 25 weeks and into the scrotum at 25 to 30 weeks.[19] Although cryptorchid testes can be located anywhere along the path of testicular descent, the most common location is in the inguinal canal.[15]

On the ultrasound scan, the undescended testis is often asymmetrically small and hypoechoic relative to a normal testis (**Fig. 12**).[4] Prepubertal orchidopexy is performed to reduce the risk of cancer in an undescended testis. After puberty, orchiectomy may be considered.[19]

Testicular Microlithiasis

These punctate hyperechoic foci arise from lamellated calcifications in the seminiferous tubules (**Fig. 13**). In past literature it was thought that testicular microlithiasis was associated with a higher risk of testicular cancer, but multiple recent longitudinal studies have questioned this association. An appropriate follow-up for patients with testicular microlithiasis, no testicular mass, and no risk factors for testicular cancer would include periodic testicular examinations. In patients with risk factors for testicular cancer, referral to urology to determine an appropriate follow-up plan should be considered.[20]

Benign Testicular Lesions

Tubular ectasia of the rete testis
The rete testis is located within the testicular mediastinum and comprises a network of seminiferous tubules that transport sperm into the efferent ductules. Obstruction of the efferent tubules may be secondary to compression by an epididymal cyst, sequela of chronic epididymitis, or postvasectomy changes, and is most common in men older than 55 years. Ectasia of the rete testis appears as dilated avascular tubular structures near the mediastinum (**Fig. 14**).

Testicular simple cysts
There are 2 types of testicular cysts, both of which are anechoic and thin-walled. Thick walls or solid nodular components should raise concern for a cystic neoplasm.[7]

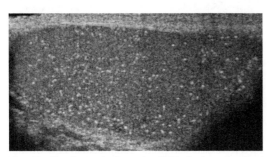

Fig. 13. Classic testicular microlithiasis. Longitudinal view of a testis demonstrates multiple punctate hyperechoic nonshadowing foci.

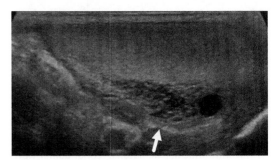

Fig. 14. Tubular ectasia of the rete testis. Longitudinal view of the testis demonstrates cystic changes along the testicular mediastinum (*arrow*).

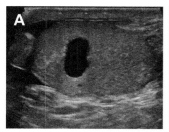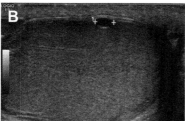

Fig. 15. Testicular simple cysts. (*A*) Longitudinal view of the testis demonstrates an intratesticular cyst. (*B*) Longitudinal view of the testis demonstrates a peripheral tunica albuginea cyst (*cursors*).

- Intratesticular cysts are most often located near the mediastinum and are rarely palpable (**Fig. 15**A). These cysts are most common in middle-aged and elderly men and are associated with spermatoceles.
- Tunica albuginea cysts are peripheral in location and are usually small, firm, and palpable (**Fig. 15**B).

Testicular epidermoid cyst

This is a rare benign lesion, representing 1% to 2% of testicular lesions.[21] On the ultrasound scan, the classic appearance is an avascular well-circumscribed lesion with alternating hyperechoic and hypoechoic rings ("onion ring" pattern) (**Fig. 16**). A peripheral calcified rim is present in some cases. This lesion is unique because it can be treated with enucleation rather than orchiectomy if (1) the lesion has a classic imaging appearance, (2) tumor markers are negative, (3) the lesion is less than 3 cm, and (4) intraoperative

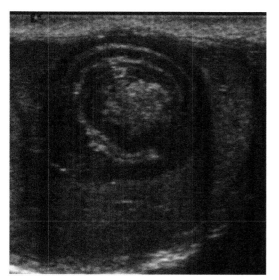

Fig. 16. Testicular epidermoid cyst. Transverse view of a testis shows an intratesticular mass with alternating hyperechoic and hypoechoic rings ("onion ring" pattern).

frozen sections confirm it is an epidermoid cyst.[6,21]

Testicular adrenal rests

Adrenal tissue trapped within the developing fetal testis results in adrenal rests.[6] These lesions are frequently associated with congenital adrenal hyperplasia and typically are small bilateral hypoechoic hypervascular nodules near the mediastinum (**Fig. 17**).[22]

Sarcoidosis

Sarcoidosis is a chronic disease with noncaseating granulomas within multiple organ systems. The genitourinary tract is involved in approximately 5% of patients.[23] The most commonly involved site within the scrotum is the epididymis, with bilateral enlargement. If the testes are involved, there typically are small, bilateral hypoechoic lesions (**Fig. 18**).

Malignant Testicular Lesions

Germ cell tumors

The vast majority of testicular tumors (90%–95%) are germ cell tumors, of which there are 2 types: seminoma and nonseminomatous germ cell tumor. Tumors may be composed of a single tumor subtype (pure) or multiple subtypes (mixed).[24]

Seminoma This is the most common pure germ cell tumor,[6] which frequently occurs at 30 to 40 years of age.[4] On the ultrasound scan, small seminomas are typically homogeneous and hypoechoic with smooth or lobulated margins (**Fig. 19**). With increasing size, the tumor may be heterogeneous. Seminomas rarely breach the tunica albuginea.[4] Even if distant metastatic disease is present, seminomas have a high cure rate because the tumor is highly radiosensitive.[25]

Nonseminomatous germ cell tumors Most of these tumors are of mixed cell type[7]; they are often heterogeneous with ill-defined margins, internal cystic spaces, or calcifications (**Fig. 20**).[4]

- Yolk sac tumors arise from totipotent germ cells and frequently elevate serum

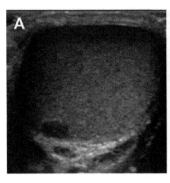
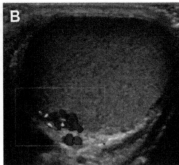

Fig. 17. Testicular adrenal rest. Transverse views of a testis shows a small hypoechoic lesion (*A*), which is hypervascular on color Doppler (*B*).

α-fetoprotein.[6] The pure form of the tumor is most frequent in children younger than 5 years.[5]

- Teratomas contain all 3 germ cell layers (endoderm, mesoderm, and ectoderm).[6] In prepubertal boys, mature teratomas are often benign. Any form of teratoma in adults is considered malignant.[4]
- Embryonal carcinoma arises from primitive anaplastic tumor cells. The tumor has a more aggressive behavior than seminoma and frequently invades the tunica albuginea.[6]
- Choriocarcinoma is composed of cyto-trophoblasts and syncytiotrophoblasts.[4,6] Its pure form represents less than 1% of testicular cancer cases and is associated with a poor 1-year survival. Hemorrhage is frequently present in both the primary lesion and the metastases. A patient with chorio-carcinoma may present with symptoms related to hematogenous metastases to the lungs, liver, or brain, rather than a palpable testicular mass. Human chorionic gonadotropin levels are elevated with this tumor.[6]

Burned out testicular tumor A rapidly growing testicular tumor can outgrow its blood supply and atrophy. The tumor remnant may be a focal calcification or a small hypoechoic lesion on the ultrasound scan (**Fig. 21**).[4,6] Patients often have extensive retroperitoneal lymphadenopathy at diagnosis.

Sex-cord stromal tumors

Approximately 4% to 5% of testicular tumors are sex-cord stromal tumors. Most of these tumors are benign, with 10% to 20% being malignant.[26] Patients may present with signs of virilization or feminization. The sonographic appearance of these tumors is variable, and there are no imaging features to reliably differentiate between sex-cord stromal and germ cell tumors.[6]

- Leydig cell tumors are the most common type of sex-cord stromal tumor and arise from interstitial (Leydig) cells, which produce testosterone (**Fig. 22**). The tumors can also produce estrogen.[26]
- Sertoli cell tumors originate within the Sertoli cells within the seminiferous tubules.[26] These

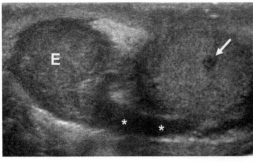

Fig. 18. Sarcoidosis. Longitudinal view of the epididymal head (E) and body (*asterisks*) show enlargement of the epididymal head. There is a small hypoechoic lesion in the testicular parenchyma (*arrow*).

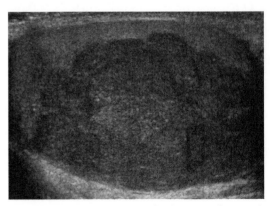

Fig. 19. Seminoma. Longitudinal view of a testis shows near complete replacement by a hypoechoic solid mass.

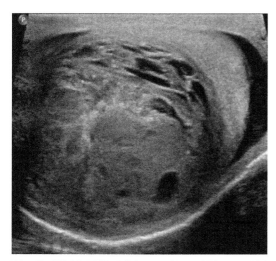

Fig. 20. Mixed germ cell tumor. Transverse view of a testis shows a solid heterogeneous solid and cystic mass.

cells produce proteins and steroids, which support the developing sperm cells.

- Other sex-cord stromal tumors are rare and include granulosa cell tumors, fibroma-thecomas, and mixed sex-cord stromal tumors. A gonadoblastoma contains both germ cell and sex-cord stromal elements.

Other testicular tumors

The testes may be involved with lymphoma, leukemia, or metastatic disease. A new testicular lesion in a patient with known malignancy may represent secondary involvement of the testis.

- Lymphoma constitutes 5% of testicular malignancies.[4] It is the most common testicular malignancy in men older than 60 years and the most common bilateral testicular neoplasm.[6,7] Secondary involvement of the testis is more common than primary testicular lymphoma. Ultrasound will demonstrate a discrete hypoechoic hypervascular testicular lesions or a diffuse infiltrative hypoechoic region (Fig. 23).[4,6] Careful evaluation of the epididymis, spermatic cord, and scrotal skin is warranted, as testicular lymphoma may extend into the adjacent structures.[27]

- Leukemic infiltration of the testes is most common in children with acute leukemia. The blood-testis barrier prevents chemotherapeutic agents from entering the testes, allowing for the testes to serve as a reservoir for residual leukemic cells and a common site of recurrent disease. The sonographic appearance is similar to that of testicular lymphoma. In a patient with leukemia, testicular hypervascularity with normal flow in the epididymis raises concern for malignancy.[20]

- Metastases within the testis are rare. The primary tumors most likely to metastasize to the testis are prostate and lung cancers.[4]

EPIDIDYMAL LESIONS
Spermatocele

A spermatocele arises from dilated efferent ductules and contains spermatozoa. It occurs almost exclusively in the epididymal head. On the ultrasound scan it is usually an anechoic lesion or may contain low-level echoes (Fig. 24).[7]

Epididymal Cyst

These simple cysts occur throughout the epididymis and are most common in the epididymal head. In contrast to spermatoceles, epididymal cysts contain serous fluid (Fig. 25). It is not possible on ultrasonography to reliably distinguish between spermatoceles and epididymal cysts.[4]

Adenomatoid Tumor

Adenomatoid tumor is a rare, benign, slow-growing lesion of mesothelial origin.[29] These tumors typically occur in men 20 to 50 years of age

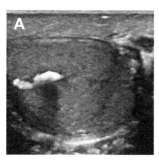

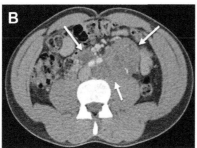

Fig. 21. Burned out testicular tumor. (A) Transverse view of a testis shows a hyperechoic shadowing macrocalcification. (B) Axial computed tomography shows extensive retroperitoneal lymphadenopathy (arrows).

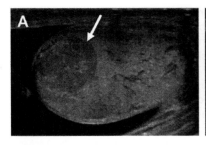
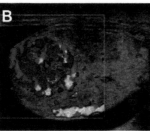

Fig. 22. Leydig cell tumor. (*A*) There is a hypoechoic solid mass in the testis (*arrow*). (*B*) On color Doppler, there is internal flow in the lesion.

and are often asymptomatic.[2] Rarely patients present with symptoms resembling epididymitis. In descending order of frequency, adenomatoid tumors arise from the epididymis, tunica vaginalis, testis, and the spermatic cord. The sonographic appearance is variable, but it is typically a solid lesion that is isoechoic to the epididymis (**Fig. 26**).[30] Excisional biopsy will confirm the diagnosis.

Sperm Granuloma

This benign lesion is seen in almost 50% of patients after vasectomy, compared with 2.5% of the general population. In the postvasectomy state, sperm is extravasated and can result in a granulomatous reaction. It is often asymptomatic, but some of the nodules are painful. A well-circumscribed solid, hypoechoic epididymal lesion is typical on the ultrasound scan (**Fig. 27**).[2]

EXTRATESTICULAR PROCESSES
Scrotolith (Scrotal Pearl)

Scrotoliths are mobile macrocalcifications with posterior acoustic shadowing. They are located within the tunica vaginalis and frequently associated with a hydrocele (**Fig. 28**).[2,4]

Varicocele

A varicocele is dilation of the pampiniform plexus and occurs in approximately 15% of the general population.[31] A varicocele is identified in 45% of men with infertility, and can result in testicular damage and arrested spermatogenesis.[32] A meta-analysis by Baazeem and colleagues[33] demonstrated that varicocelectomy can improve sperm count and mobility.

- Primary varicoceles are caused by incompetent or absent venous valves and are the most common type of varicocele.[4,7] Most varicoceles are left-sided because the left testicular vein has a longer course and drains into the left renal vein.[32]
- An isolated right varicocele or a new varicocele in an older man raises concern for a retroperitoneal mass and warrants further evaluation.[2]
- Secondary varicoceles are the result of compression of the testicular vein, renal vein, or inferior vena cava by a mass, adjacent vasculature, or thrombus.[2] Compression of the left renal vein between the superior mesenteric artery and the aorta ("nutcracker" syndrome) may lead to a left varicocele and hematuria.[34]

The sonographic appearance of a varicocele is multiple dilated serpentine structures greater than 2 mm in diameter, commonly located superior and/or posterior to the testis (**Fig. 29**). Scanning as the patient performs the Valsalva maneuver will result in augmented retrograde flow and in some cases may cause a measurable

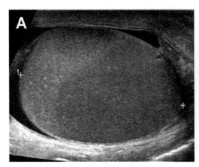
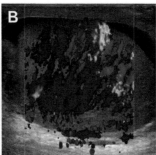

Fig. 23. Testicular lymphoma. (*A*) Longitudinal view of a testis demonstrates an area of decreased echogenicity within the inferior half of the testis. (*B*) On Color Doppler, this region is markedly hypervascular.

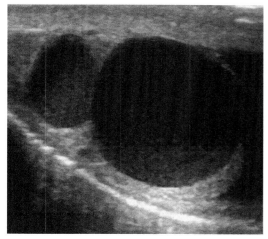

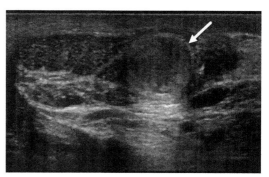

Fig. 26. Adenomatoid tumor. Longitudinal view of the epididymal body demonstrates a heterogeneous lesion with posterior acoustic enhancement (*arrow*).

Fig. 24. Spermatoceles. Longitudinal view of the epididymal head shows 2 cystic lesions with low-level internal echoes.

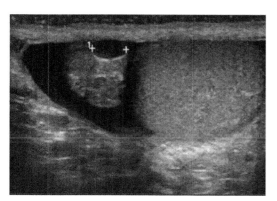

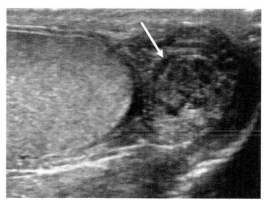

Fig. 25. Epididymal head cyst. Longitudinal view of the epididymal head demonstrates a small cyst (*cursors*) and a small hydrocele.

Fig. 27. Sperm granuloma. Longitudinal view of the epididymal tail shows a predominantly hypoechoic lesion (*arrow*) in a patient with history of vasectomy.

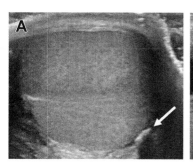

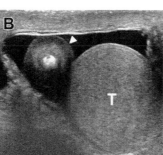

Fig. 28. Scrotoliths in 2 different patients. (*A*) Transverse view of the scrotum shows a small extratesticular hyperechoic shadowing calcification (*arrow*). (*B*) Transverse view of the scrotum demonstrates a round scrotolith with central calcification (*arrowhead*) adjacent to the testis (T).

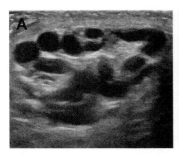
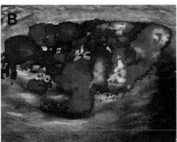

Fig. 29. Varicocele. (*A*) There are multiple dilated veins in the pampiniform plexus. (*B*) During Valsalva maneuver there is augmented flow in the veins.

increase in the size of the veins. In patients undergoing infertility evaluation, if a varicocele is not shown with supine imaging, further imaging in the upright position is recommended.[7]

Hydrocele

In the normal scrotum, there may be trace fluid in the tunica vaginalis, with larger amounts of fluid considered a hydrocele.[35] On the ultrasound scan, hydroceles are typically anechoic fluid collections surrounding the testis, although mobile low-level echoes may be present (**Fig. 30**).[2]

Complex Scrotal Fluid Collection

Blood or purulent material within the tunica vaginalis results in a hematocele or pyocele, respectively. These collections have internal septations and loculations (**Fig. 31**). Pyoceles may have surrounding hyperemia. Differentiating between a pyocele and hematocele requires correlation with history.[18]

- Hematoceles are associated with scrotal trauma or surgery. It is important to evaluate the testis for signs of trauma (ie, intratesticular hematoma or rupture). A hematocele often resolves spontaneously over time. If it does not resolve, it may develop calcifications

and present as a palpable extratesticular lesion.[5,35]

- Pyoceles result from advanced or untreated cases of epididymo-orchitis and may result in vascular compromise of the testis. Scrotal inflammation, including pain and erythema, is often present on physical examination.

SCROTAL WALL PROCESSES
Noninflammatory Edema

A variety of venous and lymphatic processes can lead to scrotal wall edema, including heart failure, liver failure, fluid imbalance, lymphatic obstruction, or filariasis. Sonography demonstrates alternating hypoechoic and hyperechoic layers of the scrotal wall without hyperemia.[3,4] In children, the differential diagnosis of scrotal wall swelling includes Henoch-Schönlein purpura, which is frequently bilateral with epididymal hyperemia, and acute idiopathic scrotal edema, which is typically unilateral without epididymal abnormality.[3,36,37]

Cellulitis

Cellulitis is often diagnosed on physical examination, as patients present with scrotal pain and a thickened, erythematous scrotal wall.[3] Predisposing risk factors include obesity, diabetes, and an immunocompromised state.[4] On the ultrasound

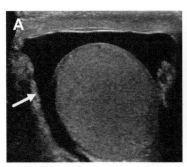
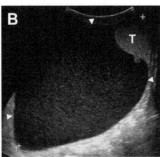

Fig. 30. Hydroceles in 2 separate patients. (*A*) There is an anechoic hydrocele within the tunica vaginalis (*arrow*). (*B*) A large hydrocele with low-level internal echoes (*arrowheads*) displaces the testis (T).

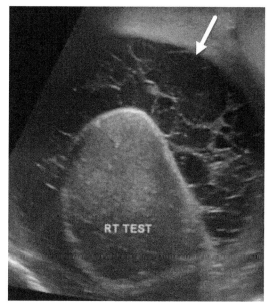

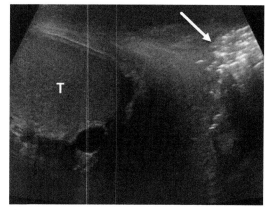

Fig. 33. Fournier gangrene. Longitudinal view of the hemiscrotum shows hyperechoic foci with dirty shadowing representing gas (*arrow*) within the scrotal wall inferior to the testis (T).

Fig. 31. Complex scrotal fluid collection. Transverse view of the right hemiscrotum shows a complex multiseptated collection (*arrow*) surrounding the right testis (RT TEST). This case represented a pyocele.

scan, the scrotal wall is thickened and hyperemic (**Fig. 32**). Ultrasound can help determine whether there is an associated inflammatory process within the testis or epididymis and evaluate for complications, such as abscess or cutaneous fistula.[5]

Fournier Gangrene

Fournier gangrene is an aggressive necrotizing polymicrobial infection of the perineum. Predisposing factors for infection include diabetes, alcohol abuse, and immunocompromised states. The imaging modality of choice is computed tomography, which is helpful in determining the extent of infection and potential complications.[3,38] On the ultrasound scan, gas within the thickened scrotal wall demonstrates multiple hyperechoic foci with dirty shadowing and/or ringdown artifacts (**Fig. 33**). Because of the rapid spread of infection, Fournier gangrene is a surgical emergency that requires intravenous antibiotics and rapid debridement.[38] Even with appropriate treatment, the mortality rate remains 20% to 50%.[39]

SUMMARY

The combination of grayscale and color Doppler ultrasound allows for differentiation among various scrotal disorders, including vascular, infectious, inflammatory, traumatic, and neoplastic lesions.

REFERENCES

1. Avery LL, Scheinfeld MH. Imaging of penile and scrotal emergencies. Radiographics 2013;33(3):721–40.
2. Woodward PJ, Schwab CM, Sesterhenn IA. From the archives of the AFIP: extratesticular scrotal masses: radiologic-pathologic correlation. Radiographics 2003;23(1):215–40.
3. Conzi R, Damasio MB, Bertolotto M, et al. Sonography of scrotal wall lesions and correlation with other modalities. J Ultrasound Med 2017;36(10):2149–63.
4. Dogra VS, Gottlieb RH, Oka M, et al. Sonography of the scrotum. Radiology 2003;227(1):18–36.

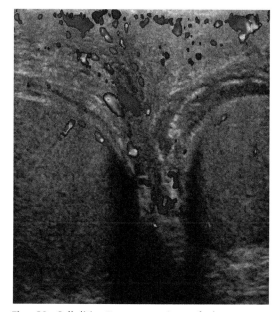

Fig. 32. Cellulitis. Transverse view of the scrotum shows skin thickening and hyperemia.

5. Bhatt S, Dogra VS. Role of US in testicular and scrotal trauma. Radiographics 2008;28(6):1617–29.

6. Woodward PJ, Sohaey R, O'Donoghue MJ, et al. From the archives of the AFIP: tumors and tumorlike lesions of the testis: radiologic-pathologic correlation. Radiographics 2002;22(1):189–216.

7. Hertzberg B, Middleton W. Lower genitourinary, . Ultrasound: the requisites. 3rd edition. Philadelphia: Elsevier; 2016. p. 146–78.

8. Middleton WD, Thorne DA, Melson GL. Color Doppler ultrasound of the normal testis. AJR Am J Roentgenol 1989;152(2):293–7.

9. Middleton WD, Bell MW. Analysis of intratesticular arterial anatomy with emphasis on transmediastinal arteries. Radiology 1993;189(1):157–60.

10. Patel AP. Anatomy and physiology of chronic scrotal pain. Transl Androl Urol 2017;6(Suppl 1):S51–6.

11. Pano B, Sebastia C, Bunesch L, et al. Pathways of lymphatic spread in male urogenital pelvic malignancies. Radiographics 2011;31(1):135–60.

12. Weatherspoon K, Polansky S, Catanzano T. Ultrasound emergencies of the male pelvis. Semin Ultrasound CT MR 2017;38(4):327–44.

13. Middleton WD, Middleton MA, Dierks M, et al. Sonographic prediction of viability in testicular torsion: preliminary observations. J Ultrasound Med 1997;16(1):23–7 [quiz: 29–30].

14. Prando D. Torsion of the spermatic cord: the main gray-scale and Doppler sonographic signs. Abdom Imaging 2009;34(5):648–61.

15. Aso C, Enriquez G, Fite M, et al. Gray-scale and color Doppler sonography of scrotal disorders in children: an update. Radiographics 2005;25(5):1197–214.

16. Mukherjee R, Sinclair AM. Epididymo-orchitis: diagnosis and management. Trends Urol Men's Health 2010;1(2):15–8.

17. Horstman WG, Middleton WD, Melson GL. Scrotal inflammatory disease: color Doppler US findings. Radiology 1991;179(1):55–9.

18. Valentino M, Bertolotto M, Ruggirello M, et al. Cystic lesions and scrotal fluid collections in adults: ultrasound findings. J Ultrasound 2011;14(4):208–15.

19. Kolon TF, Herndon CD, Baker LA, et al. Evaluation and treatment of cryptorchidism: AUA guideline. J Urol 2014;192(2):337–45.

20. Winter TC, Kim B, Lowrance WT, et al. Testicular microlithiasis: what should you recommend? AJR Am J Roentgenol 2016;206(6):1164–9.

21. Loya AG, Said JW, Grant EG. Epidermoid cyst of the testis: radiologic-pathologic correlation. Radiographics 2004;24(Suppl 1):S243–6.

22. Wang Z, Yang Z, Wang W, et al. Diagnosis of testicular adrenal rest tumors on ultrasound: a retrospective study of 15 cases report. Medicine (Baltimore) 2015;94(36):e1471.

23. Koyama T, Ueda H, Togashi K, et al. Radiologic manifestations of sarcoidosis in various organs. Radiographics 2004;24(1):87–104.

24. Kreydin EI, Barrisford GW, Feldman AS, et al. Testicular cancer: what the radiologist needs to know. AJR Am J Roentgenol 2013;200(6):1215–25.

25. Marko J, Wolfman DJ, Aubin AL, et al. Testicular seminoma and its mimics: from the radiologic pathology archives. Radiographics 2017;37(4):1085–98.

26. Dilworth JP, Farrow GM, Oesterling JE. Non-germ cell tumors of testis. Urology 1991;37(5):399–417.

27. Zicherman JM, Weissman D, Gribbin C, et al. Best cases from the AFIP: primary diffuse large B-cell lymphoma of the epididymis and testis. Radiographics 2005;25(1):243–8.

28. Mazzu D, Jeffrey RB Jr, Ralls PW. Lymphoma and leukemia involving the testicles: findings on grayscale and color Doppler sonography. AJR Am J Roentgenol 1995;164(3):645–7.

29. Amin W, Parwani AV. Adenomatoid tumor of testis. Clin Med Pathol 2009;2:17–22.

30. Akbar SA, Sayyed TA, Jafri SZ, et al. Multimodality imaging of paratesticular neoplasms and their rare mimics. Radiographics 2003;23(6):1461–76.

31. Saypol DC. Varicocele. J Androl 1981;2(2):61–71.

32. Masson P, Brannigan RE. The varicocele. Urol Clin North Am 2014;41(1):129–44.

33. Baazeem A, Belzile E, Ciampi A, et al. Varicocele and male factor infertility treatment: a new meta-analysis and review of the role of varicocele repair. Eur Urol 2011;60(4):796–808.

34. Kurklinsky AK, Rooke TW. Nutcracker phenomenon and nutcracker syndrome. Mayo Clin Proc 2010;85(6):552–9.

35. Patil V, Shetty SM, Das S. Common and uncommon presentation of fluid within the scrotal spaces. Ultrasound Int Open 2015;1(2):E34–40.

36. Klin B, Lotan G, Efrati Y, et al. Acute idiopathic scrotal edema in children–revisited. J Pediatr Surg 2002;37(8):1200–2.

37. Modi S, Mohan M, Jennings A. Acute scrotal swelling in Henoch-Schönlein purpura: case report and review of the literature. Urol Case Rep 2016;6:9–11.

38. Levenson RB, Singh AK, Novelline RA. Fournier gangrene: role of imaging. Radiographics 2008;28(2):519–28.

39. Benjelloun el B, Souiki T, Yakla N, et al. Fournier's gangrene: our experience with 50 patients and analysis of factors affecting mortality. World J Emerg Surg 2013;8(1):13.

Ultrasound in Sports Medicine

Paul J. Spicer, MD[a,b,*], Aaron D. Fain, MD[a], Steven B. Soliman, DO, RMSK[c]

KEYWORDS

• Ultrasound • Musculoskeletal • Sports • Rotator cuff • Biceps • Epicondylitis • Tendon • Ligament

KEY POINTS

- The classic rotator-cuff tear associated with overhead throwing is an articular-sided tear of the posterior fibers of the supraspinatus tendon and the anterior fibers of the infraspinatus tendon.
- Tears of the subscapularis tendon in overhead throwing athletes involve the caudal portion of the tendon at the myotendinous junction.
- Lateral epicondylitis appears as a thickened, hypoechoic, outward-bowing tendon with or without hyperemia.
- Complete tears of the distal biceps tendon occur as avulsions 1 to 2 cm proximal to the radial tuberosity with thickening of the distal tendon stump, tendon discontinuity, an effusion within the paratenon, and shadowing at the tendon stump.
- Dynamic maneuvers can help distinguish a partial-thickness from a full-thickness tear of the anterior talofibular ligament.

INTRODUCTION

Interest in imaging of sports-related injuries continues to grow as the quality of the imaging improves. This is particularly true in the area of musculoskeletal ultrasonography (US). US as a diagnostic modality for athletic injuries provides several advantages over other imaging modalities such as MRI and computed tomography (CT). These advantages include lower cost, rapid scan time, decreased metal artifact, transportability of the US unit, no radiation in comparison with CT, and the ability to compare with a potentially normal contralateral side. Patients with MRI contraindications may also be imaged with US. Finally, US offers the ability to perform dynamic imaging with direct patient interaction, which adds to its diagnostic ability.[1,2]

This article focuses on several common athletic injuries that can be diagnosed by US. The sports associated with each injury, anatomy, scanning technique, and diagnostic appearance are discussed for each diagnosis. A linear-array transducer of 10 to 15 MHz is recommended for each of these diagnoses.

SHOULDER

Rotator Cuff: Supraspinatus and Infraspinatus Tendons

Shoulder injuries are common among athletes of all ages. These injuries may involve the capsule, labrum, tendons, and cartilaginous and osseous structures. Of these, US has been shown to have sensitivity and specificity for partial-thickness rotator-cuff tears of 0.84 and 0.96, respectively; for

Disclosure Statement: The authors do not have anything to disclose regarding any commercial or financial conflicts of interest or funding sources related to this article.
a Division of Musculoskeletal Radiology, Department of Radiology, University of Kentucky, 800 Rose Street HX-315D, Lexington, KY 40536, USA; b Division of Breast Imaging, Department of Radiology, University of Kentucky, 800 Rose Street HX-315D, Lexington, KY 40536, USA; c Division of Musculoskeletal Radiology, Department of Radiology, Henry Ford Hospital, 2799 West Grand Boulevard, Detroit, MI 48202, USA
* Corresponding author.
E-mail address: paul.spicer4@uky.edu

full-thickness tears the numbers improve to 0.89 and 0.93, respectively.[3,4]

Injuries of the rotator cuff are common across a variety of sports. Carvalho and colleagues[5] evaluated 720 athletes with a combination of US and MRI, and found that 11.5% had partial-thickness rotator-cuff tears. Of those athletes with tears, the investigators determined that athletes involved in ball-throwing sports were responsible for 66% of the articular-sided partial-thickness tears, whereas those involved in bodybuilding were responsible for 75% of the partial-thickness bursal-sided tears. Tagliafico and colleagues[6] evaluated non-elite junior tennis players using high-resolution US and discovered that these young athletes only had minor shoulder abnormalities. Only 2 of 90 athletes had rotator-cuff tendinosis and none had a rotator-cuff tear. Monteleone and coworkers,[7] using US, discovered calcific tendinosis in the rotator cuff in 30% of the hitting shoulders of elite Italian beach volleyball players. Rodeo and colleagues[8] used US to examine Olympic swimmers and found that 96% of the 46 shoulders evaluated had rotator-cuff tendinosis. McMahon and coworkers[9] used US to evaluate athletes at the Summer National Senior Games and discovered that in athletes older than 60 years, full-thickness rotator-cuff tears were similar in frequency (21%) to the general population of a similar age (25%), whereas partial-thickness tears were more common (48%) than in the similarly aged general population (25%).

Of the many sports whose athletes suffer shoulder injuries, those involving overhead throwing are associated with extreme forces placed on the shoulder. Loads on the shoulder of up to 108% of body weight and humeral angular velocities of 7000°/s have been recorded.[10] These sports include tennis, volleyball, javelin throwing, American football, and baseball, among which baseball pitching is the most studied activity in the literature.[11]

The throwing motion of a baseball pitcher comprises 6 phases: windup, stride, cocking, acceleration, deceleration, and follow-through. The phases most relevant to shoulder injuries are the final 4 phases, cocking through the follow-through. The classic rotator-cuff tear associated with pitching is a partial-thickness, articular-sided tear of the posterior fibers of the supraspinatus tendon and the anterior fibers of the infraspinatus tendon (**Fig. 1**). This tear is the result of internal impingement, which occurs between the late cocking phase and the early acceleration phase. In the late portion of the cocking phase the shoulder is in maximum external rotation. The transition from the late cocking phase to the early

acceleration phase is also the time of maximal forces and angular velocity on the shoulder. The result is that the articular surface of the supraspinatus and infraspinatus tendons may suffer internal impingement between the labrum and the humeral head. This impingement, as well as tendon tensile failure resulting from overload of the rotator-cuff capsular attachment, may result in the classic articular-sided tear of the supraspinatus and infraspinatus tendons.[10,11]

There are multiple described methods for scanning the supraspinatus and infraspinatus tendons. In this article, the modified Crass position is described. The patient is seated on a stool facing the imager. The patient places the ipsilateral hand on the ipsilateral hip or buttock while pointing the elbow posteriorly. This position brings the supraspinatus and infraspinatus tendons out from under the acromion so that they can be visualized. To image the supraspinatus tendon in the longitudinal plane or long axis, begin initially by placing the probe slightly anterior to the greater tuberosity. This will place the probe over the rotator interval, which ensures that the anterior fibers of the supraspinatus tendon are evaluated. From this location, scan the probe posteriorly over the entire greater tuberosity. This will span approximately 2 to 2.5 cm and will include both the supraspinatus and infraspinatus tendons. After evaluating the tendons in long axis, rotate the probe 90° to image the tendons in the transverse plane or short axis.[12]

Injuries of the supraspinatus and infraspinatus tendons may include tendinosis or tears. Tendinosis is characterized by a hypoechoic, thickened tendon, which may demonstrate hyperemia on power Doppler. Tears of the tendon may be partial thickness or full thickness. A partial-thickness tear may be articular, bursal, or intrasubstance. Articular-sided tears begin as an anechoic defect within the articular surface of the tendon, adjacent to the hyaline cartilage overlying the humeral head, and extend into a portion of the tendon. Bursal-sided tears begin on the subacromial subdeltoid bursal side of the tendon and extend into a portion of the tendon. Alternatively, intrasubstance tears begin within the tendon and do not extend to either the articular or the bursal side of the tendon. Full-thickness tears, on the other hand, extend through the entire thickness of the tendon from the articular to the bursal surface. The classic tear associated with baseball pitching is an articular surface tear involving the posterior fibers of the supraspinatus tendon and the anterior fibers of the infraspinatus tendon. It should be noted, however, that many asymptomatic pitchers have rotator-cuff tears, and treatment should be based on a combination of imaging and clinical findings.[10,11]

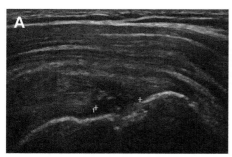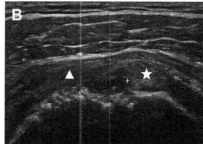

Fig. 1. A classic tear in an overhead throwing athlete. The tear is noted as the hypoechoic to anechoic area between the calipers in the long-axis image (*A*) and the short-axis image (*B*). The tear involves the articular surface of the tendon, best seen on the long-axis image, and involves the posterior fibers of the supraspinatus tendon (*star*) and the anterior fibers of the infraspinatus tendon (*triangle*), best seen on the short-axis image.

Rotator Cuff: Subscapularis Tendon

An additional rotator-cuff tear associated with baseball pitchers is a tear of the subscapularis tendon. In the general population, most tears of the subscapularis occur at the cranial border of the tendon insertion onto the lesser tuberosity. However, in baseball pitchers the tear is typically along the caudal portion of the tendon near the myotendinous junction (**Fig. 2**). This is thought to occur in pitchers who are not able to achieve sufficient external rotation of the shoulder, which shortens the throwing arc. Therefore, to achieve the same velocities with a shorter throwing arc, they must produce greater force by the subscapularis muscle as the tendon fibers are stretched along the anterior glenohumeral joint. This increased force predisposes the tendon to injury.[13]

To image the subscapularis tendon, the patient places the ipsilateral hand in his or her lap with the palm facing upward. The transducer is placed horizontally over the anterior shoulder, specifically along the lesser tuberosity. The patient should then externally rotate the shoulder, bringing the subscapularis tendon out from under the coracoid process. The tendon will be seen in the longitudinal plane or long axis. The tendon should be imaged from cranial to caudal in this position to ensure that the entirety of the tendon is visualized. The transducer can then be rotated 90° vertically to visualize the tendon in the transverse plane or short axis.[12]

Injuries of the subscapularis tendon are described similarly to that discussed for the supraspinatus and infraspinatus tendons. These injuries include tendinosis, partial-thickness tears, and full-thickness tears. Particular attention should be given to the caudal portion of the tendon near the myotendinous junction.[14]

ELBOW
Tennis Elbow

Tennis elbow, the result of injury to the common extensor tendon,[14] is a common term used to describe lateral epicondylitis, or epicondylosis, and is the most common cause of elbow pain.[14–16] This tendon comprises the extensor carpi radialis brevis, extensor digitorum, extensor digiti minimi, and extensor carpi ulnaris tendons as they attach to the lateral epicondyle of the humerus.[15] Of these tendons, the extensor carpi radialis brevis is typically involved, followed by the extensor digitorum communis.[14]

Lateral epicondylitis in athletes is associated with throwing and tennis, particularly in athletes older than 35 years.[16] It has been estimated that approximately 50% of recreational and competitive tennis players will develop lateral elbow pain during their tennis careers.[17] This is the result of repetitive loading and overuse of the common extensor muscles, which leads to mucoid degeneration, microtears, and angiofibroblastic hyperplasia within the tendon.[14–16] Clinically this presents as focal tenderness at the lateral epicondyle with reduced strength with a resisted grip. The diagnosis is usually made on the basis of clinical examination; however, imaging may be used in cases refractory to therapy or when the diagnosis is uncertain.[14,15]

To visualize the common extensor tendon with US, first identify the lateral epicondyle of the humerus in the longitudinal plane. In this position, the tendon becomes visible as a beak-shaped hyperechoic tendon between the subcutaneous tissues and the underlying radial collateral ligament.[16,18] The deepest tendon is the extensor carpi radialis brevis and the most superficial is the extensor digitorum.[16] After evaluating the tendon in the longitudinal plane, rotate the probe 90° to visualize the tendon in the transverse plane.

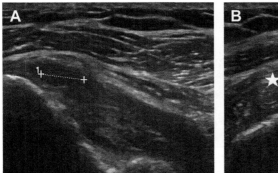
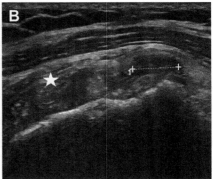

Fig. 2. A tear of the subscapularis tendon in a throwing athlete. The tear is noted as the hypoechoic area delineated by calipers. The tear is somewhat atypical in that it is near the lesser tuberosity footprint instead of the myotendinous junction as seen in the long-axis image (A), whereas the tear is noted along the caudal margin of the tendon as seen in the short-axis image (B). The star on the short-axis image represents the cranial portion of the tendon.

In this orientation, the extensor carpi radialis brevis is the most anterior tendon and muscle.[18]

With US, lateral epicondylitis appears as an outward-bowing, thickened tendon with a heterogeneous echotexture (Fig. 3). Fluid may be noted between the tendon and the underlying lateral epicondyle. With power Doppler, hyperemia may be detected because of the angiofibroblastic reaction inside the tendon.[14] Additional findings include irregularity of the osseous tendon attachment at the lateral epicondyle, calcification within the tendon, or small tears within the substance of the tendon.[15]

Distal Biceps Tendon

Injuries of the distal biceps tendon are much less common than those of the proximal long head of the biceps tendon, accounting for approximately 5% of all biceps tendon disorder and 3% of all biceps tendon tears.[14,15] In the general population, tears of the distal biceps tendon are most commonly seen in men aged 40 to 60 years, and rates are reported as 1.2 per 100,000 persons per year. These tears result from an extension force of the anterior forearm while the elbow is in a flexed position, typically while lifting a heavy object.[19] In athletics, this injury is most commonly seen in weightlifters, footballers, or gymnasts.[14,16,20]

This distal biceps tendon is approximately 7 cm in length and inserts on the medial surface of the radial tuberosity. It originates from the 2 muscle bellies of the biceps brachii muscle and in most individuals there are actually 2 tendons, 1 from each muscle belly, which collectively form the distal biceps tendon. The tendon from the long head of the biceps brachii muscle inserts proximally while the tendon from the short head inserts distally. The distal portion of the tendon is covered by an extrasynovial paratenon and the bicipitoradial bursa.[18] Proximally, the distal biceps tendon is adjacent to the brachial artery. At this location, the lacertus fibrosis provides an aponeurotic attachment to the tendon while traversing from lateral to medial to ultimately fuse with the superficial flexor fascia.[21] This is an important landmark for reporting tendon retraction in full-thickness tears.

Multiple approaches to imaging the distal biceps tendon have been described including anterior, lateral, medial, and posterior approaches.[18,22,23]

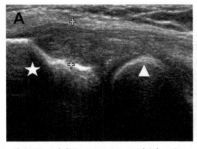
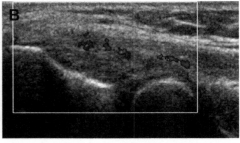

Fig. 3. Lateral epicondylitis appears as thickening and outward bowing of a hyperechoic tendon (A) with associated hyperemia, as noted by the increased vascularity (B). The star denotes the lateral epicondyle and the triangle denotes the radial head.

The most common approach is an anterior or anterior-oblique approach. The images acquired with this approach most closely mimic those obtained with MRI. The arm is extended and maximally supinated. The transducer is placed transverse, or short axis, at the level of the elbow crease, and the tendon is followed to the radial tuberosity. To image the tendon longitudinally, or in long axis, turn the probe 90°. The tendon will be found lateral to the brachial artery. Increased pressure should be applied over the distal tendon at its radial tuberosity insertion to minimize the effect of anisotropy artifact.[18]

Tears of the distal biceps tendon may be partial-thickness tears, complete tears of 1 of the 2 tendons, or a complete tear of both tendons. Complete tears of the tendon and the lacertus fibrosis leads to tendon retraction and a straightforward clinical diagnosis. However, when the lacertus fibrosis remains intact and tendon retraction does not occur, clinical diagnosis and palpation of the tendon become more limited, particularly in the presence of swelling and hematoma formation.

US has been shown to have sensitivity for complete tears of 98% in one study of 65 cases,[19] and sensitivity of 95% and accuracy of 91% for differentiating complete from partial-thickness tears in another study of 45 patients.[20] Partial-thickness tears display contour waviness, irregularity, and partial disruption of the distal 2 to 3 cm of the tendon fibers.[14,19] Hematoma formation and fluid within the paratenon may also be seen. Dynamic maneuvers using flexion-extension and pronation-supination may be helpful to differentiate the intact fibers from the torn fibers.[19] Complete tears typically occur as avulsions 1 to 2 cm proximal to the radial tuberosity where the tendon is hypovascularized.[19] These tears demonstrate thickening of the distal tendon stump, absence of the tendon at its normal location, tendon discontinuity, and an effusion within the paratenon. An additional important finding in complete tears is shadowing at the tendon stump, which has been reported with sensitivity of 97%, specificity of 100%, and accuracy of 98% for differentiating a complete tear from a normal tendon (Fig. 4). This finding suggests that the lack of shadowing may exclude a complete tear, although it does not exclude a partial-thickness tear.[20] The lacertus fibrosis is most easily visualized in the transverse plane or short axis. In complete tendon tears with an intact lacertus fibrosis, the distance of the retracted tendon stump from the radial tuberosity should be reported.[19]

ANTERIOR TALOFIBULAR LIGAMENT

Whereas tendinous injuries often relate to overuse, ligaments are most often injured following an acute injury.[24] Injury of the lateral ligament complex of the ankle is the most common injury in sports.[25,26] There are an estimated 850,000 new ankle sprains occurring each year in the United States, not including a 70% re-injury rate at the ankle.[26] Ankle sprains occur in approximately 1 of every 10,000 persons per day and account for up to 45% of all sports-related injuries.[27] Specifically, the anterior talofibular ligament (ATFL) is the most common injured ligament because it is the weakest ligament in the lateral ligament complex of the ankle. Approximately two-thirds of ankle sprains are related to isolated injuries to the ATFL. Injury to the ATFL is most commonly related to an ankle inversion injury,[25] most often sustained in sports that involve running, jumping, cutting, or contact with other players, including soccer, basketball, football, volleyball, gymnastics, and cheerleading.[28–30]

The ATFL is located at the lateral aspect of the ankle as part of the lateral ankle ligament complex.

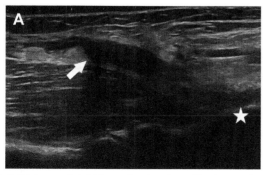
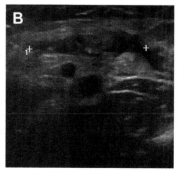

Fig. 4. A full-thickness distal biceps tendon tear. The long-axis panoramic image (A) shows the retracted, torn distal biceps tendon stump (arrow) creating shadowing artifact. The star denotes the radial tuberosity. The short-axis image (B) demonstrates hematoma formation and an effusion within the otherwise empty paratenon, as noted between the calipers.

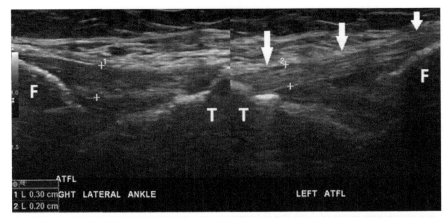

Fig. 5. Sonographic image of the normal left ATFL in a 52-year-old woman demonstrates the normal taut fibrillar pattern (*arrows*) extending from the distal fibula (F) to the talus (T). The patient had a history of a remote ankle sprain on the right where the ATFL appears asymmetrically heterogeneous and thickened (*calipers*).

There are 3 distinct ligaments forming this complex: the ATFL, the calcaneofibular ligament, and the posterior talofibular ligament. The ATFL extends from the anterior rim of the lateral malleolus at the distal fibula to the anterior aspect of the talus and is approximately 2 mm wide. Its function, along with the remainder of the lateral ankle ligaments, is to prevent excessive varus inward movement.[27] Tears more commonly occur at the fibular attachment of the ATFL rather than the talar attachment.[25]

US is excellent for imaging the ATFL and has been shown to have a high specificity and sensitivity for evaluating both acute and chronic tears.[31] Both US and MRI have a reported greater than 90% accuracy in identifying injuries to the ankle, including the ATFL.[26] In one study using arthroscopy as the reference standard, US demonstrated 91% accuracy in diagnosing ATFL injuries.[32] Sonographic evaluation of the ATFL is also performed using a high-frequency linear-array transducer, typically 12 MHz or higher. A higher-frequency compact linear transducer may be beneficial to evaluate the small ATFL and allows easier maneuvering at the lateral malleolus with minimal loss of contact. For an ATFL scan, the patient should be positioned with the foot placed on a flat surface. The probe is placed in the transverse plane (parallel to the sole of the foot) at the lateral ankle, at the level of and anterior to the palpable lateral malleolus. The ATFL will be seen as a band-like structure extending from the talus to the distal fibula.[27,33] Similar to a tendon, the normal ATFL by US appears taut with a uniform size and a fibrillary and homogenous hyperechoic appearance (**Fig. 5**).[1]

Ligament injuries can be classified as grades I, II, and III. A grade I ATFL injury represents interstitial tears, often from acute trauma, without macroscopic disruption. In grade I injuries the ligament may appear normal on US, although there is often adjacent fluid. A grade II injury is a partial-thickness tear with thickening and partial disruption of the fibers. On US the ATFL will manifest as a thickened heterogeneous ligament with focal or diffuse areas of decreased echogenicity disrupting the typical fibrillar pattern, and often with adjacent hypoechoic or anechoic fluid, but no discontinuity (**Fig. 6**). Hyperemia may also be present. Finally, in a grade III injury there is a full-thickness tear with discontinuity and associated edema or hemorrhage (**Fig. 7**).[1,24,27] If an associated avulsion fracture is present, this can also be identified by US as an adjacent echogenic shadowing focus corresponding with the avulsed fracture fragment, most often adjacent to the fibular

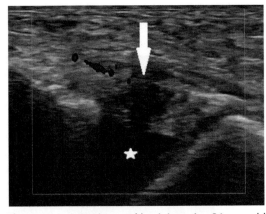

Fig. 6. An inversion ankle injury in 34-year-old woman shows an enlarged heterogeneous ATFL and adjacent hypoechoic fluid (*star*) consistent with a grade 2 injury. There is an associated partial-thickness tear (*arrow*) and slight hyperemia.

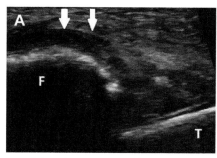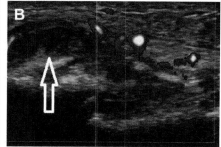

Fig. 7. A soccer injury in a 27-year-old man. (*A*) Discontinuity at the fibular attachment of the ATFL (*arrows*) consistent with a full-thickness tear. (*B*) Hyperemia and complex fluid (*open arrow*) consistent with associated hemorrhage.

attachment of the ATFL.[25] Patients with sprains or tears will often complain of pain when the ATFL is being scanned. In patients with a history of a remote ankle sprain, the ATFL will also appear thickened and heterogeneous but without adjacent fluid or hyperemia (see **Fig. 5**).[26]

Dynamic maneuvers can be used to help differentiate between a partial-thickness and a full-thickness tear,[1,27,32] by scanning the ATFL with one hand and simultaneously applying posterior downward pressure on the distal tibia with the same hand. With the other hand the heel is grasped and pulled anteriorly, therefore creating an anterior drawer test maneuver, which can displace the 2 stumps of an otherwise nondisplaced full-thickness tear. Alternatively, if another person is available, a 2-person technique can be performed with one scanning while the other performs the anterior ankle-drawer test.[1]

SUMMARY

As the quality of the transducers improves, US continues to expand as a diagnostic tool for evaluating sports injuries. As described in this article, US offers high-resolution imaging of many ligamentous and tendinous structures. US offers many advantages over other imaging modalities, particularly the ability to perform dynamic imaging and comparison with the contralateral normal side. These advantages increase the diagnostic capabilities of US. With ongoing research, diagnostic US and its role in athletic injuries will continue to evolve.

REFERENCES

1. Zbojniewicz AM. US for diagnosis of musculoskeletal conditions in the young athlete: emphasis on dynamic assessment. Radiographics 2014;34: 1145–62.
2. Lesniak BP, Loveland D, Jose J, et al. Use of ultrasonography as a diagnostic and therapeutic tool in sports medicine. Arthroscopy 2014;30(2):26–70.
3. Smith TO, Back T, Toms AP, et al. Diagnostic accuracy of ultrasound for rotator cuff tears in adults: a systematic review and meta-analysis. Clin Radiol 2011;66.1030–48.
4. Artul S, Habib G. Ultrasonographic clues for acuity/chronicity of rotator cuff tear. Eur J Rheumatol 2017; 4:260–3.
5. Carvalho CD, Cohen C, Belangero PS, et al. Partial rotator cuff injury in athletes: bursal or articular? Rev Bras Ortop 2015;50(4):416–21.
6. Tagliafico A, Cadoni A, Bignotti B, et al. High-resolution ultrasound of rotator cuff and biceps reflection pulley in non-elite junior tennis players: anatomical study. BMC Musculoskelet Disord 2014;15:241.
7. Monteleone G, Tramontana A, McDonald K, et al. Ultrasonographic evaluation of the shoulder in elite Italian beach volleyball players. J Sports Med Phys Fitness 2015;55(10).1193 9.
8. Rodeo SA, Nguyen JT, Cavanaugh JT, et al. Clinical and ultrasonographic evaluations of the shoulders of elite swimmers. Am J Sports Med 2016;44(12): 3214–21.
9. McMahon PJ, Prasad A, Francis KA. What is the prevalence of senior-athlete rotator cuff injuries and are they associated with pain and dysfunction? Clin Orthop Relat Res 2014;472:2427–32.
10. Shaffer B, Huttman D. Rotator cuff tears in the throwing athlete. Sports Med Arthrosc Rev 2014; 22:101–9.
11. Lin DJ, Wong TT, Kazam JK. Shoulder injuries in the overhead-throwing athlete: epidemiology, mechanisms of injury, and imaging findings. Radiology 2018;286(2):370–87.
12. Jacobson JA. Shoulder US: anatomy, technique, and scanning pitfalls. Radiology 2011;260(1):6–16.
13. Polster JM, Lynch TS, Bullen JA, et al. Throwing-related injuries of the subscapularis in professional baseball players. Skeletal Radiol 2016; 45(1):41–7.
14. Konin GP, Nazarian LN, Walz DM. US of the elbow: indications, technique, normal anatomy, and pathologic conditions. Radiographics 2013;33: E125–47.

15. Radunovic G, Violeta V, Mihaela CM, et al. Ultrasound assessment of the elbow. Med Ultrason 2012;14(2):141–6.

16. Bucknor MD, Stevens KJ, Steinbach LS. Elbow imaging in sport: sports imaging series. Radiology 2016;279(1):12–28.

17. Chung KC, Lark ME. Upper extremity injuries in tennis players: diagnosis, treatment, and management. Hand Clin 2017;33(1):175–86.

18. Tagliafico AS, Bignotti B, Martinoli C. Elbow US: anatomy, variants, and scanning technique. Radiology 2015;275(3):636–50.

19. de la Fuente J, Blasi M, Martinez S, et al. Ultrasound classification of traumatic distal biceps brachii tendon injuries. Skeletal Radiol 2018;47(4):519–32.

20. Lobo Lda G, Fessell DP, Miller BS, et al. The role of sonography in differentiating full versus partial distal biceps tendon tears: correlation with surgical findings. AJR Am J Roentgenol 2013;200(1):158–62.

21. de Maeseneer M, Brigido MK, Antic M, et al. Ultrasound of the elbow with emphasis on detailed assessment of ligaments, tendons, and nerves. Eur Radiol 2015;84:671–81.

22. Brasseur JL. The biceps tendon: from the top and from the bottom. J Ultrasound 2012;15(1):29–38.

23. Smith J, Finnoff JT, O'Driscoll SW, et al. Sonographic evaluation of the distal biceps tendon using a medial approach. J Ultrasound Med 2010;29:861–5.

24. Purohit NB, King LJ. Ultrasound of lower limb sports injuries. Ultrasound 2015;23(3):149–57.

25. Kumai T, Takakura Y, Rufai A, et al. The functional anatomy of the human anterior talofibular ligament in relation to ankle sprains. J Anat 2002;200(5):457–65.

26. Kathy L, Geoff G, Todd R, et al. Increased ligament thickness in previously sprained ankles as measured by musculoskeletal ultrasound. J Athl Train 2015;50(2):193–8.

27. McKiernan S, Fenech M, Fox D, et al. Sonography of the ankle: the lateral ankle and ankle sprains. Sonography 2017;4(4):146–55.

28. Swenson DM, Collins CL, Fields SK, et al. Epidemiology of US high school sports-related ligamentous ankle injuries. 2005/06-2010/11. Clin J Sport Med 2013;23(3):190–6.

29. Woods C, Hawkins R, Hulse M, et al. The football association medical research programme: an audit of injuries in professional football: an analysis of ankle sprains. Br J Sports Med 2003;37:233–8.

30. Fong DT, Hong Y, Chan LK, et al. A systematic review on ankle injury and ankle sprain in sports. Sports Med 2007;37(1):73–94.

31. Hua Y, Yang Y, Chen S, et al. Ultrasound examination for the diagnosis of chronic anterior talofibular ligament injury. Acta Radiol 2013;53(10):1142–5.

32. Battaglia PJ, Craig K, Kettner NW. Ultrasonography in the assessment of lateral ankle ligament injury, instability, and anterior ankle impingement: a diagnostic case report. J Chiropr Med 2015;14(4):265–9.

33. De Maeseneer M, Marcelis S, Jager T, et al. Sonography of the normal ankle: a target approach using skeletal reference points. Am J Roentgenol 2009;192(2):487–95.

Ultrasound of Soft Tissue Masses and Fluid Collections

Jason M. Wagner, MD[a],*, Kristin Rebik, DO[a],
Paul J. Spicer, MD[b]

KEYWORDS

- Ultrasound • Soft tissue mass • Sarcoma • Lipoma • Abscess • Hematoma • Hernia

KEY POINTS

- Sonography allows characterization of many superficial soft tissue masses and identification of fluid collections.
- Many soft tissue masses are hypovascular and Doppler assessment requires careful technique to optimize sensitivity.
- Masses larger than 5 cm or deep to the fascia generally require further imaging or tissue sampling.
- There is substantial overlap in the sonographic appearance of hematoma and sarcoma. The diagnosis of soft tissue hematoma should be made with caution.
- Real-time imaging during compression and release of compression is key to detection of soft tissue abscesses.

 Video content accompanies this article at http://www.radiologic.theclinics.com.

INTRODUCTION

Soft tissue masses and fluid collections are frequently encountered in sonographic practice, either as the principal indication for a diagnostic examination or as an incidental finding during an examination performed for other indications. The estimated incidence of soft tissue tumors is 3 per 1000 per year, about 98% to 99% of which are benign, mostly lipomas.[1–3] Additionally, there are many nonneoplastic causes of a superficial mass, including fluid collections, epidermal inclusion cysts, fat necrosis, and foreign bodies.[4–6]

The challenge of managing patients with a soft tissue mass is to avoid excessive evaluation in the large number of patients with benign pathology while avoiding delayed diagnosis in the small number of patients with malignancy.[7] Although some superficial masses are effectively diagnosed and managed based on history and physical examination, clinical evaluation is difficult because of the nonspecific presentation of soft tissue masses, necessitating imaging for further evaluation.[8]

When imaging of soft tissue masses is indicated, ultrasound is an attractive modality because of its low cost, lack of ionizing radiation, and high spatial resolution. Ultrasound also offers the ability to assess blood flow without contrast administration, evaluate for compressibility/mobility of structures,

Disclosures: None.
[a] Department of Radiological Sciences, University of Oklahoma Health Sciences Center, Garrison Tower, Suite 4G4250, Oklahoma City, OK 73104, USA; [b] Department of Radiology, University of Kentucky, 800 Rose Street, HX-315D, Lexington, KY 40536-0293, USA
* Corresponding author.
E-mail address: jason-wagner@ouhsc.edu

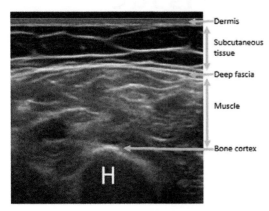

Fig. 1. Transverse view of the upper arm demonstrating the major tissue layers. The H indicates the humeral shaft.

and correlate with palpation.[1] We only advocate ultrasound as an initial imaging evaluation if the soft tissue mass is believed to be less than 5 cm in size and superficial in location. If the mass is large or deep to the fascia, MR imaging without and with contrast is generally regarded as the best imaging study.[3,9]

ANATOMY

The major soft tissue layers observed with ultrasound are the dermis, subcutaneous tissues, deep fascia, and muscle (**Fig. 1**). A key step in characterization of a soft tissue mass is localizing the lesion within a tissue layer (**Fig. 2**).

ULTRASOUND TECHNIQUE

Sonographic imaging performed for evaluation of a possible soft tissue mass is generally a targeted examination focused on the area of symptoms or palpable abnormality. Although these examinations can generally be performed rapidly, careful attention to technique is critical. A key part of the examination is obtaining a targeted history regarding the possible mass, when the mass was first noticed, change in size of the mass, pain at the site, drainage from the site, prior trauma, and history of malignancy. A brief physical examination should also be performed, assessing for firmness, mobility, and tenderness of the mass, and overlying skin changes. Imaging of a palpable mass should be confirmed by simultaneous palpation.[1]

Sonography of a superficial abnormality should generally be performed with a high-frequency linear transducer and a generous mound of coupling gel. It is important to use the highest possible frequency that provides adequate deep visualization (**Fig. 3**). In the thicker portions of the body, particularly the trunk and thigh, it is important to also use a lower frequency transducer to visualize deep tissues (**Fig. 4**). In the thigh, we use visualization of the femoral shaft as confirmation that visualization of the deep tissue was sufficient. Extended field of view imaging is helpful to visualize large superficial masses (**Fig. 5**).

Doppler interrogation of a soft tissue mass allows noninvasive evaluation of blood flow, but requires careful attention to technical detail, because many soft tissue neoplasms are hypovascular. The following steps should be followed to produce high-quality color (or power) Doppler images and maximize detection of slow flow:

- Use the highest frequency transducer that provides adequate visualization.
- Use an application/preset (eg, musculoskeletal or scrotal) that maximizes visualization of slow flow in soft tissues. If a soft tissue

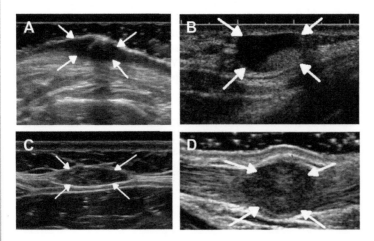

Fig. 2. Mass localization. (*A*) Intradermal squamous cell carcinoma (*arrows*). (*B*) Subcutaneous epidermal inclusion cyst (*arrows*). (*C*) Intrafascial lipoma (*arrows*). (*D*) Intramuscular metastasis (*arrows*) from lung carcinoma. This patient was cachectic and the subcutaneous tissue are very thin (*asterisk*).

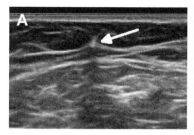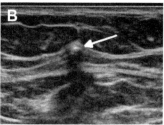

Fig. 3. Importance of using high-frequency imaging for superficial structures. Although this subcutaneous implanted contraceptive device (Nexplanon, *arrows*) is visible at 12 MHz (*A*), the device and the associated deep acoustic shadowing become more visible at 15 MHz (*B*).

mass is discovered during a vascular examination, it is helpful to switch to low-flow settings.

- Minimize the size of the color box to maximize frame rate.
- Support the weight of the transducer with your hand so that it barely rests on the skin surface. Only a small amount of pressure applied through the transducer can reduce or eliminate detectable flow in a superficial structure.[1]
- Decrease the color Doppler scale (pulse repetition frequency).
- Increase the color Doppler gain until there is diffuse flash artifact and then slowly decrease the gain. In our opinion, a color Doppler image intended to show that no flow could be detected in a soft tissue mass should have some artifactual color Doppler signal in the surrounding tissues.
- If color Doppler signal is found within a mass, use spectral Doppler to confirm that the signal actually represents blood flow (**Fig. 6**).

NEOPLASMS
Lipoma

Lipoma is the most common benign soft tissue tumor with an estimated incidence of 1/1000 per year.[8] Lipomas are most frequently encountered between the ages of 40 and 60. Although lipomas are occasionally encountered in teenagers and young adults, soft tissue lipomas are rare in children.[10] Approximately 5% of patients presenting with a lipoma have multiple lipomas.[10]

On clinical examination, lipomas tend to be soft or rubbery, nontender, and mobile. Angiolipoma, a frequent benign variant of lipoma, may be tender to palpation.[11] The sonographic features of lipoma are listed next with examples given in **Fig. 7**.[1,4,11]

- Smoothly marginated oval or lobulated mass that is wider than tall.
- Frequently isoechoic or hypoechoic to normal subcutaneous fat and contain wavy echogenic lines.
- Some lipomas, and most angiolipomas, are hyperechoic and, when hyperechoic, are often homogeneous without the wavy echogenic lines seen in less echogenic lipomas.
- No acoustic shadowing.
- Minimal or no Doppler signal.

Can ultrasound make the diagnosis of lipoma? This question has been extensively debated in the literature, with varying results and opinions.[1,3,4,12–14] It is our opinion that the diagnosis of subcutaneous lipoma can be made for a mass

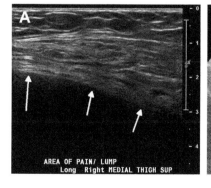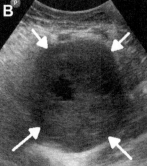

AREA OF PAIN/ LUMP
Long Right MEDIAL THIGH SUP

Fig. 4. Importance of deep imaging. A 43-year-old woman who presented with a proximal thigh mass. (*A*) Initial imaging with a high-frequency transducer failed to appreciate the large mass that is suggested by the abnormal deep tissue interface (*arrows*). (*B*) Subsequent imaging with a low-frequency curved transducer demonstrates a large mass (*arrows*), which was found to be a poorly differentiated sarcoma.

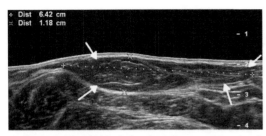

Fig. 5. Extended field of view imaging provides visualization of a large superficial lipoma (*arrows*).

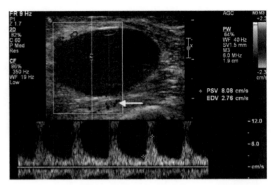

Fig. 6. Doppler technique. The color box is minimized allowing a frame rate of 9 Hz. The color scale is minimized and the color gain is adjusted to have some artifactual signal (*arrow*). Color Doppler signal in the mass is interrogated with spectral Doppler to confirm that it is arterial blood flow.

that is no more than 5 cm in greatest dimension, meets all of the previously mentioned criteria, and has no concerning imaging or clinical features. When we make the diagnosis of a superficial lipoma with ultrasound, we recommend clinical follow-up with repeat evaluation if there is any concerning change. Masses that are larger than 5 cm, deep to the fascia, or have any atypical features generally need further evaluation. In our opinion, the major risk of misdiagnosing a soft tissue malignancy as a benign condition lies not with the diagnosis of subcutaneous lipoma, but with the diagnosis of intramuscular hematoma.

Benign Neoplasms Other than Lipoma

There are numerous benign neoplasms and neoplastic-like conditions that occur in the soft tissues. Although specific diagnoses can sometimes be suggested based on location, clinical features, and sonographic appearance, many benign neoplasms present as nonspecific hypoechoic solid masses and require biopsy or excision for definitive diagnosis (**Figs. 8** and **9**).[5]

Neural origin masses are a frequent cause of a benign soft tissue mass. With careful inspection, a nerve can sometimes be visualized entering or exiting the mass (**Figs. 10 and 11**).

Neurofibromas are typically central within a nerve and schwannomas are typically eccentric to the nerve.[5]

Vascular lesions, such as hemangiomas, are seen in children and adults.[15,16] In adults, hemangiomas tend to present as ill-defined mixed echogenicity lesions with high vessel density and phleboliths that may be visible with ultrasound or radiograph (**Fig. 12**).[1,5]

Malignant Neoplasms

Primary soft tissue malignancies represent 0.8% of all cancers, with an incidence of 3.4 per 100,000 per year and an expected 13,040 new cases in the United States in 2018, 50% of which occur in the extremities.[17] Sarcomas commonly present as solid or mixed solid and cystic intramuscular masses in the extremities with variable echogenicity and vascularity. The most common types of primary soft tissue sarcomas are pleomorphic sarcoma and liposarcoma (**Figs. 13** and **14**).[5]

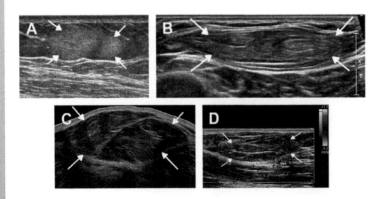

Fig. 7. Lipomas. (*A*) Lipoma of the chest wall (*arrows*) in a 53-year-old man. This lipoma is hyperechoic and essentially homogeneous without curvilinear hyperechoic lines. (*B*) Lipoma of the lateral neck (*arrows*) in a 54-year-old man. (*C*) Lipoma of the midline low back (*arrows*) in a 53-year-old man. The lipomas in *B* and *C* are essentially isoechoic and contain curvilinear hyperechoic lines. (*D*) Lipoma of the thigh (*arrows*) in a 65-year-old woman showing no internal Doppler signal.

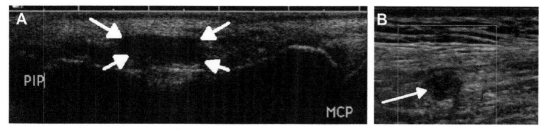

Fig. 8. Benign soft tissue masses in characteristic locations. (A) Giant cell tumor of the tendon sheath (arrows) in a 38-year-old man, along the flexor tendon sheath near a finger proximal phalanx. (B) Endometriosis of the abdominal wall (arrows) in a 28-year-old woman, located adjacent to an incision from prior cesarean section.

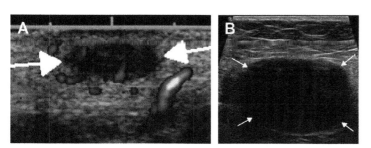

Fig. 9. Nonspecific benign soft tissue masses. (A) Pilomatricoma in the hand (arrows) of a 10-year-old girl. (B) Benign fibromatosis of the anterior abdominal wall (arrows) of a 28-year-old woman.

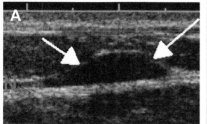
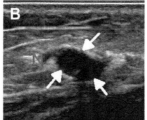

Fig. 10. Neural origin superficial masses (arrows) with visible nerves (orange N). (A) Neurofibroma in a 29-year-old man. (B) Post-traumatic neuroma in a 78-year-old woman occurring several years after surgery in that location for a sarcoma.

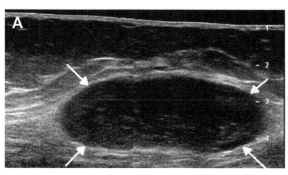
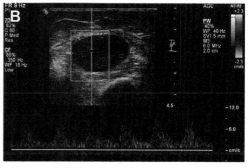

Fig. 11. Schwannoma in the thigh of an 82-year-old woman. (A) Mostly solid, smoothly marginated, intramuscular mass (arrows). An entering or exiting nerve could not be visualized. (B) Low-velocity internal arterial flow.

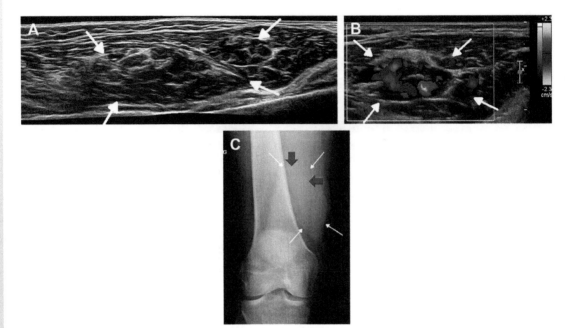

Fig. 12. Low-flow vascular lesion (*white arrows*) near the knee of a 50-year-old man. An extended field of view image (*A*) demonstrates an intramuscular mass with mixed hyperechoic and hypoechoic components. Color Doppler image (*B*) demonstrates low velocity flow anechoic portions of the mass. Flow was augmented with gentle compression of the mass. Anterior-posterior radiograph of the knee (*C*) demonstrates the mass (*white arrows*) and small calcified phleboliths (*red arrows*).

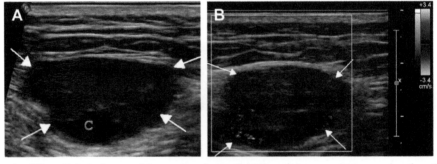

Fig. 13. Poorly differentiated pleomorphic sarcoma (*arrows*) in the gluteus maximus muscle of an 83-year-old man. (*A*) The mass was predominantly solid, but had a few small cystic spaces (orange C). (*B*) The mass (*arrows*) was hypovascular with essentially no internal blood flow identified with color Doppler.

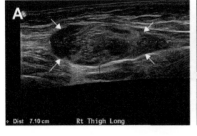

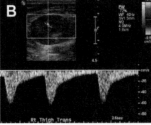

Fig. 14. (*A, B*) Intramuscular liposarcoma (*arrows*) in the thigh of a 59-year-old woman. Although this mass has a few curvilinear echogenic lines as is seen in benign lipoma, the mass is deep, larger than 5 cm, and has vigorous internal blood flow, all features that should prompt further evaluation.

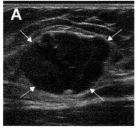
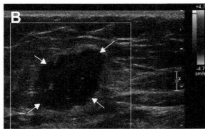

Fig. 15. (A, B) Primary subcutaneous synovial sarcoma (*arrows*) in the groin of an adult woman. On presentation to another institution, this lesion was initially diagnosed as a hematoma, leading to delayed therapy.

Although most superficial masses less than 5 cm are benign, superficial sarcomas do rarely occur (**Figs. 15** and **16**).[8] In our practice we encounter superficial malignancy related to widespread metastasis far more commonly than primary superficial soft tissue malignancy. Lymphoma occasionally presents as a primary soft tissue mass (**Fig. 17**). Soft tissue malignancies can have an ultrasound appearance that mimics a fluid collection, producing a potential pitfall (**Fig. 18**). The following features raise concern that a soft tissue mass may be malignant and should prompt further evaluation:

- Size greater than 5 cm
- Intramuscular/deep location
- Infiltrative border
- Violation of tissue planes
- Rapid growth
- Pain
- Potential fluid collection without a good clinical explanation

FLUID COLLECTIONS
Hematoma

Superficial and intramuscular hematomas can occur for a variety of reasons including trauma, invasive procedures, and complications of anticoagulation. Soft tissue hematomas may be smoothly marginated or irregular in shape. Hematomas may be hyperechoic in the acute phase, but are generally hypoechoic with a variable degree of internal linear echoes

(**Fig. 19**).[1,18] A hematoma should not have internal Doppler signal, unless there is active bleeding (**Fig. 20**).

There is substantial overlap between the sonographic features of hematoma and some soft tissue neoplasms.[14,19] When an incorrect sonographic diagnosis contributes to delayed diagnosis of a sarcoma, hematoma is the most common incorrect diagnosis.[7,20] Additionally, some high-grade sarcomas are internally hemorrhagic, which poses a significant diagnostic challenge for ultrasound and MR imaging (**Fig. 21**).[21,22] In our opinion, the diagnosis of soft tissue hematoma requires a good clinical explanation and we are suspicious of any potential hematoma without a clear cause.

Abscess

Soft tissue infections are a common reason for patients to seek medical attention and it is important to determine if the patient has only cellulitis or an abscess is present. This differentiation is difficult without imaging and ultrasound is an excellent option to evaluate the superficial soft tissues.[23] Cellulitis typically presents as expanded and hyperechoic adipose tissue with variable degrees of hypervascularity and nonloculated perifascial fluid (**Fig. 22**). The sonographic findings of cellulitis are similar to noninfectious edema, requiring correlation with patient presentation.

Abscesses may be well-defined or ill-defined with contents that vary from anechoic to hyperechoic. Superficial soft tissue abscesses

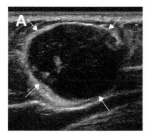
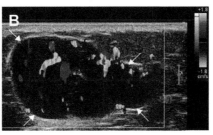

Fig. 16. (A, B) Dermatofibrosarcoma protuberans (*arrows*) in the arm of a 36-year-old woman.

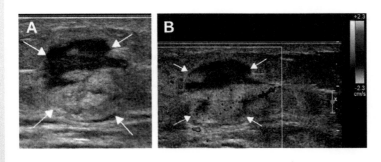

Fig. 17. (*A, B*) Extranodal lymphoma (*arrows*) in the anterior thigh subcutaneous tissues of a 58-year-old man. This mass has hyperechoic and hypoechoic components, ill-defined borders, and essentially no detectable internal blood flow by color Doppler imaging.

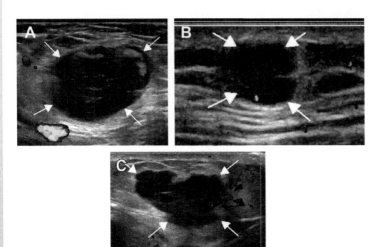

Fig. 18. Superficial malignant masses (*arrows*) that mimic fluid collections. (*A*) Histiocytic sarcoma in the groin of a 53-year-old woman. (*B*) Metastatic melanoma in the gluteal region of a 36-year-old man. (*C*) Metastatic high-grade neuroendocrine tumor in the abdominal wall of a 51-year-old woman. All of these masses have deep acoustic enhancement and essentially no detectable internal blood flow by color Doppler imaging.

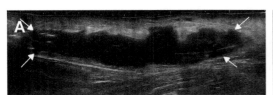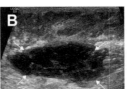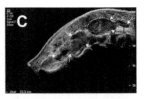

Fig. 19. Soft tissue hematomas (*arrows*). (*A*) Subcutaneous hematoma in the thigh of a 50-year-old man after vascular surgery. (*B*) Intramuscular hematoma in the gluteus maximus muscle of a 33-year-old man after tumor resection. (*C*) Extensive gluteal muscular hematoma after a bone marrow biopsy in a 53-year-old man with thrombocytopenia.

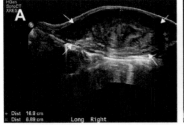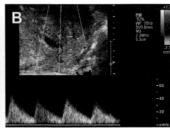

Fig. 20. Actively bleeding rectus sheath hematoma (*arrows*) in a 76-year-old woman who was anticoagulated for a cardiac catheterization procedure. (*A*) Extended field of view images shows the acute hematoma to be predominantly echogenic. (*B*) Spectral Doppler image identified the active bleeding arising from the inferior epigastric artery.

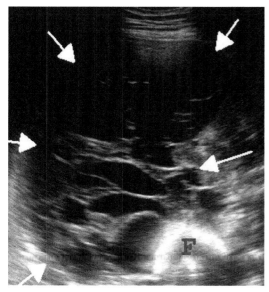

Fig. 21. Spindle cell sarcoma (*arrows*) in the thigh of a 76-year-old man. The mass has a large internal hemorrhagic component and extends deep to the femoral shaft (*red F*).

generally have mobile contents that are observed with real-time sonography during gentle compression and release of compression (**Figs. 23** and **24**; Videos 1 and 2). We regard compression to assess for mobile fluid as a critical part of an ultrasound for potential abscess. In the setting of soft tissue infection, it is critical to look for soft tissue gas, which could indicate necrotizing fasciitis, a surgical emergency (**Fig. 25**).

The common sonographic features of soft tissue neoplasms and fluid collections are summarized in **Table 1** with examples of compression provided in Videos 1–5.

Ganglion Cyst

Ganglion cysts occur adjacent to a joint or tendon sheath and account for 60% of wrist

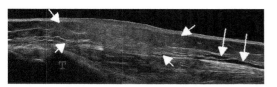

Fig. 22. Cellulitis. Longitudinal extended field of view image of the lateral superior aspect of the calf of a 19-year-old woman. The area of cellulitis (*short arrows*) is manifested by focal thickening and hyperechogenicity of the subcutaneous adipose tissue. Inferior to the area of cellulitis, there is perifascial edema (*long arrows*). The proximal tibia is visible deep to the cellulitis (red T).

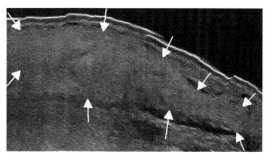

Fig. 23. Large abscess (*arrows*) with contents that are isoechoic to the adjacent tissues and easily missed on static ultrasound. Video 1 shows compression of this collection.

and hand masses.[24] Ganglion cysts are typically anechoic with deep acoustic enhancement, but may have internal septations and debris (**Fig. 26**). A connection to an adjacent joint is visible in many cases.

NONNEOPLASTIC CAUSES OF SOFT TISSUE MASSES
Epidermal Inclusion Cysts

Epidermal inclusion cysts commonly occur in hair-bearing areas of the body and contain keratin debris surrounded by a wall of stratified squamous epithelium.[25] Epidermal inclusion cysts are typically subcutaneous but contact the dermis, with extension into the dermis commonly observed (**Fig. 27**). These lesions typically are well defined and avascular with deep acoustic enhancement and diffuse internal echoes (pseudotestis pattern). A ruptured epidermal inclusion cyst may have irregular borders and surrounding hypervascularity (**Fig. 28**).[26]

Fat Necrosis

Fat necrosis in the subcutaneous tissue may present as a palpable, possibly painful, nodule caused by focal aseptic saponification, with a variable history of trauma.[27] Fat necrosis has a variable sonographic appearance, from a well-defined isoechoic mass to poorly defined areas of hyperechogenicity. There may be acoustic shadowing caused by calcification (**Fig. 29**). Given the variable sonographic appearance, fat necrosis may require MR imaging or biopsy for confirmation.

Foreign Body

Sonography is sensitive and specific for the detection of foreign bodies.[28] Foreign bodies are

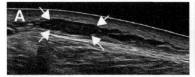
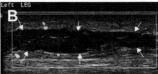

Fig. 24. (*A, B*) Deep subcutaneous abscess (*arrows*) that could be confused for confluent perifascial edema. Video 2 demonstrates mobile internal material visible during compression.

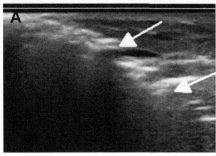
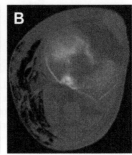

Fig. 25. Necrotizing fasciitis in a 54-year-old man with poorly controlled diabetes. (*A*) Transverse ultrasound of the popliteal fossa demonstrates extensive gas (*arrows*) with dirty shadowing. (*B*) The patient was taken emergently to the CT scanner to confirm the diagnosis and determine the extent of soft tissue gas for surgical planning. Despite emergent surgical debridement, the patient expired the next day of overwhelming sepsis.

Table 1
Comparison of sonographic features of soft tissue neoplasms, hematomas, and abscesses

	Neoplasm	Hematoma	Abscess
Clinical	Gradual enlargement, but may be noticed after minor trauma	Rapid onset Should have a good explanation	Signs and symptoms of infection
Location	Sarcoma, typically intramuscular Lipoma, typically subcutaneous Mets, anywhere	Variable	Variable
Echogenicity	Variable	Acute, hyperechoic/isoechoic Chronic, hypoechoic or heterogeneous	Variable
Shape	Sarcoma, variable Lipoma, wider than tall Met, variable	Often elongated Multiple collections/ multiloculated	Irregular/variable Multiple collections Multiloculated
Compression	Lipomas are soft, otherwise neoplasms are usually minimally compressible	Often deformable, with limited internal mobility	Mobile internal contents
Doppler	Vessels helpful if present, but may not be detectable	No internal flow, but may surround vessels Peripheral flow variable	No internal flow Peripheral hypervascularity

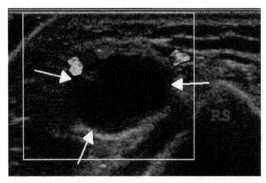

Fig. 26. Ganglion cyst (*arrows*) of the wrist adjacent to the radial artery and vein and the radial styloid (RS).

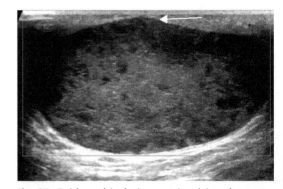

Fig. 27. Epidermal inclusion cyst involving the posterior trunk of a 44-year-old man. The mass has deep acoustic enhancement, no internal color Doppler signal, and focal extension into the dermis (*arrow*).

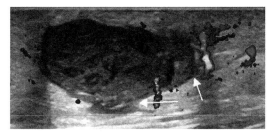

Fig. 28. Ruptured epidermal inclusion cyst involving the thigh of a 65-year-old man. The mass has irregular borders (*arrows*) and prominent surrounding vascularity.

typically echogenic and may produce acoustic shadowing (see **Fig. 3**). Wooden or other biologic foreign bodies frequently have a hypoechoic halo of granulation tissue (**Fig. 30**).

Hernias

Ultrasound is an excellent imaging modality to evaluate for suspected hernia, with upright imaging and real-time assessment for tissue motion during Valsalva maneuver and compression.[29,30] Upright imaging is particularly important because some hernias are only present or only contain bowel when the patient is upright.

The most common locations of abdominal wall hernias are:

- Epigastric: near the midline above the umbilicus
- Umbilical (**Fig. 31**, Video 6)
- Hypogastric: near the midline below the umbilicus
- Spigelian: near the lateral border of the rectus abdominus muscle at the semilunar line (**Fig. 32**, Video 7)
- Lumbar: near the posterolateral border of the internal and external oblique muscles

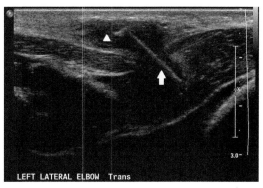

Fig. 30. Foreign body caused by a thorn near the elbow of a 19-year-old man. The actual foreign body (*arrow*) is an echogenic line, which is surrounded by hypoechoic granulation tissue (*triangle*).

- Incisional
- Parastomal

Groin hernias occur in the following locations:

- Indirect inguinal hernias traverse the deep inguinal ring to enter the inguinal canal (**Fig. 33**). The hernia neck is superior and lateral to the inferior epigastric vessels and herniated tissue courses superficial to the inferior epigastric artery.
- Direct inguinal hernias are the result of weakness of the transversalis fascia at Hesselbach triangle and enter directly into the inguinal canal without traversing the deep inguinal ring. The hernia neck is medial and inferior to the inferior epigastric vessels.[31,32]
- Femoral hernias occur within the femoral canal inferior to the inguinal ligament and are typically located medial to the common femoral vein. Femoral hernias are more

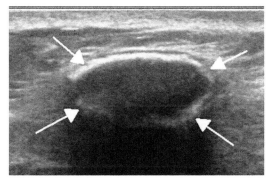

Fig. 29. Fat necrosis (*arrows*) with peripheral calcification in the gluteal subcutaneous tissues of a 64-year-old woman with a history of a horse bite in that location.

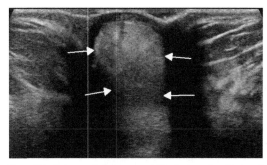

Fig. 31. Fat containing umbilical hernia (*arrows*) shown on a transverse image of the anterior abdomen of a 54-year-old man. Acoustic shadowing at the margins of an umbilical hernia is common. Video 6 demonstrates mobility of the herniated tissue with compression.

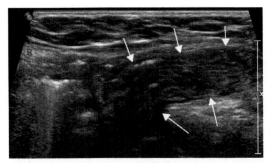

Fig. 32. Spigelian hernia (*arrows*) containing bowel on a transverse image of the left lower quadrant of 50-year-old woman. The lateral portion of the left rectus abdominus muscle is visible (red R). Video 7 demonstrates mobility of the hernia with Valsalva maneuver.

common in women and are the most common type of groin hernia to strangulate.

The sonographic appearance of a hernia is variable and dependent on the hernia contents. Mesenteric fat, small bowel, and colon are frequently seen in hernias. Sonographic findings of herniated bowel include intraluminal gas manifested by hyperechoic foci with dirty shadowing and peristalsis.[31,32]

A potential complication of a hernia is strangulation. This occurs when the blood supply to the herniated abdominal contents is compromised. Strangulated bowel is aperistaltic with wall edema and adjacent free fluid. The bowel wall is hyperemic or avascular, depending on if it is an acute or late process, respectively.[32]

SUMMARY

Sonography is a good first-line imaging modality to evaluate small superficial masses. Real-time dynamic imaging during compression and Valsalva maneuver is a unique advantage of ultrasound.

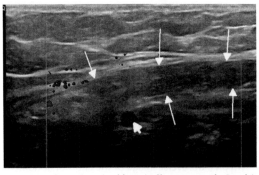

Fig. 33. Indirect inguinal hernia (*long arrows*). On this longitudinal image oriented along the inguinal canal, the herniated tissue courses superficial to the inferior epigastric artery (*short arrow*).

Doppler imaging provides noninvasive assessment of blood flow, but requires careful attention to technique. Sonography can provide a specific diagnosis for many superficial masses and triage other masses to further evaluation with MR imaging or tissue sampling. Sonography can successfully identify soft tissue fluid collections, but the diagnosis of hematoma should be made with caution to avoid delayed diagnosis of a significant neoplasm.

SUPPLEMENTARY DATA

Supplementary data related to this article is found at https://doi.org/10.1016/j.rcl.2019.01.013.

REFERENCES

1. Wagner JM, Lamprich BK. Ultrasonography of lumps and bumps. Ultrasound Clin 2014;9(3): 373–90.
2. Fletcher CDM, Rydolm A, Singer S, et al. Soft tissue tumours: epidemiology, clinical features, histopathological typing and grading. In: Fletcher CDM, Unni KK, Mertens F, editors. World Health Organization classification of tumours: pathology and genetics of tumours of soft tissue and bone. Lyon (France): International Agency for Research on Cancer; 2002. p. 12–8.
3. Lakkaraju A, Sinha R, Garikipati R, et al. Ultrasound for initial evaluation and triage of clinically suspicious soft-tissue masses. Clin Radiol 2009;64(6): 615–21.
4. Wagner JM, Lee KS, Rosas H, et al. Accuracy of sonographic diagnosis of superficial masses. J Ultrasound Med 2013;32(8):1443–50.
5. DiDomenico P, Middleton W. Sonographic evaluation of palpable superficial masses. Radiol Clin North Am 2014;52(6):1295–305.
6. Crundwell N, O'Donnell P, Saifuddin A. Non-neoplastic conditions presenting as soft-tissue tumours. Clin Radiol 2007;62(1):18–27.
7. Brouns F, Stas M, De Wever I. Delay in diagnosis of soft tissue sarcomas. Eur J Surg Oncol 2003;29(5): 440–5.
8. Balach T, Stacy GS, Haydon RC. The clinical evaluation of soft tissue tumors. Radiol Clin North Am 2011;49(6):1185–96, vi.
9. Datir A, James SL, Ali K, et al. MRI of soft-tissue masses: the relationship between lesion size, depth, and diagnosis. Clin Radiol 2008;63(4):373–8 [discussion: 379–80].
10. Nielsen GP, Mandahl N. Lipoma. In: Fletcher CDM, Unni KK, Mertens F, editors. World Health Organization classification of tumours: pathology and genetics of tumours of soft tissue and bone. Lyon

(France): International Agency for Research on Cancer; 2002. p. 20–2.

11. Bang M, Kang BS, Hwang JC, et al. Ultrasonographic analysis of subcutaneous angiolipoma. Skeletal Radiol 2012;41(9):1055–9.

12. Inampudi P, Jacobson JA, Fessell DP, et al. Soft-tissue lipomas: accuracy of sonography in diagnosis with pathologic correlation. Radiology 2004;233(3): 763–7.

13. Hung EH, Griffith JF, Ng AW, et al. Ultrasound of musculoskeletal soft-tissue tumors superficial to the investing fascia. AJR Am J Roentgenol 2014; 202(6):W532–40.

14. Carra BJ, Bui-Mansfield LT, O'Brien SD, et al. Sonography of musculoskeletal soft-tissue masses: techniques, pearls, and pitfalls. AJR Am J Roentgenol 2014;202(6):1281–90.

15. Paltiel HJ, Burrows PE, Kozakewich HPW, et al. Soft-tissue vascular anomalies: utility of US for diagnosis. Radiology 2000;214:747–54.

16. Widmann G, Riedl A, Schoepf D, et al. State-of-the-art HR-US imaging findings of the most frequent musculoskeletal soft-tissue tumors. Skeletal Radiol 2009;38(7):637–49.

17. Progam NCIS. SEER cancer stat facts. 2018. Available at: https://seer.cancer.gov/statfacts/html/soft.html. Accessed August 3, 2018.

18. Jain N, Goyal N, Mukherjee K, et al. Ultrasound of the abdominal wall: what lies beneath? Clin Radiol 2013;68:85–93.

19. Taieb S, Penel N, Vanseymortier L, et al. Soft tissue sarcomas or intramuscular haematomas? Eur J Radiol 2009;72(1):44–9.

20. Coates M. Ultrasound and soft-tissue mass lesions: a note of caution. N Z Med J 2003;116(1187):1–2.

21. Ward WG, Rougraff B, Quinn R, et al. Tumors masquerading as hematomas. Clin Orthop Relat Res 2007;465:232–40.

22. Kontogeorgakos VA, Martinez S, Dodd L, et al. Extremity soft tissue sarcomas presented as hematomas. Arch Orthop Trauma Surg 2010;130(10): 1209–14.

23. Adhikari S, Blavias M. Sonography first for subcutaneous abscess and cellulitis evaluation. J Ultrasound Med 2012;31:1509–12.

24. Freire V, Guerini H, Campagna R, et al. Imaging of hand and wrist cysts: a clinical approach. AJR Am J Roentgenol 2012;199(5):W618–28.

25. Kim HK, Kim SM, Lee SH, et al. Subcutaneous epidermal inclusion cysts: ultrasound (US) and MR imaging findings. Skeletal Radiol 2011;40(11): 1415–9.

26. Jin W, Ryu KN, Kim GY, et al. Sonographic findings of ruptured epidermal inclusion cysts in superficial soft tissue. J Ultrasound Med 2008;27:171–6.

27. Robinson P, Farrant JM, Bourke G, et al. Ultrasound and MRI findings in appendicular and truncal fat necrosis. Skeletal Radiol 2008;37(3):217–24.

28. Jacobson JA, Powell A, Craig JG, et al. Wooden foreign bodies in soft tissues: detection at US. Radiology 1998;206:45–8.

29. Stavros AT, Rapp C. Dynamic ultrasound of hernias of the groin and anterior abdominal wall. Ultrasound Q 2010;26(3):135–69.

30. Wagner JM, North JC. Ultrasound of the abdominal wall. Ultrasound Clin 2014;9(4):775–91.

31. Cabarrus MC, Yeh BM, Phelps AS, et al. From inguinal hernias to spermatic cord lipomas: pearls, pitfalls, and mimics of abdominal and pelvic hernias. Radiographics 2017;37(7):2063–82.

32. Revzin MV, Ersahin D, Israel GM, et al. US of the inguinal canal: comprehensive review of pathologic processes with CT and MR imaging correlation. Radiographics 2016;36(7):2028–48.

Moving?

Make sure your subscription moves with you!

To notify us of your new address, find your **Clinics Account Number** (located on your mailing label above your name), and contact customer service at:

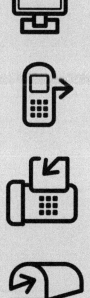

Email: journalscustomerservice-usa@elsevier.com

800-654-2452 (subscribers In the U.S. & Canada)
314-447-8871 (subscribers outside of the U.S. & Canada)

Fax number: 314-447-8029

**Elsevier Health Sciences Division
Subscription Customer Service
3251 Riverport Lane
Maryland Heights, MO 63043**

ELSEVIER

Printed and bound by CPI Group (UK) Ltd, Croydon, CR0 4YY

08/05/2025

01864745-0011